DEPRESSION IN JAPAN

DEPRESSION IN JAPAN

Psychiatric Cures for a Society in Distress

Junko Kitanaka

PRINCETON UNIVERSITY PRESS

PRINCETON AND OXFORD

Copyright © 2012 by Princeton University Press

Published by Princeton University Press,
41 William Street, Princeton, New Jersey 08540
In the United Kingdom: Princeton University Press,
6 Oxford Street, Woodstock, Oxfordshire OX20 1TW
press.princeton.edu

Library of Congress Cataloging-in-Publication Data

Kitanaka, Junko, 1970–
  Depression in Japan : psychiatric cures for a society in distress / Junko Kitanaka.
    p. ; cm.
  Includes bibliographical references and index.
  ISBN 978-0-691-14204-3 (hardcover :alk. paper) — ISBN 978-0-691-14205-0 (pbk. : alk.
paper) 1. Depression, Mental—Treatment—Japan. 2. Psychotherapy—Japan. I. Title.
  [DNLM: 1. Japan. 2. Depressive Disorder—psychology. 3. Depressive Disorder—
therapy. 4. Patient Acceptance of Health Care. 5. Psychiatry—trends. 6. Suicide—
psychology. 7. Workload—psychology. WM 171]
  RC537.K536 2012
  616.85'2706510952—dc23   2011012706

British Library Cataloging-in-Publication Data is available

This book has been composed in Sabon

Printed on acid-free paper. ∞

Printed in the United States of America

10 9 8 7 6 5 4 3 2 1

To Chris and Rick

Contents

List of Illustrations

Acknowledgments

THIS BOOK IS A PRODUCT of my engagement with three fields—medical anthropology, psychiatry, and medical history—that have profoundly shaped my thinking over the years I've spent in Japan and in North America. Margaret Lock has been a constant source of inspiration. Her vision of medical anthropology was what drew me to this field in the first place, and her deep compassion and unfailing support have kept me going. I have learned much from years of enriching conversations with Allan Young, whose incredible depth of knowledge, underlying passion for social justice, and great sense of humor I so respect and admire. Ellen's Corin's brilliant insights and willingness to engage deeply with my own thinking have helped me give shape to the ideas that really mattered to me. And I can never fully thank Laurence Kirmayer for helping me navigate through fieldwork in both Canadian and Japanese psychiatries, and enabling me, through his incisive comments on my writing, to raise my work to a higher level.

Over the last decade, I have been fortunate to have met many superb psychiatrists, who have been open to far-ranging discussions with an anthropologist. In particular, I'm deeply indebted to my Japanese mentor in medical anthropology, Dr. Eguchi Shigeyuki, without whose generous help this research would not have been possible. (Japanese names are written in the order of family name followed by given name.) Special thanks go to Dr. Katō Satoshi, who has exemplified the blending of critical intellectualism and passionate commitment to clinical practice. Dr. Noda Fumitaka introduced me to the fascinating world of cultural psychiatry. Doctors Kanba Shigenobu and Kuroki Toshihide have opened my eyes to historically informed, critical biological psychiatry. I've enjoyed talking with such brilliant scholars-cum-clinicians as Doctors Ōtsuka Kōichiro, Noguchi Masayuki, Abe Takaaki, Tsujiuchi Takuya, Kobayashi Toshiyuki, and Okajima Yoshirō. I'm also grateful to Doctors Hayashi Akiko, Ogiwara Chikako, Maeda Keiko, Suzuki Kunifumi, Hayashi Naoki, Tajima Osamu, and Ōmae Susumu. I have felt privileged to learn from depression and suicide experts such as Doctors Utsumi Ken, Takahashi Yoshitomo, and Ōno Yutaka, as well as Morita specialists such as Doctors Nakamura Kei, Kitanishi Kenji, and Kondō Kyōichi. I've also benefited from dialogue with psychologists Ichikawa Kyōko, Yamashita Mayu, Tsuruta Nobuko, and Ehara Yumiko. I've appreciated many conversations with Doctors Pierre-Henri Castel, David Healy, Sing Lee, and Dominic T. S. Lee. I want to thank numerous other doctors who so generously allowed me into their clinical practices and shared their time and thoughts in interviews.

Without the help of the brilliant historian Professor Suzuki Akihito, who invited me to participate in the research group on premodern senses of the body at the International Research Center for Japanese Studies (Nichibunken), I could not have delved as deeply into the historical aspects of depression. Professor Suzuki's work on English and Japanese psychiatries sets a standard that I hope to achieve some day. Thanks also go to Professors Waltraud Ernst, Clark Lawlor, Elizabeth Lunbeck, Jonathan Metzl, Mark Micale, Thomas Müller, Christian Oberlaender, and David Wright, all of whom so generously shared their expertise with a nonhistorian. I'm honored to have worked with Professor Kuriyama Shigehisa, who has showed me what it means to do medical history with an anthropological edge. I'm also indebted to medical historians Doctors Hiruta Genshirō, Sakai Shizu, Omata Waichirō, and Okada Yasuo, as well as Professors Shirasugi Etsuo, Kitazawa Kazutoshi, and Kōzai Toyoko.

I've learned so much from years of engaging dialogues with my dear friend Dominique Béhague, whose work on Brazilian psychiatry continues to inspire me. I also thank Sean Brotherton, Steve Cohen, Stephanie Lloyd, Sadeq Rahime, Audra Simpson, and Christina Zarowsky for stimulating conversations and friendship. Professor Adriana Petryna has given me many insights and warm encouragement. I've benefited greatly from my conversations with Professors Kal Applbaum, Alan Harwood, Bill Kelly, Lenore Manderson, Karen Nakamura, and Chikako Ozawa-de Silva. Professsror Amy Borovoy has engaged deeply with my work and given me much support over the years. In Tokyo, Professors Ogawa Kōichi, Takei Hideo and Miyaji Naoko, as well as Kobayashi Kayo and Hashimoto Yōko gave me valuable comments. My colleagues at Keio University, particularly Professors Mitsui Hirotaka and the late Fujita Hiroo provided a wonderfully congenial environment in which to work. Special thanks go to Professor Miyasaka Keizô, whose creative anthropological reflections have encouraged me to think beyond conventional disciplinary borders. I am indebted to Adam Lock for his diligent editorial work and moral support as well as Teruyama Junko, from whose research assistance I benefited greatly. I also want to thank Fred Appel, senior editor at Princeton University Press, for his kindness and professionalism throughout the process of completing the book.

Needless to say, I will forever be indebted to the people suffering from depression who agreed to participate in my research. They taught me far more than I was able to convey in my writing—through their profound reflections on the nature of depression, and the quiet, inner strength they drew upon in trying to overcome their difficulties. I'm truly grateful for their kindness and the trust they gave me—for so generously opening themselves up and sharing what was undoubtedly one of the hardest, most vulnerable times in their lives. I sincerely hope that this book will contribute in some way to ease, and not aggravate, the pain of those who experience depression.

The research was generously funded and supported at different stages by grants from the Canadian government, McGill University, the Wenner-Gren

Foundation for Anthropological Research (Grant #6682), the Japan Foundation, the International Research Center for Japanese Studies, Keio University, the Japanese Society for the Promotion of Science, and the Global COE program of the Japanese government.

I am grateful to my parents, Kenji and Keiko Kitanaka, and my sister, Makiko. I thank the O'Boyles as well as Margie and Jim Oliver for always being there for me. Finally, I could not have come this far without the love, help, and inspiration from my husband, Chris Oliver.

Versions of the following chapters were published previously:

Chapter 2. Reading Emotions in the Body: Translating Depression at the Intersections of Japanese and Western medicines. In *Transnational Psychiatries. Social and Cultural Histories of Psychiatry in Comparative Perspective, c. 1800–2000*, eds. Thomas Müller and Waltraud Ernst. Newcastle: Cambridge Scholars Publishing, 2010. Published with the permission of Cambridge Scholars Publishing.

Chapter 7. Diagnosing Suicides of Resolve: Psychiatric Practice in Contemporary Japan. *Culture, Medicine, and Psychiatry*, vol. 32, no.2, (June 2008). Published with kind permission from Springer Science+Business Media: *Culture, Medicine and Psychiatry*.

Chapter 9. Questioning the Suicide of Resolve: Disputes Regarding "Overwork Suicide" in 20th Century Japan. In *Histories of Suicide: International Perspectives on Self-Destruction in the Modern World*, eds., John Weaver and David Wright. Toronto: University of Toronto Press, 2008. Reprinted with permission of the publisher.

DEPRESSION IN JAPAN

CHAPTER ONE

Introduction:
Local Forces of Medicalization

> A Typus Melancholicus, at a big corporation, working
> harder for three months after being promoted . . . develops
> a clear case of depression. After taking antidepressants
> and time off for half a year or so, he returns to work fully
> recovered. . . . This is a typical depression in Japan.
>
> —Kasahara Yomishi in Kasahara, Yamashita,
> and Hirose, *Utsubyō* (*Depression*) (1992:29)

> When I first came to the hospital, I felt so liberated from my
> work and my family that I immediately got better. But now
> that I've started thinking about going back to work and
> about what might await me upon my return . . .
>
> —(a forty-three-year-old salaryman; a recovering
> patient who became depressed again immediately
> after receiving a call from his boss)

The Rise of Depression

IN JAPAN, THE TERM *karōshi*, or death from overwork, was coined in the 1980s to describe cases where people have essentially worked themselves to death. In the late 1990s, when Japanese began to see suicide rates skyrocket, other similar terms emerged and gained currency in the national media. These were *karō ji-satsu*, or overwork suicide, referring to the suicide of people who are driven by excessive work to take their own lives, and *karō utsubyō*, or overwork depression, clinical depression that is seen to underlie such an act. The concern about overwork suicide and overwork depression heightened in 2000, when Japan's Supreme Court ordered Dentsū, the biggest advertising agency in the country, to compensate the family of a deceased employee with the largest amount ever to be paid for a worker's death in Japan. While Dentsū argued that the employee's suicide was an act of free will, the Supreme Court determined that it was a product of *depression* that had been caused by chronic and excessive overwork. After the precedent-setting verdict, a number of similar legal victories have followed, increasingly by workers who contend that their depression is work-induced. Alarmed by these legal disputes and the rising number of the depressed in society at large, the government has installed new mental health measures and launched a series of labor policy changes aimed at taking on stress-induced mental illness as a significant national problem.[1]

While this outcome has often been discussed as a triumph of the workers' movement, I want to call attention to the fact that it has also signaled the beginning of broad-scale medicalization of suicide and depression in Japan, in which psychiatry and psychiatrists have played a key role.[2] Psychiatrists, through the above-mentioned legal disputes and mental health initiatives, are persuading Japanese that those who break down under tremendous social pressure may be victims of depression (*utsubyō*), an illness that until fairly recently had remained largely unknown among lay Japanese. Amidst the prolonged economic recession since the 1990s, psychiatrists have been urging people, with increasing effectiveness, to recognize their sense of fatigue and hopelessness in terms of depression. They have also linked depression to suicide at a time when Japanese have faced disturbingly high numbers driven to self-killing—more than 30,000 annually for twelve consecutive years (which is three to six times the number of traffic-accident deaths per year). Spurred on by aggressive pharmaceutical marketing of antidepressants during the 2000s, this process of medicalization has resulted in a rapid increase in the number of patients diagnosed with depression: between 1999 and 2008, the number grew by a multiple of 2.4 (*Yomiuri Shimbun* [*Yomiuri*], January 6, 2010). Depression is now one of the most frequently cited reasons for taking sick leave. Depression has thus been transformed from a "rare disease" to one of the most talked about illnesses in recent Japanese history. Psychiatry, as part of this transformation, is increasingly called upon to provide a cure for a society in distress.

This book thus examines how, at the turn of the twenty-first century, depression has suddenly become a "national disease" in Japan, and how psychiatry has emerged as a new vehicle for remedying the ailing social order. These changes are remarkable first of all because Japanese, until recently, had long resisted psychiatric intrusion into everyday life. While psychiatry was adopted from Germany and has been institutionally established in Japan since the 1880s, its use had been reserved for the severely ill. Because of its stigmatizing role in confining "deviants," psychiatry's expansion into the realm of everyday distress had been greatly limited. Its growing influence in Japan in the 1960s was soon disrupted by what came to be known as the antipsychiatry movement, when psychiatry was criticized as being an insidious tool for social management. Psychotherapy as well, though introduced to Japan in 1912 (Okonogi 1971), had been "viewed with deep suspicion" (Lock 1980:258, Ohnuki-Tienery 1984, Ozawa 1996, Doi 1990); some psychiatrists wondered whether the absence of a

---

[1] These include establishing criteria for diagnosing mental illness in the workplace in 1999 as well as implementing the Basic Laws on Suicide Countermeasures and national incentives for "Building Mental Health" in 2006 (Kōsei Rōdōshō 2010: see chapter 9).

[2] Medicalization refers to the process of the expanding jurisdiction of biomedicine over life problems (Fox 1979, Conrad and Schneider 1980).

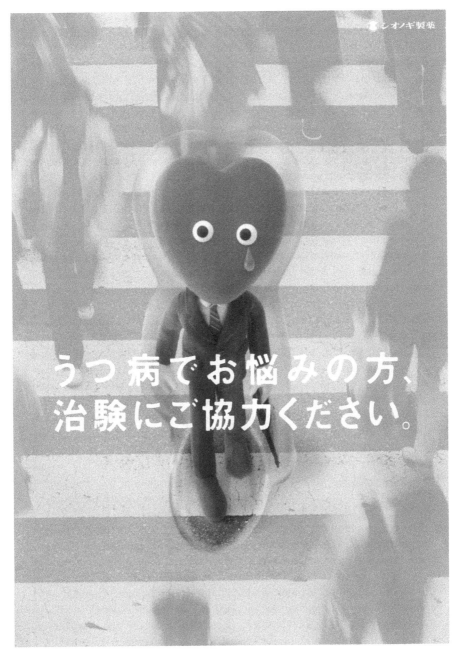

Figure 1.1. An image of depression; a 2007 pharmaceutical company advertisement seeking research volunteers for an antidepressant clinical trial (courtesy of Shionogi & Co., Ltd.).

psychiatric proliferation in the realm of everyday life problems attested to Japan having attained a modernity without the degree of alienation found in "the West" (e.g., Machizawa 1997). Depression in particular was regarded as "rare" in Japan, prompting some psychiatrists to speculate whether Japanese—who (they claimed) "aestheticize" rather than "pathologize" depressive moods— might have been largely spared the experience of depression (Kimura 1979). Such assumptions about cultural differences were so firm that psychiatric experts dissuaded Eli Lilly & Co. from promoting and selling Prozac in Japan for lack of a market (Applbaum 2006, Landers 2002). All of this has taken a radical turn since the late 1990s, as an unprecedented number of Japanese have begun to suffer "depression" and to seek psychiatric care for it.

While psychiatrists might generally regard their growing influence as a sign of scientific progress, in North America critics have been concerned with how the rise of depression has correlated with the advent of new antidepressants; they warn that it is instilling a form of individualized biological reductionism. This line of criticism draws upon the "medicalization critique" to argue that the rise of depression globally exemplifies a process whereby a problem of living— indicating social origins and social contradictions—comes to be redefined as a problem of individual biology. North American critics who take this view have argued that this biologization of depression constitutes a fundamental assault on the self, which, in the guise of a quick cure via the prescription of antidepressants, silences people's dissent and diminishes their capacity to reflect upon the social and political roots of their affliction (cf. Illich 1975). Some have argued that such biological reductionism may further lead to biological surveillance, depoliticization, and decreased autonomy (see Rose 2007). Another line of criticism asserts that the medicalization of depression has brought to North America a "loss of sadness" (Horwitz and Wakefield 2007), whereby people are losing their capacity for tolerance, patience, suffering, and grief. Noting how emotional life is being transformed by the act of taking "happy pills," some scholars suggest that this form of medicalization is creating moral anxiety— seen as impoverishing the cultural resources with which people have traditionally confronted the hardships of life (Elliott and Chambers 2004).

Given the outpouring of such concerns and criticisms in North America, and given that this kind of global medicalization is often equated with "Americanization," one may wonder why similar concerns have not been voiced as much in a society like Japan, where psychiatry has certainly been accused of this type of individualized biological reductionism in the past.[3] How has Japanese psychiatry overcome strong lay resistance to the intrusion of psychiatry into everyday life? How exactly is it incorporating biological reasoning into its understanding and treatment of depression? Has it succeeded in providing a biological explanation that is somehow acceptable, perhaps even liberating, for

---

[3] As during the antipsychiatry movement of the 1960 through the 1980s (see chapter 3).

those in distress? Have Japanese somehow found a different path of medicalization from that which has developed in North America—and, together with it, an alternative vision of happiness?

Building from recent anthropological analyses of medicalization and medical practices, this book investigates how psychiatry has come to provide Japanese with a new understanding of "depression" and asks what kind of political subjects this gives rise to. In contrast to the view of medicalization as a tool of top-down biomedical domination and homogenization, anthropologists have of late come to examine this process as grounded in the local, historical contexts of social controversies and political movements. Instead of assuming that medicalization uniformly leads to depoliticization, they have illuminated the way in which it is a generative and politically charged process where local actors come to articulate competing views on the nature of their distress (Lock 1993, 1999, 2002, Young 1995, Cohen 1998, Kleinman 1986, 1995, Scheper-Hughes 1992, Todeschini 1999a, 1999b, Martin 2007). Building upon this approach, I investigate not simply how psychiatry subjugates but rather how it generates new subjects via new or altered norms, knowledge, concepts, and a way of talking about problems of living—or what I refer to here as "psychiatric language."[4] I show how psychiatric language is essential in constituting the reality that it seeks to represent (Foucault 1973, 1975, Hacking 1995), particularly for those who are seeking psychiatric care for an "illness" that, in significant ways, previously did not exist as such in Japan.

From this perspective, I argue that psychiatry has largely overcome Japanese resistance by creating a new language of depression that closely engages with—in fact reappropriates—cultural discourse about the *social* nature of depression. Particularly through the medico-legal debates regarding overwork depression, psychiatrists have provided powerful descriptions of the depressed, explaining how, for instance, their patients' self-sacrificing devotion to the company is no longer rewarded in the deepening recession and the crumbling system of lifetime employment. Focusing on what some psychiatrists have termed "Japanese-style fatigue-induced depression" (Kasahara, Yamashita, and Hirose 1992), they have concretely demonstrated how depression is not only a pathology of the individual brain but is also rooted in the Japanese culture of work itself. In so doing, they have elevated depression to a symbol of collective distress faced by many Japanese in times of economic uncertainty. Through this "socializing" language of depression, psychiatrists have emerged as unlikely agents of *liberation*: they are now successfully altering the way Japanese think about the borders of normality and abnormality, health and illness,

---

[4] The term "language" is not meant to exclude practices (cf. Bourdieu 1977), nor is it an attempt to extract some deep symbolic structure (cf. Levi-Strauss 1963a). Rather, I use it in part to stress a departure from the previous *silence* in Japan surrounding mental illness and a movement toward ways of talking about "depression."

and reshaping cultural debates about how society should deal with individual subjects of social distress.

The book thus explores how this different form of medicalization in Japan has come about, and what consequences it brings. My analysis of the emergence of a psychiatric language of depression in Japan is based upon anthropological research that stretches from 1998 to early 2010, a decade that covers before and after the onset of the medicalization.[5] I began my preliminary fieldwork in the summer of 1998, when depression was still relatively unknown in Japan. I carried out the main fieldwork from 2000 to 2003, just when a new generation of antidepressants (selective serotonin reuptake inhibitors or SSRIs) was being introduced to the Japanese market and people were learning how to talk about "depression." While observing the changing depression scenes from Tokyo throughout the 2000s, I also did follow-up fieldwork in 2008 and 2009 by returning to the same hospitals that I had previously conducted participant observation. During the 2000s, the Ministry of Health, Welfare, and Labor made a number of important changes in its health and labor policies, which have provided institutional/material reality to the idea that depression is rooted in social conditions. These policy changes have also led industry to begin dealing with depression as a collective risk, to be prevented and treated through close management. By the last phase of my fieldwork, the notion of depression had become deeply entrenched in the lives of ordinary Japanese; everyone that I talked to seemed to know people afflicted with depression, including those who had taken sick leave because of it. With the growing number of depressed in society at large, however, there has also emerged new public anxiety about the therapeutic efficacy of psychiatry and the nature of the "remedy" it actually offers. Thus, throughout the book I explore whether psychiatry, as it expands further into the realm of everyday life, may end up constituting a new form of domination by subjecting people to further surveillance and biological management; or, if it instead helps to give rise to subjects who reflect on, and act to resolve the social roots of their predicaments, thereby allowing their dissent to become a motor for social transformation.

---

[5] Research in mental health poses ethical issues that should not be compromised. I presented my research plan and obtained official approvals for my research from the ethic committees of the two psychiatric institutions (a university hospital and a private mental hospital) where I conducted most of my fieldwork. At a psychosomatic clinic, where there was no formal ethics committee, I was given permission from the doctors in charge. With all the patients I interviewed, I first explained the aim of my research, the measures I would take to protect their privacy, and made sure they knew that they had the right to withdraw from participating anytime they wished. It was only then that I obtained their written informed consent. Patients' health and well-being always is a concern that must be given top priority, and I avoided seeking any interviews with people who were under severe distress, and consulted closely with psychiatrists before asking any patients for an interview. Any information that might reveal their identity (including their names and sometimes their occupation) has been changed in order to protect their privacy. As well, most of the psychiatrists who appear in this book are also given pseudonyms.

The Production of Psychiatric Subjects as Reflexive Agents

The proliferation of psychiatry has been cited as a hallmark of modernity (Rieff 1966, Giddens 1991) and a sign of the changing nature of governance, political surveillance, and possible forms that agency can take in contemporary society (Marcuse 1970, Foucault 1975, Rose 1996). The first generation of critical studies of biomedicine created a forceful polemic against the teleological view of its history as governed by the principles of progress and humanitarianism. Defining works in medical sociology provoked scholars to conceptualize biomedicine in ideological terms that reproduce the dominant social order and power structures (Goffman 1961, Scheff 1966, Zola 1972), while establishing a medical monopoly (Freidson 1970, Illich 1975). Psychiatry in particular has been criticized for having served as a state apparatus for excluding those deemed unfit to fully participate in the social order by labeling them as "mentally ill" (Becker 1960) and justifying its position by claiming the "scientific" neutrality of its knowledge. Central to this scientific ideology is a conceptualization that locates the cause of madness within individual biology/psychology, rather than in a set of social relations (Laing 1969, Szasz 1974, Cooper 1967, Ingleby 1980). By defining depression as a matter of brain anomalies, for example, psychiatry is said to shift people's attention away from the social conditions that may have given rise to alienation in the first place. According to these analyses, psychiatry serves to silence social contradictions by pathologizing people to the extent that they are denied a voice with which to speak back.

Similarly, scholars of Japanese psychiatry have examined psychiatry mainly as a means of oppression. Because earlier studies commenced under the influence of the antipsychiatry movement of the 1960s, many scholars have drawn upon Marxist critiques in order to expose the ways in which psychiatry has functioned as an arm of the modern state, suppressing alternative forms of healing, classifying and standardizing subjects, and depriving people of the authorship of their own illness experience. They have shown how psychiatry has abused scientific categories to confine people deemed as "unproductive" and concealed its underlying economic rationality. Moriyama (1975, 1988), for instance, has illuminated the long-term history of how psychiatric institutions developed in Japan as part of the expansion of the modern state; Tomita (1992) has demonstrated how the number of psychiatric confinements fluctuated accordingly with the patterns of local economies; and Asano (2000) has analyzed the historical disputes surrounding occupational therapy and the charge against it that it has functioned as an imposed form of labor in the guise of treatment (also see Yamada 2000, Itsumi et al. 1970). While there are other, nuanced ethnomethodological studies, one of which closely analyzed communication breakdowns in a mental hospital (Nomura and Miyamoto 1996), the overall effect of the critique of psychiatry has been to portray it as a monolithic, repressive enterprise. Though the importance of these previous critical studies must not be minimized, it is also evident that their vision of psychiatry fails to explain the current documented rise of depression or why so many people are suddenly, and *voluntarily*, seeking out psychiatric care.

In order to understand psychiatry's changing forms of power, more recent works on the history of psychiatry (particularly in Europe and North America) have analyzed how both an institutional and conceptual transformation of subjects into "mentally ill" have been made possible at all. They have elaborated on the microscopic technologies by which people are conditioned to understand their distress in biological or psychological terms (Foucault 1975, Atkinson 1995). In place of earlier emphasis on experts' domination, these investigations have illuminated the process of *normalization*, whereby certain sets of ideas become produced, naturalized, and stabilized as "facts" or "truth" (Rose 1996, Nye 1984, Turner 1996). This perspective has proved particularly pertinent for analyzing psychiatry as it moves beyond asylums and penetrates deeper into everyday life through social institutions such as schools, the military, and industry (Castel et al. 1982, Rose 1985, Nolan 1998, Herman 1995, Henriques et al. 1984, Still and Velody 1992, Lutz 1997, Turkle 1992). The working of psychiatric power here is no longer conceptualized as top-down oppression and coercion, but as persuasion, incorporation, and habituation (Foucault 1977, Althusser 1971). Through localized and routinized practices, the language of psychiatry becomes, in other words, power *internalized*—intrinsically woven into the voice of the "lifeworld" of subjects (Foucault 1973, Armstrong 1983, Osborne 1994, Crawford 1984, Eguchi 1987, Miwaki 2000, Corin 1990, Lutz and Abu-Lughod 1990, Battaglia 1995, Sampson 1989, Sawicki 1991). As we see in the emergent discourse about depression and suicide in Japan, this new regime of psychiatry does not so much silence people as it encourages them to share and speak in its own terms—to undertake self-discipline.

In examining how psychiatry is entering the everyday lexicon of Japanese, it is important to understand the institutional and conceptual transformations that psychiatry has gone through in the last few decades. First of all, with policy changes, psychiatrists are no longer secure in their role as society's gatekeepers in mental hospitals. Particularly after the vehement antipsychiatry movement from 1969 on, younger generations of psychiatrists have sought to dismantle the old system by shifting their focus from asylums to community, and in the process they have become much more receptive to the idea of treating a wider range of mental distress than before (often referred to as a shift from mental illness to *mental health*). In addition, the global impact of American psychiatry—in the form of DSM-IV and psychopharmaceutical influences—encouraged Japanese psychiatrists to broaden their definition of depression (Healy 2004). It is in this context that psychiatrists are beginning to include in their practice not only psychotic depression (which was the main interest of psychiatrists before) but also more broadly defined mood disorders in general. In other words, Japanese psychiatrists, no longer confined by their traditional nosology, are redrawing the borders of what are considered psychiatric problems as opposed to mere problems of living. The fact that the state itself has shown much interest in adopting psychiatry on a much larger scale, for treating mental health in workplaces and preventing suicide, suggests that this medicalization signals an important change for Japanese psychiatry in its attempts to transform itself as a medicine for ordinary Japanese.[6]

The Biological and Social Causes of Depression

Within this context, psychiatrists are beginning to popularize depression by disseminating in the media two contrasting—yet complementary—languages of depression. One is grounded in the biological, which depicts depression as a disease affecting both the physical and mental condition of individuals, and emphasizes that its cause first and foremost lies in the brain. Biopsychiatrists who use this language write and speak about depression in a manner that differs little from that of American psychiatrists. Often in collaboration with the pharmaceutical industry, they have widely circulated the self-diagnostic list for depressive symptoms, telling Japanese to understand that depression can be a serious illness—possibly leading to suicide—if not properly treated by antidepressants. The other is the social language of depression, promoted mainly (but not only) by socially and phenomenologically oriented psychiatrists (Shiba 1999, Takaoka 2003). Appealing to public anxiety about rising rates of suicide, they have asserted that depression is not only about individual chemical imbalances but foremost about socially caused pathologies. Drawing upon the traditional psychiatric theory of melancholic premorbid personality or "Typus Melancholicus" (Tellenbach 1980[1961], Shimoda 1941), these psychiatrists have popularized the idea that it is the kind of people who have been most valued in corporate Japan—who selflessly devote themselves to the collective good—that are now being driven in great numbers to depression and suicide. They point out how Japanese society no longer rewards or protects those who have internalized the tradition of a work ethic. For them, conceptualizing depression only at the level of individual biology misses the point: the alarming suicide rate requires that psychiatry—and Japanese society as a whole—start thinking about depression in social terms.

[6] Of late, anthropologists of Japan have increasingly turned to analyzing how psychiatry is beginning to enter the realm of everyday distress as a new technology of social management (Lock 1988, 1993, Borovoy 1995, Breslau 1999, Ozawa 1996, Ozawa-de Silva 2006). Though the depression discourse is the latest venture in these developments, what is significant is that it involves the intervention of the state, which has historically employed various means for shaping how ordinary Japanese should think and behave (Rohlen 1974a, 1974b, Kelly 1993, Kondo 1990, Garon 1997, Kinzley 1991, Gordon 1998).

Thus, unlike earlier medicalization in the West where its effect was assumed to be biologizing and individualizing, psychiatry in Japan is gaining influence by questioning the social order in which the depressed must live. Socially aware psychiatrists, in particular, turn depression into not only a symbolic token for the anguish of workers living in a recession but also a practical means of obtaining long-term sick leave and economic compensation. Thus, for those involved in workers' movements, the psychiatric diagnosis of depression has become an indispensable tool. What is notable is that these psychiatrists have opened up the etiology of depression to legal, public debates, turning it into a political battleground for disputing whether the responsibility of an individual's breakdown lies in their biological vulnerability or in the social environment. In retreating from the traditional genetic determinism of Japanese psychiatry, psychiatry seems to be trying to shed itself of the potential criticism that it is a tool of social management, serving as a means of individualizing dissent and reproducing docile workers (c.f. Miwaki 2000). Even so, there is an apparent tension in the way the psychiatric language is being used, on the one hand, by dejected workers and their supports as a channel for vocalizing their dissent, and on the other hand, by the state and industry as a potential means of controlling and quieting such sentiment.

Psychiatry's new political subversiveness in Japan perhaps signals a triumph of social concern, but if we consider the ways in which biomedicine has attempted to incorporate the "social" under its rubric, we would do well to ask if such optimism is warranted. Anthropologists and sociologists who have analyzed reformist biomedical practices elsewhere have often pointed out the alarming developments when the social is translated into individualizing biomedical concepts such as "stress" (Young 1980), "lifestyles" (Comaroff 1982, Armstrong 1983), or "family life" (Silverman 1987). They have repeatedly shown how psychiatry and psychology have found ways to fragment these potentially social factors into individual biological/psychological attributes. In the pathbreaking ethnography of medicalization, Arthur Kleinman (1986) demonstrates how the discourse about "neurasthenia" emerged in 1980s China as a state-sanctioned mode of expressing people's social suffering caused by the injustices of the Cultural Revolution. Kleinman shows that, despite its potentially emancipatory implications, the biomedical form of liberation ends up disempowering those who voiced their political dissent in this way, as they are often left pathologized and further isolated (Kleinman 1995). Allan Young (1995) examines the rise of PTSD (Post Traumatic Stress Disorder) and its adoption by Vietnam veterans, who have drawn upon it in order to assert their victimhood, obtain public recognition of their plight as a group, and gain governmental compensation. Despite its political effectiveness, however, Young also shows the emotional, moral price that the veterans have had to pay in adopting the PTSD discourse for expressing their pain because it ultimately deprives them of the historical, political implications of their experience and trivializes the moral meanings of their *anger*. Furthermore, Young shows how, with the re-biologization of psychiatry (as in the rising dominance of neurobiology), patients' ailments are now increasingly reinterpreted in terms of biological vulnerabilities within individuals.

In order to understand the distinctive politics that characterizes the "socializing" forms of medicalization in Japan, it is important to recognize that the "social" and the "biological" map onto different ideological terrains depending on the historical and political contexts. For instance, biological reductionism is often criticized as the hallmark of American biomedicine; as historian of science Hiroi (1996) points out, this preoccupation in the United States cannot be understood apart from the history in which biological determinism has often been linked to racist discourse (Hiroi 1996:151–56). In Japan, where such biological determinism has not gained the same level of ideological power, what is evoked instead is the image of pathology as a metaphor for "'social dilemma' or upheaval . . . , rather than as a label of individual aberration" (Borovoy 1995:7). This socializing discourse in Japan, it has been suggested, derives from an ideology of "socio-somatics," a Confucian-derived political vision of society in which the health of individuals is believed to depend on a harmonious social order (Lock 1987). This cultural ideology has been given further institutional backing by the Japanese state, which has done much to maintain political stability by cultivating a network of family and corporate welfare as the basis of social life (Gordon 2009). Thus, examining the medicalization of socially withdrawn children, Lock (1986, 1988) has shown that socially oriented medical discourse in Japan is not necessarily liberating, but can be moralizing and hegemonizing in the way that it overdetermines the meaning of people's distress (see also Lock 1993).[7] She has explored how this notion has been used to shift the focus from individuals' actual ailments and the possibilities of change to abstracted notions about a collective predicament from which one cannot easily escape. Borovoy (2008) has also shown how this kind of socializing discourse has been used to help legitimize a social (environment-based) interpretation of children's disabilities at the expense of failing to recognize their individual needs.

Thus, while popular discourse and legal disputes are important sites where the meanings of depression are contested, I will in addition examine how depression is talked about in actual clinical practice. Given that the aim of clinical practice is not to voice social critique but to provide a remedy for the disruptions in people's lives, How do psychiatrists direct people's awareness about the nature of their affliction?

---

[7] Some Japanese psychiatrists I have interviewed have also expressed caution about explicit socializing rhetoric that intrudes into—and seeks to speak for—the experience of patients (cf. Foucault 1973, Armstrong 1983). Such socializing discourse, they suggest, homogenizes patients and thus reduces the complexity of clinical realities (see chapters 6 through 8).

Therapeutic Encounters as Sites of Persuasion

The current medicalization in Japan, it seems to me, needs to be examined at the level of internal persuasion, if we are to understand how psychiatry has overcome Japanese resistance from understanding everyday distress in psychiatric terms. This proliferation of psychiatric terminology could certainly not have happened while Japanese psychiatry was operating by means of materialistic domination. Until relatively recently, psychiatry in Japan was able to maintain its authority not because its knowledge was accepted as cultural commonsense (far from it), but because it was able to control and monopolize medical knowledge and exercise its jurisdiction for treating those diagnosed as mentally ill even without their consent. In practicing such a brutal form of power, there was no need for psychiatrists to persuade patients about the naturalness of the psychiatric worldview or expect them to understand it—let alone internalize it. By contrast, the emergent form of psychiatric practices of today, most clearly represented by its depression discourse, is seeking to operate at the conceptual level (cf. Althusser 1971); for people to voluntarily see themselves as depressed and in need of medical care, psychiatry, it would seem, has to begin to perform as an "internally persuasive discourse." Its subtle coercion requires individuals' own "ideological becoming" (Bakhtin and Holquist 1981:342) of psychiatric subjects (cf. Lunbeck 1994).

Yet, this presupposition seems to present immediate difficulties not only because "consciousness" is a notoriously difficult thing to scrutinize but also because, despite what critical theorists have insinuated, psychiatry's conceptual hold on people is often shown to be far from complete (see Young 1982a, 1983). Ethnographers have repeatedly illuminated how psychiatric therapeutic encounters are not places of epiphanic conversions but rather sites of contestations (Corin 1998a, Corin and Lauzon 1992, Taussig 1980, Estroff 1981, Saris 1995), where patients' voices are often dismissed, discredited, or simply "pushed to the margins of 'reasoned' discourse" (Young 1982b:275). Without achieving the kind of conceptual transformation that psychiatry's hegemony would seem to require, psychiatrists are often left to strive for the minimum of shared understanding of the "mental disorder" by staying away from the realm of social meanings associated with the distress. In this regard, Robert Barrett (1996) has given a nuanced analysis of how experts encourage a patient to co-produce a psychiatric narrative about "schizophrenia" by selectively incorporating parts of a patient's own accounts of the experience. Other scholars have turned to examining how people come to constitute themselves as pragmatic agents of medicalization, without necessarily accepting a psychiatric framing of their distress (Nichter 1998, Lupton 1997, Good et al. 1992). Thus, ethnographic examinations of psychiatry leave much uncertainty as to how it may work at all at the level of conceptual, symbolic transformation (Kirmayer 1993, Comaroff 1982).

In examining how psychiatry may begin to operate at the conceptual level, I show how Japanese psychiatry successfully converges the biological and the social in its particular construction of depression, providing a generic framework that translates individual misery into signs of collective suffering (cf. Kleinman 1986, Kleinman, Das, and Lock 1997). Psychiatrists achieve this first of all by urging patients to objectify their bodies and systematically cultivate an awareness of how fatigued and alienated their body has become. Particularly for those who are preoccupied with the meanings of their dejection and anger, psychiatrists try to defuse such emotions by urging them instead to focus on bodily recovery. At the same time that their intense emotions are tamed and transformed into objects of biological management, psychiatrists emphasize the social pressures that drove their patients to a breakdown, thereby illuminating their *victimhood*. By emphasizing overwork—not just the salaried labor of (often male) workers but also the emotional labor of housewives—psychiatrists achieve what biomedicine has always done best: liberation of the afflicted from the self-blame and moral responsibility to which they might otherwise be subjected (Sontag 1978). In such ways, they are able to help patients reproduce narratives with surprising uniformity and consistency, not because they have thoroughly persuaded and transformed their consciousness, but because they intentionally leave much unexplored. They carefully stay away, for instance, from in-depth explorations of how—through their unreflexive overconformity—patients might have played a part in structuring their own affliction, or what they can do to change it (Suzuki 1997). The resulting language of depression, while it certainly serves as a means of legitimizing individual suffering, is also curiously devoid of individual agency (see chapter 6).

This pronounced lack of interest on the part of psychiatrists to determine individual agency in connection with depression is above all contested in connection with attempted suicide. While most depressed people seem to accept, at least on the surface, the biological language of depression without much protest, some of the patients who have attempted suicide in Japan clearly resist medicalization by evoking the dominant cultural notion of suicide (to be elaborated on in chapter 7). Insisting that suicide be seen as an act of free will rather than as a product of pathology, some patients explicitly question the implications of adopting the biological language. Some psychiatrists try to go beyond this biological reductionism by incorporating the cultural notion of suicide, emphasizing how the patients are victims of societal problems. While this suggests new possibilities for psychiatric dialogues, the resulting depiction of the suicidal as passive victims might serve to take people's attention away from the specificity of individual angst to the abstracted notions about collective predicaments (cf. Lock 1986, 1988). And, by eluding its psychological and existential aspects, psychiatric discourse—particularly for those who wish to explore the individualized meaning of their behavior and ways of changing their lives— falls short of becoming an internally persuasive, *experiential* language.

What is Depression?

In terms of psychiatry's effects on people's experience, what concerns me in the end is the fundamental criticism of psychiatry, not uncommon in Japan itself, that it assembles an inchoate mass of realities as an illness, cultivates perpetual anxiety in people, and thus creates the problem that it purports to cure. Though this claim comes in different forms, the alleged fact that Japanese rarely suffered depression before modernity, and the alleged fact that they are now suffering en masse, urges us to seriously confront the potential ill-effects of medicalization. Could it be that medicalization is impoverishing the Japanese "cultural self," that, according to some scholars (Kimura 1979, cf. Obeyesekere 1985), has allowed people in Japan to tolerate and even aestheticize depression to the extent that it protected them from regarding it as a pathological experience?

Surprisingly, during my fieldwork, I found criticisms against the ongoing medicalization coming from the most unlikely sources—the Japanese psychiatrists themselves. As noted above, they believed initially that there would not be a sizable market for Prozac in Japan. Even after 2000, when SSRI's were introduced and were becoming widely prescribed, I heard many Japanese psychiatrists proclaim that the sudden rise of depression was largely due to the "conspiracy of pharmaceutical companies." Indeed, as these psychiatrists criticized it, some pharmaceutical companies initially tried to market antidepressants by "altering the language" (Landers 2002)—that is, they adopted the phrase "*kokoro no kaze*" ("cold of the heart" or "the soul catching a cold") for talking about utsubyō (depression) in order to give it a more positive connotation. Psychiatrists were also critical of the way these companies were presenting it as an illness that could affect anyone at any time. Apparently, they were uncomfortable treating patients who did not have what these doctors considered "real" psychiatric problems, and were alarmed by the way their own profession was expanding its jurisdiction over problems of living by blurring the accepted distinction between normality and abnormality. Even given the fact that most of the prominent depression experts I interviewed became doctors at the height of the antipsychiatry movement in the 1970s, and knew how to talk critically of their own profession to an anthropologist, such critiques were remarkably frequent and most psychiatrists seemed genuinely concerned. They worried that people were being "duped" into believing that they have a disease easily cured by medication, when in fact, so many of them might end up becoming chronic patients, seeking a cure for social/existential/psychological problems for which biomedicine can only offer temporary relief.

While the psychiatrists' own skepticism adds complexity to our understanding of the competing forces for medicalization, what I want to emphasize is the fact that the conceptual control of clinical "depression"—traditionally tightly held by psychiatrists—is now beginning to break down. Depression as it is being talked about is no longer a biomedical monopoly but a bundle of concepts whose meanings are constantly negotiated and redrawn by various actors—including pharmaceutical companies, physicians, and public administrators, as well as lawyers and judges who are playing a part in this medicalization (cf. Lock 1997, 2002, Cohen 1998, Clarke and Montini 1993). And it is in this context—where the meaning of depression itself is in flux—that people are beginning to "recognize" depression and possibly claim different things by it. This leads me to wonder what exactly depression is for most Japanese today. And, second, had the idea of depression (and of psychiatry as a profession) not been so stigmatized previously, might not Japanese have experienced depression differently as early as a century ago, and even sought out medical care for a condition from which they wished to be liberated?

For us to start examining these questions in greater depth, previous historical claims made about depression by cultural psychiatrists may have been too ideologically drawn, it seems, and were based on radically dichotomized notions about the West and the Rest (e.g., Ōhira and Machizawa 1988). Before its currently reported rise worldwide, depression had often been talked about as a quintessentially Western experience. Melancholy, the predecessor to depression, is said to have a long history in the West, dating from when Aristotle claimed it to be an illness of geniuses (Jackson 1986, Radden 2000). Along this line of thought, the symptoms of depression—particularly sadness, a sense of guilt, and self-blame—were regarded as signs of maturity, even of adult selfhood. Later claims were made in the 1960s that Westerners suffered depression because of their Christian notion of guilt, which gave them a sense of interiority and an ability to reflect upon themselves. By contrast, non-Westerners, it was claimed, did not possess reflexive selves and were unable to suffer from depression because their immature and nonautonomous selves did not have a capacity for introspection (see Littlewood and Dein 2000). Japanese psychiatrists have examined, from the 1950s, the claim made by Ruth Benedict (based on Japanese detainees in California during World War II) that Japanese have a cultural self that is based not on guilt but rather on shame (Benedict 1946). They have considered the further implication of this argument and wondered if the absence of depression in Japan might be because the Japanese self was heavily dependent on adherence to external authority and a so-called "relational self." Indeed, it is against this highly Western-centric discourse that some Japanese psychiatrists such as Kimura Bin began to assert an alternative argument. Kimura adopted the notion of "cultural self" only to invert it to argue that the absence of depression in Japan testified not to an immature self but rather to the strength of their cultural tradition. Unlike "Westerners" who find in depression "something unnatural and abnormal," Japanese, Kimura argued, maintain a high level of tolerance for, and even find aesthetical dimensions of, depression (Kimura 1979).[8]

---

[8] The essence of this cultural argument was crystallized in Gannath Obeyesekere's (1985) work

Miyamoto Tadao (1979) as well urged other scholars to start examining why it is that Japanese had not apparently perceived depression as a medical condition prior to the introduction of Western psychiatry in the nineteenth century. From these perspectives, the current rise of depression documented in Japan might be regarded as yet another example of the encroachment of the West into the intimate realm of the sense of self.[9]

By going back to the time prior to the advent of psychiatry in Japan in the late nineteenth century, however, I have uncovered that there was—and has remained—a rich undercurrent of alternative medical language that recognized "depression" as a form of pathology (see chapters 2 through 5). Contrary to the common claims made by Japanese psychiatrists, traditional medicine, at least since the sixteenth century onward, had a concept of depression as an illness of emotions. In fact, the modern Japanese term for depression—utsubyō—came directly out of traditional medicine, when the term was adopted in the nineteenth century as the Japanese translation of melancholia. Utsubyō[10] or *utsushō*, as it was formerly called, had strikingly similar characteristics to the Western notion of melancholia: Both referred to the physical and mental condition of stagnation in vital energy—*ki* in the case of Japanese utsushō and a humor in the case of Western melancholia. They both accounted for how people might feel "depressed" from the complex interplay between social events, emotional experiences, and physiological changes in the body. Adopted in popular writings and plays, they respectively carried cultural and moral meanings that were far beyond the narrow medical definitions of a "disease." What partly brought an epistemological break to the premodern notion of utsushō in Japan was, I suggest, the adoption of German neurobiological psychiatry in the nineteenth century, which turned this condition into a matter of a diseased brain, while thoroughly erasing for Japanese its social, cultural, and psychological mean-

---

on depression in Sri Lanka; he argued that culture interprets the negative affect as a religious experience to the extent that the depressed are saved from being pathologized and socially excluded as mentally ill. These perspectives are important in illuminating the "work of culture" (Obeyesekere 1985) as a mediating force, and examining how certain affects become bestowed with much anxiety in some societies more than others (also see Gaines 1992, Kleinman and Good 1985).

[9] In the postwar period, Japanese psychiatry has paid relatively little attention to milder forms of mental illness in the population at large. A well-known psychiatrist who specializes in depression, Ōhara (1981), suggests that there was a near-absence of depression in the war periods. A leading psychoanalyst, Nishizono (1988:265), notes his amusement at the popularity of depression in the West in 1964. This is not so surprising if we realize that until the 1960s, when antidepressants were introduced, depression was considered—even in the United States—a "rare" disease (Healey 1997). But even after the 1980 introduction of DSM-III, Japanese psychiatrists continued to state that the American concept of major depression is far too inclusive (Honda 1983), and not applicable to Japanese. However, the exclusive focus on academic psychiatry misses, as we will see in chapter 4, the flourishing interest in mental illness in popular culture from the early twentieth century.

[10] The historical origin of this term will be closely examined in chapter 2. Many medical terms were newly invented in the eighteenth and nineteenth century, when scholars were translating a massive number of Western medical texts into Japanese.

ings. Furthermore, modern psychiatry created not just categories of disease but, as Ian Hacking (1986) has argued, "kinds of people"—in this case, the manic-depressive whose brain was assumed to be inherently different from others." Psychiatry, in other words, no longer listened to narratives about the depression of ordinary Japanese.

Indeed, one may even argue that the history of modern psychiatry in Japan is characterized by this radical disconnection with subjective pain (Foucault 1975, cf., Duden 1991, Yamaguchi 1990, Porter 1985). Japanese psychiatry, similar to psychiatric practices in other countries, has asserted its scientific authority by determining what is a medically recognized, legitimate "disease" as opposed to an unclassified and undiagnosable (mere) complaint. Moreover, its history started as an importation of Western-born categories, with the result that psychiatrists have paid more attention to making everyday reality fit preexisting classifications rather than exploring the chaotic realities presented by their patients. By adopting the neurobiological language of German psychiatrist Emil Kraepelin, which replaced the authority derived from patients' subjective accounts with the experts' objective observation (Hoff 1996, Radden 2000), Japanese psychiatry may have done much to discredit people's experience. And it is by means of this selective attention and particular construction of mental illness that Japanese psychiatrists have claimed that Japanese did not suffer from depression. Thus, the new psychiatric language of depression might, in fact, re-cultivate people's awareness of the interconnectedness of the social with the body and emotions. But this could also serve as a "colonization of the lifeworld" (Habermas 1987), if it begins to function as the authoritative, monolithic language that overdetermines the meanings of subjective experiences (Good 1994).

As one arena where psychiatry exposes its limits as a language of experience, I will examine people's own narratives about how they have recovered from depression and illuminate the gaps and discrepancies that so often exist between what is reported from psychiatrists and patients. At another level of analysis, I will examine why, statistically, until recently Japanese males were as likely, if not more so, to suffer depression as women—a striking difference from the West, where women are twice as likely as men to suffer depression (these figures have changed rapidly with the current medicalization of depression: see chapters 8 and 10). Through Japanese men's narratives, I show how psychiatric language might effectively provide a way of understanding—and legitimizing—their distress as a product of overwork. By contrast I show how the same language seems to have often failed to speak in a satisfactory way about women's "depression," and how much difficulty women seem to have had, and continue to have at times, in having their profound distress even recognized. By illuminating the gendered structuring of depression (cf. Hubert 2002), I raise the possibility that psychiatrists may listen more attentively to the suffering of certain people to the exclusion of others. And in so doing, I ask for whom this language may be particularly liberating, and for whom it may be subjugating (Abu-Lughod 1990, Comaroff 1985, Scott 1985, 1990). Whether medicalization results in more diversified articulation of individual suffering, and if these new-found voices serve to counter the effects of medicalization that dominate individual subjectivity, are questions that will be examined throughout this book.

Importantly, I also want to call attention to the pivotal role psychiatrists have played in transforming fragmented individual testimonies of social injustice into a *public language* of pain by focusing on the psychopathology of work (chapter 9). This kind of biomedical validation of suffering—such as a PTSD diagnosis for war veterans (Young 1995) or a medical certificate of disability for the victims of Ukrainian nuclear disaster (Petryna 2002)—has become an indispensable tool for people in contemporary societies demanding economic compensation for their social distress (cf. Kleinman 1986). Also, it is partly because Japanese psychiatrists have portrayed typical depressed patients as hardworking salarymen that they have been persuasive. Both in the media and in psychiatric literature, they have done much to create a strong association between depression and people suffering overwork, loss of employment, bankruptcy, and overwork suicide. Psychiatrists, by providing powerful testimonies for depressed workers, have come to redefine the depressed as victims of both biological and social forces. By emphasizing work as an important cause of depression and by portraying the depressed as subject to the brutal forces of economic restructuring that Japanese society is going through, they have successfully promoted depression as a social problem worthy of political, economic, and legal intervention. It is in this sense that psychiatrists have had their most liberating effects well beyond the narrow clinical domains—and have begun to have a public voice in the political sphere (see chapters 9 through 11). I thus demonstrate the conceptual and institutional links psychiatrists have made between depression, work stress, and recession in order to demonstrate how the difference in medicalization stems in part from particular political and economic concerns that are driving the medicalization of depression in Japan.

PART ONE

Depression in History

WHEN SPEAKING IN North America and Europe about the sudden rise of depression in Japan, I have frequently been asked whether Japanese did not suffer from depression previously and why it is that Japanese have become susceptible so suddenly. Some scholars have asked me whether the Japanese experience is another case of the transfer of the "Western" concept to—and Americanization of—Japan, or if there were equivalent (or alternative) understandings of depression that are somehow unique to Japanese society. While there are no simple answers to these questions, my historical investigation of depression in Japan, drawing on medical texts and other printed works dating back to the sixteenth century, sheds some light on the fact that depression is not merely a recent import.

From my investigation into premodern notions of utsubyō (or its predecessor, utsushō), I discovered that, contrary to the assertion made by some psychiatrists, this term has had long historical roots in Japanese traditional medicine (chapter 2). Originally imported from China and incorporated into Japanese medical knowledge by the sixteenth century, utsushō was a category that indicated pathological stagnation leading to a wide range of symptoms, including lack of energy, dejection, and social withdrawal. After the mid-seventeenth century when lay people began to seek medical care for it, utsushō gradually took on polarized moral meanings, later used by intellectuals to connote an illness caused by both excessive use of the mind and of idleness. Tracing the shifting meanings given to utsushō, I examine in what ways premodern Japanese employed this term to express their sense of the body, ways of being, and the social environment in which they lived. I also point out certain parallels between this notion and melancholia in the West, as they were both used to express the intimate connection between mind and body.

In chapter 3, I suggest that what partly created this historical discontinuity in Japanese medical knowledge of depression was the epistemological break brought by the official installation of biomedicine in the late nineteenth century. Adopting German neuropsychiatry in the 1880s, Japanese psychiatrists began to discard traditional medical ideas by arguing that psychopathology—including utsubyō—was a matter of individual neurological defects existing independently of social environment. Utsubyō became further detached from its former cultural meanings when it was reclassified as a form of psychosis (manic depression), which signified genetic abnormality. I thus provide in this chapter a broad sketch of the history of Japanese psychiatry to show that the reemergence of utsubyō as a popular category of illness today cannot be understood apart from the historical transformation that Japanese psychiatry itself has gone through—from a biologically oriented discipline reserved for the severely ill to an expanding web of medical practice that encompasses treatment of people's everyday distress.

Despite the seeming obscurity of depression in the official discourse of early twentieth century Japanese academic psychiatry, a shift in vantage point allows us to discover rich terrain where Japanese continued to express anxiety over everyday distress and sought medical care for it. As discussed in chapter 4, this is manifested in the "epidemic" of neurasthenia that swept through the United States and Europe in the late nineteenth century and spread to Japan at the turn of the twentieth century. While this epidemic was a global concern at the time, it took a distinctive form in Japan as it helped familiarize Japanese with Western concepts of the nervous system and the brain. As an early case of broadscale medicalization, that discourse about neurasthenia retained many parallels with the current discourse around depression, most notably in the public debates over its causality—that is, whether neurasthenia was a result of overwork or of individual biological weakness. I further show in this chapter how psychiatry relentlessly expanded the neurasthenia concept, only to later stigmatize those who had resorted to it and internalized this illness category.

The neurasthenia discourse of the 1900s through the 1930s created a mold from which Japanese psychiatrists came to shape their distinctive language of depression from the 1930s on. In chapter 5, I examine the emergence of this psychiatric language by focusing on local medical theories about premorbid depressive personality. These theories, which were further developed by psychiatrists of the post–World War II era as an attempt to overcome prewar biological reductionism, show the personality of depressed Japanese in a normative light (serious, hardworking, considerate, and responsible), while also calling attention to overwork and fatigue as important social causes for depression. By tracing the shifting interpretations of this premorbid depressive personality, I show how psychiatrists' reinterpretations of the "biological" have been essential for redefining depression as social pathology warranting legal, economic, and political intervention.

By providing an overview of the changing history of depression in Japan—an area that has remained largely unexplored to date—I show how Japanese psychiatrists have successfully transformed depression into one of the most talked about illnesses today. Also by illuminating the recurrent theme of overwork and fatigue in Japanese medical discourses about depression, I explore how they have come to construe a particular understanding of the depressed as legitimate victims of both biological and social forces lying beyond their control.

CHAPTER TWO

Reading Emotions in the Body:
The Premodern Language of Depression

> When doctors in the Neijing subsequently spoke of *qi*
> rising in anger, sinking in fear, sweeping away in sorrow,
> they weren't so much trying to explain emotions,
> objectively, as relating what they knew from their own
> bodies, describing what they felt, subjectively, within
> themselves. In anger, a sudden, explosive surge; in grief, a
> draining away. It was the intimate everyday familiarity of
> such sensations that made the traditional discourse of
> vital flux so compelling. The deepest certainties about *qi*
> were rooted in knowledge that people had of the body
> because they *were*, themselves, bodies.
>
> —Kuriyama (on Chinese traditional medicine),
> *The Expressiveness of the Body* (1999:103)

The Historical Absence of "Depression"?

ANTHROPOLOGISTS OF MEDICINE have long asked how it is that some medical concepts travel well—and become integrated into local knowledge—while others, when transferred to another culture, seem to remain alien, experience-distant, even incommensurable. While anthropologists have traditionally interpreted a failure of translation as a sign of fundamental cultural difference, more recently they have questioned the cultural essentialism lurking behind such a claim and instead begun to explore the issue of power in translation. By investigating initial moments of concept transfer historically, anthropologists have asked what forces are at play in adopting a certain medical concept—or a language—and how such moments of transfer can be read as sites of power struggle among competing medical languages, each of which is used to represent, even construe, different modes of reality.

In this regard, the "rise" of depression in Japan since the late 1990s presents an intriguing case because, despite the nineteenth-century transfer of the psychiatric concept of depression from Germany, Japanese psychiatrists have long been puzzled about the seeming rarity among Japanese. While the depression concept itself is firmly entrenched in professional psychiatric knowledge in Japan, it seems to have had little salience or explanatory power among most Japanese for understanding their experiences, thereby suggesting a failure in translation. Some psychiatrists have thus speculated that, unlike in the West where depression—or its precedent melancholia—has had a long history, depression essentially did not exist in Japan before the advent of modern psychiatry (Miyamoto 1979). Other prominent scholars such as Kimura Bin (1979) have also argued that a Japanese traditional tolerance for—or even aestheticization of—depressed feelings might have kept Japanese from seeing depressive-like moods as pathological. Psychiatrists in Japan were thus confounded to find depression suddenly emerging from the 1990s as an everyday idiom of distress, with the media calling it a "national disease."

How can we interpret this sudden rise and the alleged historical absence of depression? On the one hand, Kimura and other Japanese psychiatrists may be pointing to a salient difference when they state that, unlike in the West, where the notion of melancholia achieved an evocative, symbolic status not only in medicine but also in religion, philosophy, and literature, there was no equivalent of melancholia-like insanity in the history of Japanese medicine. On the other hand, however, if we broaden the notion of depression to include its milder forms, psychiatrists may have been too presumptuous in thinking that Japanese simply aestheticized—and rarely pathologized—depressed emotions. My research into the history of depression has revealed that not only did the same term that Japanese now use for depression—utsubyō (鬱病)—exist in premodern Japan but that its antiquated forms—utsushō (鬱症／鬱証) and ki-utsubyō (気鬱病) —began to appear in popular literature by the eighteenth century as illness categories characterized by gloomy mood, lack of energy, and social withdrawal. In fact, when the concept of melancholia was transferred from Dutch medicine in the late eighteenth century, some variants of "utsu" terms (such as utsubyō or utsuyūbyō) were eventually adopted as its standard translation. Why is it then that Japanese psychiatrists have come to assume that premodern Japanese had no concept of depression?

By drawing upon recent historiographies of the body in Japanese medicine by Kuriyama Shigehisa (1997, 1999) and others (Shirasugi 1997), and using traditional medical texts and popular literature, I want to attempt a kind of semantic historiography of depression. Instead of starting with a strictly defined cluster of depressive symptoms as we understand them today and examining how such a disease entity moved across history under different times, I want to trace the term "utsu" itself and examine what meanings and conditions were implicated at different moments of concept transfer. In so doing, I hope to illuminate how the previous psychiatric discussions about premodern depression have not fully taken into account that the kind of epistemological break that Foucault has described with regard to French modernity (Foucault 1973) happened in Japan with far more decisive force—particularly in medicine (e.g., Garon 1997). By the late nineteenth century, Japanese had come to largely abandon traditional ways of understanding themselves and instead adopted an entirely new language,[1] a language that began to constitute the modern self. This new, "global" medical language introduced to lay Japanese notions like "nerves" (which was unknown in Japan until introduced from Europe) and the brain (an organ previously thought to have little importance) as the locus of control. This language further introduced the neuropsychiatric concept of depression as an abstracted reality that exists in and of itself (cf. Zimmermann 2008), while serving to invalidate the traditional language for reading emotions in the body, of which the premodern notion of *depression* was a part. Illuminating how Japanese experienced the body and mind differently at different times, I will ask how it is that "depression" as people talked about it in the Edo Era had, via the nineteenth-century concept transfer of depression from German neuropsychiatry, become so unfamiliar, so obsolete for most Japanese that psychiatrists even came to assume that such an illness experience hardly existed.

Utsushō as an Illness of *Ki*-stagnation

A contemporary Japanese who hears that there existed an illness term called *utsubyō* or *utsushō* might readily assume that depression must have existed in premodern Japan. *Utsu* is a common term that has long been used to connote a gloomy mood, and *shō* and *byō* respectively indicate symptom and illness. Yet, this seeming transparency is actually deceiving when we look at the original meaning of utsushō. Before there was the medical concept of utsushō, utsu was an ordinary word that already had a long history. Utsu has dual meanings: first of all, as the character utsu (鬱) is graphically made up of trees "densely growing together," the term signifies a physiological state where things are rampant, densely overgrown, or stagnated. Second, in both Chinese and Japanese literature, utsu has also been used from the early time as an expression for gloominess, sorrow, and pensiveness (Morohashi 1984: 13261–65). What united these seemingly separate meanings was the premodern belief in the phenomenon called ki (*qi* in Chinese). Ki was an essential aspect of the premodern Japanese thought—the idea that not only all the living things but also the world, and the cosmic itself, are filled with this life energy (Arima 1990, Maebayashi et al. 2000). Ki was invisible and intangible, and yet it could be felt in the form of wind when it moved in the atmosphere and in the form of breath when exhaled by the human body. As something that was constantly circulating, ki would alter and was altered by both external and internal forces, one of which was the movement of emotions. Thus when premodern Japanese talked about utsu, presumably it was ki itself that was being stagnated in the physiological sense,

[1] The modern state officially adopted "Western medicine" and effectively de-legitimized traditional medicine in 1874, though the latter has certainly survived into the twenty-first century (see Lock 1980).

while the same ki—causing blockage in the human body—was thought to give rise to a psychologically depressed state. In fact, premodern literature is rife with such words that referred to utsu in these dual meanings, suggesting the idea that ki surging in anger, draining away in sorrow, knotted and blocked in prudence, was indeed part of the common wisdom in premodern Japan, which accounted for the sensations arising both in the mind and body (cf. Kuriyama 1999).

While the word *utsu* itself had these two meanings, "utsushō" (sign of utsu) as a medical concept seems to have started with its first connotation, that is, to simply denote various sorts of pathological stagnation, before it came to acquire a predominant image of an illness of emotions. The concept was transferred from China at the turn of the sixteenth century by Tashiro Sanki (1465–1544). According to Tashiro, there were, under the category of utsushō, six different kinds of utsu, depending on what was stagnating: that is, stagnations of ki, moisture, heat, phlegm, blood, and food. Ki-utsu would produce "sharp, stinging pain" in the chest, dizziness and headaches, or "swelling in the auxiliary region" (Tashiro 1979:151); phlegm-utsu would cause shortness of breath; blood-utsu would cause limbs to lose their energy and produce red feces (see Manase Dōsan 1979:15–17). Because such stagnation was thought to be underlying various physical pains, doctors were able to make diagnoses of what kind of utsu a patient had by examining the manifested physical symptoms. Tashiro's famous disciples, Manase Dōsan (1507–94) and Gensaku (1549–1631), who helped establish Gosei School of Medicine, further instilled this notion in medicine by using it in their case books. For instance, Yodogimi (a mistress of the ruler of Japan at the time) was diagnosed with utsushō in her thirties when she showed the symptoms of headaches, insomnia, and congested and aching chest. Emperor Goyōzei was also diagnosed with utsushō at the age of twenty-eight and successfully treated with herbal medication when he suffered sudden dizziness, lost consciousness, and rapidly fell into a critical condition (Manase Gensaku 1979:93–94, 98). The third Shōgun of the Edo Era, Tokugawa Iemitsu, also suffered the illness of ki-utsu in his thirties (Hattori 1978:686–92). As these cases suggest, utsushō as a medical diagnosis was originally a broadly defined concept that indicated the internal blockages of all kinds. The fact that the traditional medical notion of "shō" merely indicates a symptom, even a shifting phase of an illness, makes it even more difficult to equate it with the modern notion of depression as a disease.

While such essential differences exist between utsushō and depression, it is notable that when Japan's first medical dictionary was published in 1686, utsushō came to be succinctly defined as an illness of seven emotions (Ashikawa 1982). *Ki-utsushō* (the illness of ki-utsu) in particular became a common category, interchangeably used with utsushō to indicate an illness of lack of energy and gloomy mood. Perhaps this was not surprising given the fact that ki was the most essential element of health, the very thing that made possible the circulation of other substances throughout the body. And because ki was also thought to govern emotions, ki-utsu became the most essential feature of utsushō, and took on both the physiological and psychological meanings. Utsushō was conceptualized as a state in which ki would lose its normality, becoming stagnated and blocked, unable to dissipate (Tashiro 1979), and as such would be caused by both external and internal forces, such as climate, diet, sleep, and lifestyle. Yet, what seems to stand out in these medical texts as an important cause for utsushō, was the movement of *emotions*. When a person experienced sudden and intense emotions, ki was thought to gather in one place and become stagnated. Ki-stagnation could also occur from chronic emotional distress, when there was a long-term discord in interpersonal relationship or one's relation to the environment. For instance, Tashiro writes: "when a man or woman has his/her spirit knotted in pensiveness, is unable to fulfill their amorous longing, or rages in jealousy, ki in the chest would go wild, losing its order, rising in its intensity" (Tashiro 1979:40). Stagnated ki could become a knot, gradually form a blockage in the body, at times causing sharp pain around the stomach and the heart, which were, in traditional Japanese thought, the location of the *soul*. One may say that, for Japanese, in accordance with Chinese traditional thought, what "control[s] and regulate[s] the body and its various energies" was the "flowing mind" (cf. Ishida 1989:67). Such descriptions of utsushō continued to appear in medical textbooks throughout the Edo period, suggesting that, when premodern Japanese talked about the illness of ki-utsu, presumably it was ki itself that was being stagnated in the physiological sense, while the same ki—causing blockage in the human body—was thought to give rise to a psychologically gloomy state. Thus the kind of people often described in popular literature at the time—people who long for someone so deeply, so intensely that they would wither away, fall ill, even die in sorrow—could now be medically understood and treated accordingly, at least theoretically, as suffering utsushō.

What may have helped establish utsushō—particularly ki-utsushō—as a distinctive illness category was the increasing attention to *psychological*, emotional distress as a cause of illness in seventeenth-century medicine. This was a time when the Edo government brought more than two hundred years of political stability and economic prosperity, which encouraged medical practice to become more widely available as a form of commercial enterprise. Medical theories also came to be deeply engrained in lay people's lives, as they began to read how-to books on health and to seek out wide-ranging treatments—including herbal medication, acupuncture, moxibustion, massage, and hot springs (Shirasugi 1997). Influential doctors such as Gotō Konzan, who helped establish the Kohō School of Medicine in opposition to the Manases' Gosei School, chose to practice among lay people rather than catering to the wealthy few and ardently promoted the idea that people can cultivate their own health by maintaining a smooth circulation of ki (Liang 1997). Based upon his clinical practice, Gotō observed that, paradoxically in a time of peace and prosperity, "more and more people are suffering from *ki-utsu*" (Gotō, cited in Shirasugi 1997:71). Gotō argued that in the Tokugawa Regime, when people no longer had to suffer from serious external injuries (as they did during previous wars), they were instead beginning to suffer from altogether different kinds of illnesses. This was because, he asserted, people no longer "moved their bodies" but "used their mind, seeking to fulfill their desires." What they now had was "internal torment and a hundred illnesses," which, according to Gotō, stemmed from the condition of ki-utsu (Gotō cited in Shirasugi 1997:71). The secret to health was thus to prevent ki-stagnation by going out and moving their bodies and nurturing one's ki. Through Gotō's formulation, ki-utsu came to represent a ubiquitous and overarching theory of illness, while utsushō and ki-utsushō were often used to connote psychological, emotional distress that underlined physical symptoms (Gotō 1971: 395).

Ki-utsu became an important theme for doctors across competing schools of medicine, as they began to preach how severe stagnation of ki would not occur in a day or two but indicated that days, months, even years were spent in the kind of life that would produce ki-utsu. The presence of stubborn ki-utsu thus reflected the habit of the body and one's way of living, or as Kuriyama puts it, "the weight of one's past" (Kuriyama 1997:58). As to what kind of "past" they were referring to, there emerged, in the discourse of ki-utsu, two polarized moral meanings, with gradations in between. On the one hand, as Katsuki Gyūzan (1656–1740), a contemporary of Gotō noted, the kinds of people who would develop ki-utsu were thought to be "a formerly affluent person who fell into poverty, a woman who does not get along with her in-laws or husband, and a samurai who works far from home" (Katsuki 1981:361). In other words, they were the kinds of people whose social, moral, and psychological agonies were manifested through ki-utsu—as an inscription of suffering onto the body. On the other hand, however, ki-utsu was also a sign of moral failure for those who lead an unproductive life. Kaibara Ekiken (1630–1714), one of the most important neo-Confucianist scholars in the Edo period who also produced influential self-help books, described ki-utsu as a sign of idleness, particularly afflicting women. In his widely read book, *Yōjōkun* (Theory of Health), published in 1713, he says: "Women are more prone to *ki-utsu*—and illnesses in general—because they tend to stay inside. They should make sure to use their body and labor" (Kaibara 1928:103). Behind this new health consciousness about ki-stagnation may lie, as Kuriyama has argued, the protocapitalist transformation that Japan was experiencing from the seventeenth century, which brought an increasing demand on human labor. The work ethic born out of this so-called "industrious revolution" was, he suggests, inseparable from the discourse of health that was being advocated by medical theorists of the time. The new sensibility and anxiety about ki-stagnation may have paralleled the rise of the sociopolitical discourse on the smooth flow of goods and currency in the new economic order (Kuriyama 1997).[2]

---

[2] Note that the dual moral meanings of sorrow and idleness are also pronounced in the history

These polarized moral meanings of ki-utsu seem to have also penetrated the popular imagination of the Edo Era. The first prototypical utsushō patient that appeared in popular books was an intellectual who adopted the notion of the illness of ki-utsu for describing his own condition as an embodiment of excessive contemplation and long-term emotional agonies that he silently suffered. For instance, Tachibana Nankei (1753–1805), a doctor and a popular essayist of the Edo period, cites his friend's words that "[p]eople today are suffering from the illness of ki-utsu and, even after they rest, remain dejected. They have poor complexion, lack ki-energy, and become thin." Tachibana agrees with his friend, however, that "the kind of people who do not even suffer ki-utsu are generally fools" (Tachibana 1927:28), which suggests that the illness might have carried a certain moral weight of social legitimacy for those who suffered. Also, Rai Shunsui, the father of Rai Sanyō who later became one of the most influential historians of the Edo period, wrote in his diary on June 8, 1798 that his son was suffering "utsushō." During the same month, Shizuko, Sanyō's mother, repeatedly noted in her diary that her son was feeling dejected and withdrawn, for which he was treated with medication and moxibustion as well as taken out for walks (Rai Shizuko 1931–32:129–30). Rai Sanyō apparently went through depressed phases and highly active phases (Nakamura 1971:15–25) and was rumored by his neighbors to be suffering insanity. Such a case suggests that utsushō may have served as a conveniently ambiguous and broad category used to connote insanity. Indeed, while a medical specialization in insanity began to emerge in the latter half of the eighteenth century, ki-stagnation became one of the important foundations for Japanese medical theorizing of madness. Prominent scholars such as Kagawa Shūan (1683–1755), a distinguished disciple of Gotō, began to produce a systematic classification of insanity (published in 1807) based on his clinical observations, and discussed how it could be explained by ki-stagnation (Kagawa 1982).[3]

---

of melancholia. As Stanley Jackson discusses, *acedia*, a notion that has a historical link with melancholia in the West, which implied sorrow or dejection, also came to acquire the meaning of idleness by the eleventh century (Jackson 1986:72–77).

[3] As in many other parts of the world, in Japan there were historical shifts in the way people talked about insanity from earlier, magical thought that located the pathogenic agent of insanity external to individuals (as in spirit possession) to later traditional medical thoughts that increasingly placed it internal to individual biology (cf. Young 1976). The previous term for insanity was "tabure" (deviation from others), which was treated by various forms of religious chant meant to drive the bad spirit away. Such beliefs were increasingly replaced, in the Edo Era, by the notion of *ki-chigai* (ki-discord, which, according to Kaneko [1965], originally meant one's ki becoming replaced by a wraith or a spirit of the dead) by medical doctors who came to redefine it as a loss of balance in interpersonal relations as well as in natural elements within an individual body (Oda 1998). Historians have suggested that it was in the late Edo Era that a notable specialization in insanity took shape in medical textbooks and clinical practice (Okada 2002, Omata 1998). This sudden specialization might be due, according to Hiruta (1999a), to urbanization and the development of a commerce economy that led people to look for a different rationale (and a more individualized approach) to health and illness. In addition, the high density and oversupply of doctors in the cities (e.g., 250 doctors per 100,000 people in Edo in 1819) may have prompted some doctors to seek a

The second prototypical utsushō patient, who continued to appear in popular literature from the Edo period to the Meiji, was a spoiled son or daughter of a rich family, leading a leisurely, unproductive life, who suffered utsushō as a form of love sickness. A widely read book that collected town rumors in the eighteenth century, it featured a story about a son of an affluent farmer who developed utsushō from the strong longings for a courtesan he left in the city (Negishi 1972:250). Also, in a number of stories in Ukiyozōshi, a genre of highly popular novellas for townspeople, Ejima Kiseki (1666–1735) writes about the kinds of people who were thought to have "utsushō," including a young woman who becomes pregnant without her mother's knowledge and develops a condition resembling illness. Her worried mother has this to say: "An illness like this in a girl brought up with tender care must be *utsushō*; it might develop into *rōzeki* [an illness which was later equated with tuberculosis]. Take good care of yourself and get well soon" (Ejima and Hasegawa 1989:426). In other stories, Ejima also wrote that "women are prone to *ki-utsu*," and that "if it is *ki-utsu*, then there is no need to take any medication. Go out as you would like and nurture your ki. What is important is that you do not worry about a thing" (Ejima and Hasegawa 1989:462). This seems to suggest a transformation of utsushō from the Manases' time, when their clients—mainly aristocrats whose leisurely, idle way of being would have been simply assumed rather than condemned—were seriously treated with herbal medication. As utsushō became reinterpreted by Gotō to symbolize lack of physical movement and an excess of desires, it may have acquired a certain moral ambiguity as a medical category, particularly for the rising merchant class with the new work ethic, who constituted the readership of such literature. For them, utsushō may have served as a symbolic label of mockery and blame, an illness of those who stood in opposition to the idealized, active, hardworking life where ki was constantly in flux. Utsushō signaled for them not just a psychological torment but also its unhealthy excess.

And it might have been this popularization and psychologization of utsushō that played a part in its gradual conceptual transformation—and later its historical obscuration. There are signs that, by the time the illness of ki-utsu became popularly known, it may have had lost its original meaning of vital energy being physically stagnated, a lay interpretation that doctors at the time apparently saw as a threat to their original medical formulation. Azai Teian (1770–1829), who wrote thirty-four medical textbooks, was an influential director of a tutoring school that trained over 3,000 doctors. In his lecture on utsushō, he gave an extensive criticism of the increasing gap between the technical, medical meaning and the lay interpretation of utsushō. Azai's words suggest that lay

---

new subfield (Hiruta 1999b). Thus, after Ashikawa Keishū created the classifications of insanity (such as *tenkyō*), Kagawa Shūan (1683–1755) for the first time produced systematic classification of insanity. In 1819, Tsuchida Ken wrote Japan's first treatise on insanity, discussing more than 58 such cases out of 1,000 patients he treated over ten years (Tsuchida 1979).

people at the time, even when they said they were suffering from ki-utsu, did not envision their ki to be physically stagnated:

> What we here [in this lecture] call ki-utsu is different from what today's people say, as in 'working made me ki-utsu.' Ki-utsu means that ki-breath is in a state of utsu—that is, ki-breath is unable to stretch and has become blocked. . . . In Japanese language, people use ki to refer to mind. They say they used ki when they mean they used their mind. They say they dispersed ki when they mean they refreshed their mind. What ki really means, however, is ki of breath. Thus these (usages) are entirely mistakes on the side of lay people. (Azai 1981:440–41)

This psychologized lay interpretation of ki-stagnation may have had to do with the fact that the notion of ki itself was going through a fundamental transformation during the Edo period, when, as many Japanese historians have pointed out, ki began to lose its corporeality and instead came to be used as a psychological term merely indicating mood or feeling (Nakai 1995, Maebayashi et al. 2000). Unlike Chinese who have largely retained the traditional meaning of qi, as a notion that unites mind and body,[4] Japanese have come to regard ki predominantly as a psychological notion, stripped of its former relation to the body. For modern Japanese (except in special contexts such as traditional medicine and martial arts), ki denotes little more than the mind or feeling, and while there are numerous psychological expressions that include ki, these are almost all understood to be little more than a metaphor (Doi 2000). When Japanese today talk about *"ki ga hareru"* (ki dissipating) to express feeling cheered up, *ki ga meiru* (ki depressed) or feeling depressed, they almost never imagine that there is a real physiological entity called ki doing all these movements—it is only in the mind. When depressed, they certainly would not think that it may be that their mind—as well as body—could be suffering from some kind of stagnation. No definitive studies have been conducted to trace exactly how this conceptual change happened in Japan. We do not know to what extent this was an "internal" development that signaled the beginning of Japanese modern thought (Nakai 1995) or a result of "external" stimuli brought on by the fragmented but increasing encounters with Western medicine and science. Whatever it was that created a new critical sensibility, it may well be that this psychologization and decorporealization of ki itself partly explains how utsushō became an obscure, metaphorical existence, prompting Japanese psychiatrists to assume that Japanese had rarely spoken of an illness of depressed emotions (see figures 2.1 and 2.2).[5]

---

[4] Dominic T. S. Lee, Joan Kleinman, and Arthur Kleinman (2007) have been conducting a fascinating exploration of how these traditional medical ideas about qi are expressed through a language of embodied emotion by people who suffer "depression" in contemporary China.

[5] I would like to thank Professor Kuriyama Shigehisa for drawing my attention to the existence of this print.

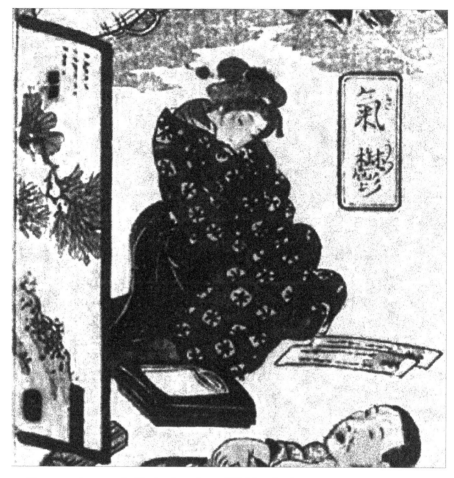

Figure 2.1. A woman in ki-utsu (courtesy of Nichibunken).

Replaced by Melancholia

> The sorrow that has no vent in tears
> makes other organs weep.
> —Henry Maudsley[6]

If utsushō had become a rather ambiguous medical category even before modernity, what made it decisively obsolete was the transfer of Western concepts

---

[6] Cited in Littlewood and Dein 2000:14

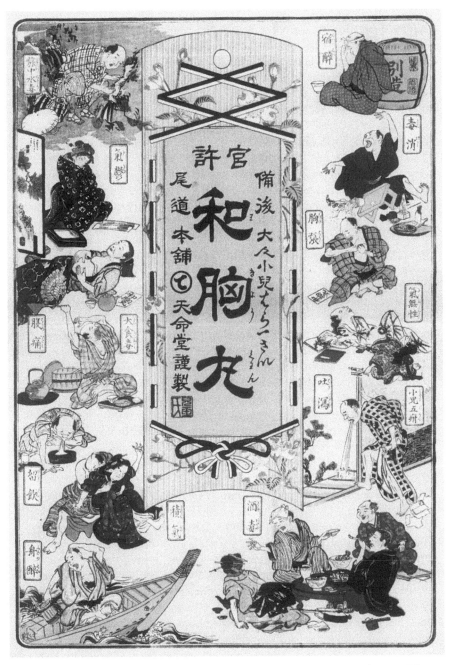

Figure 2.2. An advertisement for an all-purpose pill called Wakyōgan (Wakyōgan Hiki-fuda, courtesy of Nichibunken).

of melancholia and later depression. Yet, it is important to note that this historical transformation did not occur at once, but that it happened in two steps.

Initially, the two concepts—utsushō and melancholia—may have had more similarities than differences. First of all, both signified pathological gloom and sorrow. Second, just as utsushō was caused by stagnation of ki, melancholia was, in the eighteenth-century West, still thought to be caused by stagnation of black bile (Jackson 1986). Thus, in Japan's first textbook on Western internal medicine, by Udagawa Genzui (1755–97) published in 1792 (which was a translation of a textbook written by a Dutch doctor named Johannes de Gorter [1689–1762], a disciple of Herman Boerhaave at the Leiden School of Medicine), melancholia, though here given the name of an illness of black bile (*zoeki haikokushō*), was translated in language that closely resembled the descriptions of utsushō in traditional medical writings. The textbook explained how black bile that traveled to the brain ended up "changing the normal state of ki-spirit (Geist here translated as *sei-ki* or 'ki-spirit')" thereby causing "one's spirit and perception to become illusionary, pensive, and sad." Like utsushō, melancholia was still an extension of normality, and could thus be treated, for instance, by "discharging the black bile through feces" (Udagawa 1995:357–60). Utsushō appeared as a translation for melancholia in a widely used textbook on Western medicine published by Komori Touu (1782–1843) in 1829–34 (see Komori excerpted in Kaneko 1965:272–75), from which time on, utsushō or another variant of the term *utsu-yū-byō* (the added "yū" meaning pensiveness) became the standard translations for melancholia. A notable difference was that, in various translated Western medical texts, there was an increasing emphasis on melancholia's hereditary cause—with the diseased brain as the locus of insanity (see Komori in Kaneko 1965). However, as melancholia and utsushō still reflected holistic perspectives on health, what was important for both was, in principle, to restore the balance of the mind and body by recovering the natural circulation of the essential life force—albeit with different ideas of what constituted that life force.

If Japanese psychiatrists today are largely unaware of the conceptual affinity and even a certain historical continuity between melancholia and utsushō, it is partly because the notion of melancholia itself in the West went through significant conceptual transformations, particularly during the nineteenth century. The change of the term from melancholia to depression was in effect to cut off the philosophical and existential baggage that the holistic concept of melancholia had, and instead to emphasize the pathological physiological mechanism of the brain and the nerves. These changes brought by Western medicines and their mechanical notion of the nerve were indeed numerous and important for Japanese, who did not regard the brain as an important organ, and for whom nerves were even alien (Sakai 1982). Unlike ki, whose presence could only be felt but never seen, nerves were tangible, visible, and thus "real." Instead of being dispersed and flowing like ki, nerves were contained within one's individual body, and as such, were used by modern doctors to explicitly point to the internal physiological mechanism rather than to the external discord in interpersonal relationship or one's relationship to the environment. This opened the way for the anatomical worldview to take hold, serving to legitimate the dissection-based technology of modern medicine and to promote its ideas about the localization of disease. The new nerve discourse helped doctors trained in Western medicines to denounce traditional medicine and gradually relegate ki to the realm of superstition. It also directed psychiatrists' attention to the brain as the central governing mechanism of the mind. In other words, through their anatomical investigation of mental disorders, these psychiatrists began to redefine the brain as the new location of the soul.

The humoral explanations of melancholia continued to be seen in Henry Maudsley's textbook translated in 1876, which was widely read among early Japanese psychiatrists (Kanbe 1973[1876]). However, after psychiatry became institutionalized at Tokyo Imperial University in 1886, melancholia began to lose its premodern, holistic connotations, and was quickly replaced by the German neuropsychiatric notion of depression. As Kure Shūzō ("the father of Japanese psychiatry") introduced Kraepelinian neuropsychiatry as the official doctrine in academia in 1901, the image of depression as an inherent brain disease—with the central locus of control gone wrong—came to the fore, eclipsing the earlier humoral theory of melancholia altogether. This move was further accelerated by Kraepelinian reclassification of depression as part of manic-depression, an inherent and incurable illness characterized by automatic recurrence of psychotic attacks. This notion was distributed through Japan's first Kraepelinian psychiatric textbook published in 1906, where manic-depression was defined as one of the two major psychoses (the other being dementia praecox, later renamed schizophrenia) and that it was 80 percent hereditary-based (Ishida 1906). The clinical cases Kure discussed in the *Journal of Neurology* further served to illuminate the inherent danger of the depressed: the cases included a dejected man who suddenly began to claim himself to be an emperor and a woman who had suffered "so-called ki-utsubyō" when young, who eventually turned manic, taking off her clothes in public. She was finally brought to the psychiatric institution by the police (Kure 1914, 1915). As these cases suggest, manic-depression was considered to be one of the two major psychoses, and was highly difficult to differentiate from schizophrenia (its distinguishing feature being only a better prognosis).

The consequence of this reclassification was far-reaching. Anthropologist-psychiatrist Robert Barrett has suggested that we conceptualize an illness category as a "polysemic symbol" (Barrett 1988:375), in which "various meanings and values are condensed into a syndrome" (Lock and Nguyen 2010:73). Utsubyō, reclassified as part of manic depression with its own constellation of meanings, became an entirely different kind of polysemic symbol from what utsushō was. Depression as one pole of manic depression began to represent, to paraphrase Barrett's discussion of schizophrenia, "stigma, weakness, inner degeneration, brain disease, incurability and unpredictable danger" (Barrett 1988:375)—even if its stigma was not as severe as that of schizophrenia. Utsubyō as such signaled a hidden, dangerous psychosis, even doomed heredity, which could bring devastating effects on the afflicted individuals and their families. As an irreversible brain disease, utsubyō became further detached from the (transient) illness that used to reflect the stagnation of ki in one's mind and body. This technical reconceptualization was confirmed by not only the medical discourse but also the state, which began to use manic-depression as a basis for legal incompetence. The effect of this conceptual transformation via neuropsychiatry was so broad and profound that it led Miyake Kōichi, the third professor of psychiatry at Tokyo Imperial University, to lament in 1924 how Japanese had come to largely disregard the effect of the mind on the body:

> Just as people used to call it the illness of ki, some illnesses are caused by the mind. . . . The body and mind cannot be separated, and most diseases used to be thought to occur from mental causes. However, with the development of natural sciences and medicine, it was discovered that physical diseases are mainly caused by (external) agents such as germs and toxins. . . . People have even come to consider at times that the mind has nothing to do with illness. (Miyake 1924:336)

Disconnected from psychological, social meanings, utsubyō no longer evoked the images of accumulated sorrow, excessive contemplation, or silent endurance. Reclaimed by modern neuropsychiatry, utsubyō became an illness that was so experience-distant, so stigmatizing, that Japanese could no longer afford to suffer from it.

The Disappearance of Ki-utsu?

> Whatever [a tyrannical Shōgun] did not want to do, he
> avoided them by feigning an illness. . . . He refused to see
> people and withdrew to a dark room, only to soon deve-
> lop a real illness. . . . He became afflicted with what would
> now be called shinkeisujijaku (neurasthenia)—or what we
> used to call ki-utsushō.
> —from a classic *rakugo* story (a highly stylized
> form of comedy) by Sanyūtei Enshō (1980)

What then happened to the kind of experience that people called the illness of ki-utsu? Did the experience disappear entirely with the transformation of the word itself?[7] A hint can be found in the comparison table between Japanese and Western medical terms compiled by a military doctor in 1883, in which we find a clear distinction made between melancholia (as stark insanity) and depression (as a milder form of mental illness), respectively translated as utsuyūbyō (melancholia) and utsushō (depression or an illness of depressed ki) (Ochiai 1883). This distinction already appeared in Komori's text on Western medicine published in the 1820s–30s, in which utsuyūbyō was explained as an abnormal state of delirium, where the afflicted were in constant sorrow, fear, doubt, and avoided others. In contrast, utsushō was described by Komori as a milder form of depression, caused either by *ichōsuijaku* (gastrointestinal exhaustion) or *shinkeisuijaku* (nerve exhaustion) (Komori in Kaneko 1965). Shinkeisuijaku was later used as a term for translating neurasthenia, which became one of the most widely used categories in Japanese medicine in the early twentieth century. The relatively smooth acceptance of the notion of nerves and neurasthenia may have been due to the fact that intellectuals at the time explicitly attempted to replace the premodern notion of ki with the new idiom of nerves.

A quick glance at the newspapers of the time suggests this transition, in which the new, biomedical concept of nerves was being used by doctors, intellectuals, and later lay people, to overwrite the traditional notion of ki-utsu. An 1878 article depicting an aristocratic daughter in ki-utsu was obviously still written within the traditional framework (Yomiuri, March 23, 1878). An article appearing in the following year, however, discussed a young woman who was "shy by nature" and depressed (utsu) all the time, finally developing a "nerve disorder" (shinkei-byō) and throwing herself in Shinbashi River (Yomiuri, July 25, 1879). What we see here is the beginning of a conversion of the two notions—ki-utsu and a nerve disorder—and the penetration of the modern categories into the lexicon of lay people. Another newspaper article in 1886 even more explicitly illuminated how Japanese at the time were dealing with the transition from the old to new; it told that a daughter of an affluent family suffered from "utsuyūbyō" (melancholia). The worried family thought it was love sickness and took her to a shrine to pray, where they were told that what she really had was a "nerve disorder." The astonished family asked for prayers and exorcism, but was instead advised that simply "reasoning with her" would do to cure such a disorder. The article ended with a comic statement: "how trivial the cause of *ki-utsu* really is!" (Yomiuri, September 16, 1886). Interestingly, the meaning of nerve disorder was still diffused and unknown, treated here as little more than a metaphorical illness (that ki-utsu had become by then) despite the

---

[7] Here we find ourselves in tricky epistemological, and empirical, questions about a history of illness. Although I do not consider depression to be a thing-in-itself—a constant biological phenomenon that is merely given different names at different historical eras—I do want to point out that the rise of certain medical ideas not only give voice to preexisting anxiety about the body but also actively cultivate it.

fact that psychiatrists were beginning to warn at the time of the serious consequences that damaged nerves could bring (see chapter 4).[8] Here we find the
familiar, traditional moralization of ki-utsu, though it had become a kind of
catchall label given to an ailment of uncertain nature. The rise of the nerve discourse served medical experts to denounce traditional medicine and relegate ki
to the realm of superstition,[9] turning ki-utsu into a metaphorical existence, increasingly decorporealized and psychologized.[10]

Conclusion: The Globalization of Depression and the Thriving of Local Knowledge

Behind the puzzling discontinuity of historical knowledge about depression
lies, I have suggested, two important transformations via concept transfers:
first, the gradual conceptual change through popularization and psychologization of the traditional medical term "utsushō" and, second, the epistemological
break brought on by modern psychiatry that further accelerated this psychologization. Indeed, the Japanese adoption of German neuropsychiatry initially
started as an imposition of Western-born categories, backed up by the power of
the modern state. Psychiatrists sought to establish their medical legitimacy by
emphasizing a sharp departure from the traditional medical knowledge, while
paying more attention to making everyday reality fit Western classifications
than to exploring indigenous illness categories or the chaotic realities presented
by their patients. Psychiatrists trained in this new language asserted their scientific authority by determining what were medically recognized, legitimate "diseases" as opposed to unclassified and undiagnosable (mere) "complaints." This
initially instilled a radical disconnection between the local, subjective, and experiential idioms of distress and the universal, objective, and technical language of psychiatric disorders. It is because of this displacement of traditional
medical knowledge, selective attention to patients' distress, and particular con-

---

[8] In a 1925 novel set in the Edo Era, the kabuki writer Okamoto Kidō depicts a merchant family
in torment over the mysterious illness of their daughter: "[D]octors were unable to give a definite
diagnosis . . . and the family finally concluded that it was probably something like *ki-utsu*, which
girls of marriageable age often suffer from" (Okamoto 1999:252).

[9] Note that the German neuropsychiatry that Japanese psychiatrists imported at the time "made
no real distinction between diseases of the brain and diseases of the mind, for they held that mental
processes were always the unvarying result of underlying brain functions" (Bynum 1985:89).

[10] Interestingly, nerve-related words became quickly incorporated into traditional medicine as
well: for example, "shinkeishitsu," or nervous temperament, as a personality trait that can be caused
by "hereditary factors, overdiscipline and overprotection during childhood, and the institutionalized family structure and educational system" (Lock 1980:222). Psychosomatic medicine also took
up and elaborated on shinkei and popularized neurosis. Biomedical psychiatry retained the ambiguity of shinkei by using notions such as autonomic nervous system disorder (jiritsu shinkei
shicchōshō) that simultaneously denotes both biological and psychosocial implications.

struction of mental illness, I suggest, that Japanese psychiatrists have largely come to assume that Japanese did not have a language for describing an illness of depressed emotions.

The alleged historical absence of depression in Japan may also indicate the fact that, despite the twentieth-century dissemination of nerve discourse, psychiatry's conceptual hold on people has been far from complete. This is partly because biomedical modernity is characterized by dual discrepancies that exist not only between doctors' technical language and patients' experiential narratives but also between global scientific medicine and local clinical practices (to be elaborated upon in chapter 5). In today's medicalization, however, more aggressive attempts are being made by doctors and pharmaceutical companies to make the neurological language of depression penetrate deeply into people's lexicon. Instead of depicting depression as an isolated brain anomaly whose mechanism remains alien to the afflicted themselves, psychiatrists are now trying to articulate, using graphics and brain imaging, how psychological distress is intimately connected to the inner working of the brain. This new psychiatric language of depression does not so much silence people (by the alienating power of technical language) as it encourages them to share and speak in its own terms. Thus, on the one hand, this neuropsychiatric language may well be becoming *power-internalized* through the increasingly localized and routinized practices of psychiatry and pharmaceutical technologies. On the other hand, however, the limit of the neuropsychiatric language (evidenced by the growing dissatisfaction with antidepressants: see chapter 10) also seems to be prompting some Japanese to explore the premodern notion of ki-stagnation and herbal medication.[11] One of the effects of this may be that Japanese are increasingly turning to the traditional medical language that addresses the profound connection between the depressed body and mind, as well as between depressed individuals and the social environment in which they live. Such contemporary undercurrents of Japanese local knowledge about depression may also prompt us to wonder what happened to the way in which those in premodern Europe once talked about their stagnated body and mind in terms of the *melancholic body*.

---

[11] Notably, pharmaceutical companies are also capitalizing on these new demands by reviving traditional herbal prescriptions for depressive symptoms.

CHAPTER THREE

The Expansion of Psychiatry into Everyday Life

Three Phases of Psychiatric Expansion

RISING CONCERN OVER the increase of depression marks a new phase in the history of Japanese psychiatry, a transformation from the time when it was rarely used as a treatment for "ordinary" Japanese. In this chapter, I examine this transformation by dividing the history of psychiatry into three phases, each contributing to the expansion of psychiatry into the realm of everyday distress. The first (1870s to the 1930s) was in the prewar era, when the state introduced psychiatry as a force for modernization. The view that mental illness was a biological—and often hereditary—disease displaced the previous notion in the Edo Era that insanity was, just like any other illness, caused by a discord of ki energy (as discussed in chapter 2). The neurobiological view of mental illness proliferated through the influence of academic psychiatry, the media, and the Social Darwinist social policies that enforced private detention of the ill. Apart from literary discussion about neurasthenia as pathology of modernity (see chapter 4), psychiatry was used as an oppressive power of exclusion and stigmatization. The second expansion came at the time of the postwar reconstruction of Japan (1950s to the 1960s). Largely driven by economic rationale, the state helped establish a large number of private mental hospitals, which institutionalized those who were deemed unfit and unproductive in the new social order. Although this expansion helped solidify the infrastructure of psychiatry, the growing contradiction in the fact that psychiatry served as a gatekeeper—rather than cure-provider—of the mentally ill led to a long-lasting antipsychiatry movement beginning in the 1960s. I suggest that the attack on traditional academic psychiatry and the increasing popular attention to psychiatric discourse created both confusion in, and a temporary retreat from, academic, biological psychiatry and a proliferation of psychiatric discourse as a language of resistance and a form of social critique (see chapter 5). I argue that this transition set the conditions for the possibility of a third expansion of psychiatry (1980s to the present), when psychiatry came out of asylums and, for the first time, began to focus on the mental *health* of ordinary Japanese as a national concern.[1]

---

[1] For more extensive (and in-depth) historiographies of Japanese psychiatry, see Okada 1981, 1999, 2002, Suzuki 2003a, 2003b, 2005, Hiruta 1999a, 1999b.

The First Expansion (1870s to the 1930s)

Modernizing Japanese Bodies: From Yōjō to Eisei

It has been convincingly argued that the modern Japanese state has used the body in inscribing the political order (Bourdachs 1997, Burns 1997, Karatani 1993, Lock 1993). The institutionalization of the new medical system in Japan was clearly the product of a top-down process, motivated by the state's goal to re-create the nation as an equal competitor among the colonizing powers of the West. The Meiji state thus took it upon itself to bodily and visually modernize Japanese first by prohibiting traditional healing practices that appeared "odd" in the eyes of Westerners (for example, the Law on Minor Offenses in 1872: Narita 1995, K. Kawamura, 1990). Amidst regional opposition, the central government banned sorcery, magic, and shamanism in 1873 (Ōtsuki 1998), and further suppressed traditional medicine, instilling in its place biomedicine as a new system of knowledge and practice in 1874 (Jannetta 1997).[2] Cholera epidemics between 1858 and 1895 became, as in Europe, a battlefield upon which biomedicine won its legitimacy over folk powers and local networks of healing (Kakimoto 1991, cf. Arnold 1993, Mitchell 1988). Overcoming the recurrent local resistance, biomedicine instituted large-scale preventive measures against cholera and thereby set a model for subsequent public health interventions and urban planning (Narita 1993).[3] The success of biomedicine meant the significant retreat of traditional medicine. In 1875, most of the practicing physicians were those trained in traditional medicine; out of 28,262 practitioners, only 5,247 were registered as physicians of Western medicine (Kawakami 1961:235). This situation began to change drastically after 1876, when the government passed a regulation requiring all physicians to study Western medicine (Lock 1980:62). The Japanese-Sino War of 1894–95 further helped legitimize biomedicine as the official medicine of the modern state.

In the realm of popular ideas about general health, biomedicine brought about a radical shift from yōjō to eisei (hygiene) (Shikano 2004, Narita 1993, Kitazawa 2000). The traditional idea of yōjō—developed and popularized through texts in the Edo Era—stressed the importance of maintaining balance between individuals and the environment, rest, and safety, and defined heath as

---

[2] Though Western medicine had been imported via Portuguese traders in the sixteenth century, and the influence of Dutch anatomy was prevalent in the end of the Edo Era, it was only after 1874 that biomedicine became the official medicine in place of traditional Chinese-derived medicine.

[3] Cholera, being the most deadly and most visible disease, caused much fear as patients were carried away to a hospital under police supervision and their neighborhoods were quarantined and disinfected. Hygiene cooperatives were set up in each municipality, and slums and poverty areas were marked. This helped give rise to a network of local governance and the scientific management of the state. As in Europe, cholera epidemics served as "proof" of the superiority of Western knowledge and Western medicine.

an absence of illness (see chapter 2). In contrast to this "passive concept," the notion of eisei was introduced in the 1870s as a new health principle and suggested the need to actively cultivate health—to scientifically and systematically go about achieving it. The eisei paradigm introduced the notions that human biology is universal, that individual bodies exist independently of nature, and that individuals must learn to achieve hygiene and health by following scientific principles. Furthermore, the eisei paradigm selectively incorporated and strengthened parts of traditional medical thought: by reworking the idea of the "socio-organic" embedded in the yōjō concept, the eisei paradigm justified the linkage between individual health and the health of the state. Particularly in the 1890s, when German policy ideas were introduced, this vision further reinforced the idea that "individuals and society represented a part of a single, unitary organic whole in which each depended upon the other for continued development" (Kinzley 1991:23).[4] Hygiene thus became an urgent national project, in which individual effort was required in the state's drive to modernize, and modernize quickly—one ultimate goal being the production of strong soldiers who could ward off any military threat from the West. Institutions such as the Department of Hygiene in the Home Ministry and the Association for Hygiene of Greater Japan (partially funded by the state) were established, paving the way for a network of local governance and scientific management of health (Narita 1993, 1995, Ikeda and Satō 1995).

The Infancy of Psychiatry

In this politicized climate, neuropsychiatry was officially institutionalized in Tokyo Imperial University in 1886. The infancy of psychiatry was characterized by a number of state requests to have psychiatrists investigate peripheral regions of Japan where spirit possession had been occurring at an alarming rate (Ōtsuki 1998). Apparently, the Meiji state was concerned with the fact that incidents of spirit possession at the end of the Edo Period often led to social unrest and the birth of new religions, which had at times organized utopian movements against the status quo (N. Kawamura, 1990, Garon 1997).[5] The aim of the state in installing psychiatry was not to promote social welfare for citizens at large but to classify and exclude those who were deemed a threat to the establishment of the new social order (Omata 1998:232). This state project was also characteristically tied to private responsibility: the state created a system of psychiatric surveillance not by increasing public expenditure on asylums but by using the prevailing family ideology and making the head of the household

---

[4] This vision, undoubtedly manipulated in constructing the ideology of national polity (*kokutai*), justified legislative and regulatory responses to social problems (Gluck 1985).

[5] This objectification and policing of the folk was followed by similar attempts by psychiatrists concerning the Ainu, for instance (Ōtsuki 1998). This helped constitute a form of internal colonization at the time.

responsible for confining their mentally ill family members *at home* (Akimoto 1976, Asada 1985). In place of the massive public mental hospitals that emerged in Europe and the United States, a tightly knit network of private surveillance was created in the late 1870s under the supervision of the police and local hygiene committees. With the implementation of the Law for the Care and Custody of the Mentally Ill in 1900, the number of privately imprisoned mentally ill continued to increase between 1924 and 1941, at a rate that exceeded that of the growth of the population as a whole (Akimoto 1976). This pattern persisted in the postwar period, when the state continued to hold families responsible for institutionalizing their mentally ill in mental hospitals, which were mostly private.[6] As Nakazawa (1985) points out, mental illness was treated in the same manner as infectious disease: one can then suspect that private confinement was based on a regime of fear, shame, and secrecy—images of mental illness that were to last long into the decades to come.

Such aggressive colonization of local lifeworlds by the Meiji state, however, also triggered folk resistance. Often, people resisted in silence: folk healing and shamanistic practices survived by going underground, and the ill simply withdrew and hid themselves from government surveillance (Shikano 2004, K. Kawamura 1990, Eguchi 1987, Ōtsuki 1998). At other times, resistance became overt and powerful. Cholera revolts (*korera ikki*) took place between the 1870s and 1880s (there were twenty-four revolts in 1879 alone, involving more than 2,000 people at times); although quelled, these revolts provide a glimpse of the rich undercurrent of folk healing movements against the state that have continued since the Edo Period (Lewis 1990, Nakai 1983, White 1995). Scandals and controversies were revealed in the media. In the midst of psychiatric expansion, the Sōma case in the 1890s stirred public sentiment and resulted in what was probably Japan's first antipsychiatry movement promoted via print culture (Akimoto 1985). When a servant of a former lord of the Sōma family accused the new lord of illegitimately confining his lord to a mental hospital in order to take over the family, there was public uproar against psychiatry. A book by the servant discussing the case in detail became a best-seller, reprinted for the seventeenth time in 1893, while the court case lasted twelve years. As the news was reported overseas, the Japanese government received international criticism that it lacked a legal system sufficient to prevent unwarranted confinement. Since this reputation significantly impaired Japan's negotiation with the West to revise the "Unfair Treaties,"[7] the state ended up tightening surveillance

---

[6] This system shared the same thread of thought with the much-debated "Japanese-style welfare" policy articulated in the 1980s, where the use of the family ideology enabled low state expenditures on welfare (Garon 1997, Lock 1993, 1998, Takahashi 1997).

[7] Beginning with the Harris Treaty of 1858, Japan signed treaties with the United States and European countries—under the threat of colonization—that gave the latter the right to determine tariff rates and provided extraterritorial rights for foreigners in Japan. The Japanese government struggled to revise these treaties for three decades by implementing Westernization measures in order to be accepted as an equal by the Western powers.

by legalizing, through a 1900 law, family detention of the mentally ill (Akimoto 1985:20).

Moving beyond Confinement and the Walls of Asylums

As biomedicine began to shift its focus from acute epidemics to chronic illness in the early 1900s, psychiatry as well positioned itself to change from an oppressive arm of the state to a profession with an independent voice and broader appeal. Under the leadership, from 1901, of Kure Shūzō, one of the first professors at Tokyo Imperial University and the "father of Japanese psychiatry," psychiatry began to expand links both in public and private sectors (Ambaras 1998). Kure and his associates vigorously engaged with the public by providing lectures to governmental officials and intellectuals, and by writing articles and question-and-answer sections for popular magazines. Kure's contribution extended to five different domains: (1) establishing the Japanese Society of Neurology (renamed the Japanese Society of Psychiatry and Neurology in 1935) and its journal, *Shinkeigaku zasshi*, in 1902; (2) establishing Kraepelinian German neuropsychiatry; (3) restructuring hospital psychiatry and humanizing care by prohibiting the use of restraints; (4) promoting the mental hygiene movement; and (5) conducting epidemiological surveys on the plight of the mentally ill between 1910 and 1916 (Akimoto 1976).[8] Through this national survey, which covered one-third of Japan, Kure called attention to the misery of private detention with no medical care, particularly among the poor. Successfully campaigning for the Mental Hospital Law (established in 1919), Kure clarified the state's responsibility for providing medical care for the ill (65,000 of whom were deemed to require hospitalization).[9] However, in the economic and social unrest from the 1920s onward,[10] lacking a financial basis, the law turned out to be rather hollow in terms of real-world consequences (Nakazawa 1985).[11]

---

[8] Kure's survey report shows that there were three categories of patients: (1) those who were treated at private homes or hospitals, who were from wealthy families, (2) those who were privately detained without much medical care, and (3) those who received folk therapy such as Buddhist rituals and water therapy. Over 80 percent were men. Kure calculated that there were 23,931 mentally ill (0.05%) in 1905, 41,920 (0.075%) in 1916, and 64,941 in 1917 (Kosaka 1984).

[9] Although the lack of mental hospitals at this time is usually cited as indicating the indifference of the state, we must also remember that "hospitals" as they developed in the West were not necessarily a common form of institution in Japan in the prewar period. As Fujisaki (1995:42) points out, despite the adoption of Dutch medicine in the Edo Period, hospitals remained unpopular while small clinics (*kaigyōsho*) remained more common. This pattern persisted until the 1950s, when medical progress necessitated more expensive medical technologies and more staff.

[10] From the 1920s to the early 1930s, Japan went through various economic hardships, social unrest, and tightening of social surveillance—the Kantō Earthquake (1923); the Social Order Maintenance Law (1925); the suppression of communism in the first democratic election (1928); the Great Depression (1929); rising unemployment and labor disputes (1930); and severe famine (1931)—while national military expenditures rose to 35 percent in 1932 and 47 percent in 1936, leading to World War II in 1939 (Asada 1985, Kinzley 1991, Silberman and Harootunian 1974).

[11] This law failed to achieve its goal of establishing three or four mental hospitals per year. The

Particularly under Kure's regime (1901 to 1925), Japanese psychiatry began to establish what Castel et al. (1982 [1979]) call "transinstitutionalization"—a process by which psychiatry proliferated into broader domains by making linkages in both public and private sectors, across various institutions and actors with differing interests. This took place when, from the 1890s, there was an increasing awareness in the media of "social problems" largely caused by rapid social change. A succession of wars (the 1894 Japanese-Sino War, the 1904 Russo-Japanese War, and then World War I in 1914) sparked the Japanese industrial revolution and urbanization, and gave rise to the new middle class, but at the same time heightened class discrepancies in cities. Numerous reports were produced that informed the public about urban misery, labor movements, the plight of the working class, the problem of delinquent children, and suicide rates among workers (Ambaras 1998, Kinzley 1991). This "social problem" perspective opened up a space where experts such as psychiatrists began to collaborate with social organizations outside of academia. Particularly, the new middle class, with their desire to modernize the rest of society, helped build alliances between the state, experts, and localized networks, thereby creating conduits for social policies (Ambaras 1998). They significantly contributed to the government's success in managing Japanese society during much of the twentieth century (Garon 1997:346). Promoted by middle-class intellectuals, hygiene education as well began to take on popular appeal via various media such as textbooks, pamphlets, magazine columns, children's games (e.g., *eisei sugoroku*) and hygiene exhibitions, which evidently stirred much excitement (Tanaka 1992, cf. Mitchell 1988). The degree of excitement and popular support that existed at the time for the hygiene movement and the role it played in making the new health regime part of people's intimate, everyday knowledge, must not be underestimated (Yoshimi 1994, Kakimoto 1991, Narita 1990).

The new science of the mind, as well, succeeded in gaining appeal in the media through discussions of abnormality and pathologies of modern life. Initially, psychologists did much to cultivate interest in problems of abnormality in everyday life. They gave a series of talks to general audiences from 1909 to 1913 and later published the popular journal, *Psychological Studies* (Furusawa 1998:42, Mamiya 1998). Psychiatrists as well began to write for popular magazines, featuring health advice about mental hygiene, hysteria, and neurasthenia (K. Kawamura 1990). For instance, one of the most notable developments in popularizing psychiatry was its growing link with education. The "ignorance" of unhygenic children—and their families—under the compulsory mass education system, provided the perfect opening for psychiatrists to intervene and install their medical knowledge and authority. With the passage of the School Hygiene Law in 1897, followed by the School Infectious Disease Prevention Law in 1898, children were routinely inspected for health and cleanliness. Their fam-

---

twenty years between 1926 and 1945 saw only seven public hospitals. This law was later replaced by the Mental Hygiene Law in 1950 (Nakazawa 1985:2).

ilies as well became incorporated into this system via "home education"(Ambaras 1998). The Child Study Association was established in 1902 for the exchange of information between various experts. Psychiatry was called in at this time, when the state became concerned with the "problems" of intelligence and retardation, which required professional intervention to determine even the presence of individual deficiency. Kure and others also wrote and lectured in the 1910s on German psychiatric theories about retardation, antisocial personality, delinquency, and adolescent crime. Allied with the Home Ministry, psychiatrists were commissioned to conduct a national survey of juvenile reformatory inmates using intelligence testing (Ambaras 1998:21). Despite controversy and criticism, by the 1920s psychiatric and psychological studies of intelligence and retardation became firmly established as an administrative device (S. Takahashi 1998:177). Psychiatric technologies were also adopted for use both in industry and the military as tools for ensuring "adaptation" and efficiency of workers and soldiers in their respective roles (Kinzley 1991:103).

World War II, Eugenics, and the Origins of Biological Discourse

Psychiatry seems to have succeeded in expanding, if temporarily, into popular domains through nonacademic networks and financial support from the private sector. Yet prewar psychiatry, despite these links, and despite the humanistic bent of Kure (who was called "Pinel of Japan"), ended up fostering prejudice against mental illness and creating a split between scientific research and clinical practice—between the diseased bodies and suffering patients.[12] There are a number of reasons for this. First, in the tradition of university-based, academic psychiatry, medical science was conceptualized separately from humanistic care. For instance, Kure's public lectures (including at the Greater Japan Women's Hygiene Association) helped raise awareness of mental illness among upper-class women. But there was a division of labor that seems to have been clearly gendered and symbolic: humanistic care for the ill remained in the hands of women doing private charity work, while academic psychiatry itself was defined as a men's scientific pursuit (see Kobayashi 1972). Out of twenty-two professors of psychiatry who studied abroad in the prewar era, Okada (1999) points out that only one studied clinical practice as well, while the rest spent time on scientific research of the brain. This is not surprising given the fact that this was a time of excitement in biological research and scientific progress. Noguchi Hideyo had just discovered the causative agent of syphilis in 1913, fueling the drive of Japanese psychiatrists to find organic causes of mental illness (Asada 1985:26). No doubt most psychiatrists saw their primary role not as clinicians but as

---

[12] According to Asada, whose father worked with Kure at Tokyo Imperial University in the 1910s, it was not uncommon to hear a psychiatrist say that academic psychiatry was interesting but clinical practice was unbearable. The therapies at this time centered around "insulin shock" and electric shock (Asada 1985:26, Nishizono 1988).

scientists, helping the ill by pursuing organic causes of, and cures for, mental illnesses.

But perhaps most importantly, the biological bent in psychiatry was reinforced and justified by the ideology of Social Darwinism and the ideology of nation-as-family: that is, the idea that medicine needed to contribute to making the "body of the Japanese race" competitive enough to survive the international struggle of "the fittest" (Matsubara 1998a:188). Herbert Spencer was translated into Japanese and twenty books on the subject were published between 1877 and 1889. More works by Japanese eugenicists continued to come out in the 1910s, and specialized journals in eugenics were published in the 1920s (Ukai 1991:126, Otsubo and Bartholomew 1998). Psychiatrists as well were drawn into the racial improvement movement that emphasized heredity over environment and biology over social conditions. In a political climate in which the family—not the individual—was conceived as the basic social unit (N. Kawamura 1990), a diagnosis of mental illness also meant a judgment on the whole family. Indeed, by the end of World War II, the idea that mental illness was a serious deficiency, a hereditary disease, and thus a family responsibility, became firmly rooted in public discourse and even legally substantiated by the enactment of the Eugenics Law in 1940.

In this social context, efforts by psychiatrists to popularize psychiatry seem to have come to a halt in 1937,[13] when they were subsumed under war-effort policies organized by the eugenics section of the newly created Ministry of Health and Welfare.[14] This is not to say that psychiatry was neatly incorporated into eugenics and its ideology of racial hygiene, nor that there was harmonious collaboration with the state. Matsubara (1998b) discusses the complex negotiations that went on among psychiatrists, who either supported or rejected the eugenic discourse that defined mental illness as a hereditary aberration. Immediately before the passing of the Eugenics Law, the Ministry of Health and Welfare published a national survey report conducted on the family trees of 3,000 mentally ill patients (1,500 hospitalized, 1,500 privately confined). *Yomiuri Shimbun* headlined the result as "3,000 doomed families," including families with members suffering from retardation, schizophrenia, manic-depression, and other mental illnesses. Despite opposition from psychiatrists involved in the study (such as Professor Uchimura Yūshi of Tokyo Imperial University), who dismissed its sci-

---

[13] Academically, however, there were a number of original research projects conducted around the 1940s. Okada even points out that this was the time when Japanese psychiatry established itself as a mature and autonomous discipline (see Okada 1999).

[14] Matsubara demonstrates that sterilization of the mentally ill under the 1940 Eugenics Law did not take place to the extent that the policy demanded, partly because of the opposition from psychiatrists but mainly because psychiatry simply lacked the institutional basis for carrying out this policy (Matsubara 1998a, 1988b). For instance, in 1941, (only) 94 patients out of 750 deemed appropriate for sterilization were actually sterilized. However, such sterilization continued to be conducted in the postwar period.

entific value, the state insisted that mental illness was "proved" to be hereditary (Matsubara 1998a, Nakazawa 1985:4). Unfortunately, the influence of this wartime "psychiatric" discourse that linked family, biology, and heredity became a lasting legacy of prewar psychiatry.[15] It is this legacy that the later antipsychiatry movement fought against, and that present-day psychiatrists have to engage with in order to popularize the idea of psychiatry as providing care for the ordinary person.

The Second Expansion (1950s to the 1960s): Postwar Institutional Expansion and the Antipsychiatry Movement

> "As the GNP doubles, the number of mentally ill will quadruple," predicted Takemi Tarō, the influential director of the Japanese Medical Association from between 1957 and 1982.

There was a brief period in Japanese psychiatry in the aftermath of World War II, when the predominance of neurobiology was fundamentally shaken by the onslaught of psychoanalytic American psychiatry. In the late 1940s to the early 1950s, the American model of "mental health" was disseminated through the newly established psychoanalytically oriented university departments and the American-led National Institute of Mental Health. Popular books on neurosis were published in succession, the word "*noirōze*" (neurosis) became a buzzword of the time (Satō and Mizoguchi 1997, see also Uchimura 1954), and media eventually began to consider the widespread use of minor tranquilizers for anxiety a social problem. Healy has discussed the possibility that what is now called depression might have been widely dealt with as anxiety in the 1950s, the era of minor tranquilizers (Healy 2000). This may well have been the case in postwar Japan; if a national newspaper cartoon ("*Sazae-san*") is any indication, an ordinary salaryman seemed to be taking such pills for trivial domestic worries in the 1950s (*Asahi Shimbun* (*Asahi*), May 14, 2005). A 1965 newspaper article that discussed the danger and horror of "casual use of minor

---

[15] Some studies have documented the extent to which, in the 1970s, fear of mental illness as a genetic, hereditary disease still permeated people's minds in the countryside and in urban clinics (Nakazawa 1985, Hirose 1972). Nakazawa (1985) describes the predicament of the mentally ill in a rural area and suggests that people believed that mental illness was both incurable, hereditary, and the doomed fate of the family. Caution for generalization is needed, however. In a survey he conducted between 1963 and 1965 on popular conceptions of mental illness, Terashima (1969) found: (1) considerable regional difference in prejudice against mental illness and practices (hospitalization); and (2) contradiction between the strong persistence of the idea that mental illness was hereditary and the prevalence of a "remarkably optimistic view" on the prognosis of mental illness. This suggests that the psychiatric discourse did not spread evenly across Japan, nor was it received uniformly (for regional variations, see also Munakata 1984, 1986).

tranquilizers" suggested that their routine usage remained a prevalent problem (*Asahi*, November 21, 1965, *Asahi*, September 15, 1956), until the government made them into prescription drugs in 1972. These indicate the popular receptiveness of such psychiatric medication and the flourishing of the American model of mental health (particularly neurosis) in the domain of popular discourse.

On the academic front, however, from the early 1950s many intellectual leaders of psychiatry (who had been steeped in German psychiatry) began to express skepticism toward the American influence, and particularly those affiliated with Tokyo University soon mobilized to critique psychoanalysis and to reestablish Kraepelinian neurobiology as the official paradigm of Japanese psychiatry. In a commemorative talk for the fiftieth anniversary of the Society of Psychiatry and Neurology, Uchimura Yūshi, professor of psychiatry at Tokyo University, reflected on the postwar confusion when Japanese psychiatrists had been "knocked down" by American psychiatry. Noting how their initial responses greatly varied ("some hesitated, some averted their faces, others adopted it"), Uchimura elaborated on how psychoanalysis was "unlike anything [they] had experienced before" (Uchimura 1954:710–11). He then drew on Karl Jaspers (who had called psychoanalysis an "as-if psychology"—blind to its own limitations) to criticize the epistemological basis of psychoanalysis while admitting its potential as a therapeutic tool (Uchimura 1954).[16] Heated debates continued both within academia and in popular intellectual magazines about the nature of American "psychologism" and what direction Japanese psychiatry should take (Muramatsu 1953, Shimazaki and Ishikawa 1954, Shimazaki 1953, Doi 1954, Uchimura et al. 1957). Mainstream psychiatrists in the Tokyo area were largely successful in warding off further psychoanalytic influence. They asserted that it was psychoses and their biological mechanisms—not neurosis and its psychology—that should be the primary object of psychiatric investigation.[17] Thus neurobiology again found its way as the supreme model of mental illness in academic psychiatry.

While psychiatrists reestablished the predominance of neurobiology conceptually, institutionally they began to expand their power through the network of private mental hospitals. In fact, the institutional expansion of postwar-era psychiatry far exceeded what had been attained by academic psychiatry

---

[16] What concerned Uchimura was the multiplicity of American psychiatry (which included Freudian theories of childhood trauma, behavioral models that "overrate" the force of environment, and Adolf Meyer's holistic approach). Both Uchimura and another intellectual leader, Shimazaki Toshiki (of Tokyo Medical and Dental University) drew extensively on psychiatrist-cum-philosopher Karl Jaspers to critique the epistemological basis of psychoanalysis, translating his work and publishing it in both the psychiatric and popular intellectual journal called *Thought* (*Shisō*) (Jaspers' lectures on psychopathology was translated in 1959).

[17] In fact, as a number of senior psychiatrists pointed out to me in interviews, "neurosis" remained marginalized and was often treated dismissively as belonging to the realm of "common-sense psychology."

in the prewar era. The collapse of the *ie* (family) system under the new Civil Law of 1947 and the outlawing of private detention under the 1950 Mental Hygiene Law, created drastic changes in psychiatric care, as the place of confinement began to shift to mental hospitals.[18] As the Ministry of Health and Welfare pointed out the "shortage" of psychiatric facilities, they resorted to providing low-interest loans for building private institutions. This produced a sudden "mental hospital boom," giving rise to numerous private institutions, many with dubious medical capabilities.[19] As the number of psychiatric patients increased with the economic boom, rapid urbanization, and internal migration, the relevant clause from the 1950 law began to be flexibly applied to justify involuntary hospitalization of the "mentally ill" on the grounds of economic hardship. While most of the money from the national mental health fund was used for this purpose, there was little imperative among asylum psychiatrists to provide therapeutic treatment, or to try to return patients to the community (Kobayashi 1972, Okagami et al. 1988).

The much-awaited amendment of the Mental Hygiene Law in 1965, which was supposed to establish a policy basis for community care, was again hindered by an unfortunate incident—an assault on the popular American ambassador Edwin O. Reischauer by a mentally disturbed nineteen-year-old. The public uproar over the incident swung the pendulum back to keeping psychiatry as an apparatus of state control, as the director of the National Police Agency declared in the Diet that there were "three thousand mentally disturbed people who need regulation and surveillance" (cited in Nakazawa 1985:8). This incident further led to the strengthening of the "surveillance" component of the law, thereby guaranteeing the police much broader responsibility for registering the names of mentally disturbed citizens and arresting and hospitalizing them (Koizumi and Harris 1992:1101). In the meantime, psychiatric institutions continued to expand in the 1960s as lucrative businesses by absorbing the contradictions caused by rapid postwar economic growth (Tomita 1992). Psychiatrists were criticized for profit making by keeping the mentally ill institutionalized and accepting a stable income from national health insurance. In fact, Takemi Tarō, the powerful director of the Japanese Medical Association, even ridiculed psychiatrists by calling them "stock farmers" (Akimoto 1976:193).

---

[18] It is important to remember that the law also paved the way for community mental health by calling for mental hygiene consultation centers and family visits, and other such normalization policies. In fact, the 1950 Law was a conceptual breakthrough for community psychiatry, as it required that each prefecture build a mental hospital, and it introduced public counseling centers and home-visit treatment programs for people suffering from mental illness. These programs, mandated by law, were not implemented, however, until the amendment of the law in 1965 (Koizumi and Harris 1992).

[19] Indeed, the number of beds in mental hospitals increased rapidly (rising from 173,000 beds in 1965; 278,000 in 1975; to 334,000 in 1985 [Okagami et al. 1988]).

By the late 1960s, international criticism of Japanese psychiatry began to be heard, which culminated in the 1968 World Health Organization Clark Report that pointed out the mass-scale confining system, lack of specialized care, and profit-oriented management of Japanese psychiatry (Hirota 1981). With the accumulating criticisms, the antipsychiatry movement took off in the 1969 Kanazawa Conference of the Society of Psychiatry and Neurology. Amidst a dispute erupting over his use of lobotomy, Professor Utena of Tokyo University retired, and the psychiatric unit of Tokyo University became occupied by students, who kept the unit under their control for the next ten years (Tomita 2000, Akimoto 1976, Healy 2002). The movement soon spread to universities nationwide, and most psychiatric societies were dismantled in the coming decade. The movement also won popular appeal through the media, with *Asahi Shimbun* taking the lead by reporting on the horror of psychiatric institutions and the plight of the mentally ill (e.g., Ōkuma 1973). Despite this, the profit-based structure of the private hospitals (which, due to the government policy, constituted the bulk of mental hospitals in Japan) proved resistant to change; even in 1987, over 90 percent of the inpatients in these hospitals consisted of involuntary patients (Asai 1999:14). The struggles were long and bitter, falling to petty, personal attacks, and gradually dying off as the antipsychiatry movement became increasingly fragmented from the 1980s. Most Japanese psychiatrists still remain undecided about the meanings and consequences of this movement (Ōhigashi 1999). Its last signs were put to a symbolic end in 2001, when the psychiatry department at Tokyo University—which had been physically divided into different buildings for three decades—was reintegrated under a neurobiology professor.

I suggest that the antipsychiatry movement—and its dismantling of traditional Japanese psychiatry—was crucial for preparing the conditions for the later medicalization of depression. Conceptually, the antipsychiatry movement annihilated the dominance of neuropsychiatry and its heredity-driven paradigm, even if the effect was only temporary. The antipsychiatry movement left disruption and a conceptual vacuum in its wake, which was quickly filled by the DSM-III (1980, translated in 1982), as Japanese psychiatrists, despite their unyielding criticisms of American psychiatry, had few other alternatives with which to try to reintegrate themselves. Institutionally, the disintegration of the university-controlled hierarchical system initiated a move toward community mental health, as dissenting young psychiatrists left universities to open small clinics that provided outpatient care (Koike and Matsuda 1997, Sekiya 1997). As the 1987 revision of the Mental Health Law expanded the coverage of the national health insurance for psychiatric outpatients, the number of such patients began to rise. The emergence of the "psy-complex" (discussed by Castel et al. 1982[1979]) can thus be said to have come about in Japan out of the antipsychiatry movement, which prepared the conditions for the later medicalization of depression.

The Third Expansion (1980s to the present): Toward Current Psychiatric Discourse on Depression and Suicide

The transition from asylum psychiatry to community psychiatry has been slow and gradual despite mounting criticism over the years: unlike in the West, where most mental hospitals have been public, in Japan the system of predominantly private mental hospitals has proved resistant to radical structural change (Okada 1999, Salzberg 1994). However, interest in mental health in the workplace has come from economic concerns: the JAL airplane crash in 1982, triggered by a mentally distressed pilot, raised public awareness of mental illness among people in the workforce (Kasahara 1991). In response to the growing public anxiety, the Ministry of Health and Welfare began implementing measures for "*kokoro no kenkō zukuri*" (promoting the health of kokoro), emphasizing the care of mental health and the need for stress management (albeit with little financial backing). The 1987 Mental Health Law, followed by the 1995 Mental Health and Welfare Law, set the tone for deinstitutionalization, normalization, and rehabilitation of the mentally ill (Komine 1996). Since the 1990s, there have been an increasing number of successful lawsuits brought by families of deceased workers against corporations on the basis of psychiatric diagnoses regarding overwork suicides (to be discussed in chapter 9).[20]

Given the economic imperatives (e.g., fear of legal compensation for overwork depression and suicide)—combined with growing public sentiment about the lack of mental health care (Kawakami 2000), the increasing competition from other professions,[21] and the aggressive promotion of antidepressants by

[20] In 2000, the Japanese government announced that one-third of the working-age population was suffering from chronic fatigue syndrome (far more than the 4 to 8 percent in the United States). According to the *New York Times*, these Japanese patients are treated with antidepressants, biofeedback, and counseling. The article also notes that "in Japan, where the condition appears to be far more prevalent, the experts lean toward explanations that emphasize societal mutations far more than their American counterparts," it is foremost associated with "the stresses placed on this society since it began its dramatic economic slide more than 10 years ago." The doctor cited in the article lists a variety of changes—from eating habits, environmental problems, housing, urban alienation, overwork, and changing family relationships—all of "which produce stress" (French 2000). The media presents the view that Japanese lack a secure sense of what kind of "society" or "tradition" the afflicted are to be returned to. It thus remains to be seen how psychiatry is going to help constitute a place of return for these people.

[21] An interest in mental health is being cultivated by forces other than psychiatry as well. First of all, rebuilding clinical psychology from the fragments of the antipsychiatry movement from 1974, Kawai Hayao and his associates created a new psychological association that was able to establish a licensing system for its members in 1988 (Murase 1995). Through links with the Ministry of Education, since 1992 clinical psychologists have gone to public schools nationwide to work as school counselors, and psychologists are also negotiating with the government for a national licensing system (Maruyama 1998). Secondly, since the 1960s, Ikemi Yūjiro and his associates have been appropriating ideas from psychiatry and traditional medicine to create their own brand of psychoso-

the psychopharmaceutical industry (New Current 1999)—psychiatry in Japan seems for the first time to be preparing for a significant expansion into the domains of everyday distress. Another notable factor for change is the introduction of DSM-III and the re-Americanization of Japanese psychiatry (Okada 1999, Klerman 1990, Tajima 2001). At the time that I was conducting other research on psychiatry in 1997, hardly any psychiatrists I interviewed at prestigious institutions claimed that they consulted DSM regularly. In 2000, when I began my fieldwork, most depression experts admitted using the DSM alongside their traditional diagnosis, but were still openly skeptical and critical. Toward the end of my fieldwork, the DSM had become a fact of everyday clinical practice, there to stay, despite the lingering criticism. The full impact of the DSM on Japanese psychiatry is yet to be known, but I suspect it will be profound. Unlike the psychoanalytic American psychiatry that flooded Japan in the 1950s, the current American influence—as exemplified by the DSM's neo-Kraepelinian paradigm and descriptive approach—has been highly congenial to Japanese psychiatrists' neurological understanding of mental illness (for the reaction to the DSM, see Honda 1983). At the same time, the DSM—with its "operational diagnosis"— is indirectly familiarizing Japanese psychiatrists and their patients with the idea that the vast range of what used to be mere life problems can now be regarded as manifestations of psychopathology. This seems to be achieving what American psychoanalysis tried but failed to do in the 1950s Japan; that is to say, the DSM may be breaking down the previous Japanese resistance against medicalization by collapsing the previously tightly held boundary between normality and abnormality. Particularly through the concept of depression—which lies uneasily in between the two—some Japanese psychiatrists are now aggressively attempting to expand their influence into the realm of everyday distress, and seem to be succeeding in this endeavor.

---

matic medicine (shinryō naika). They have reintroduced and invigorated the notion of neurosis from the 1960s (Ohnuki-Tierney 1984), and have become successful in attracting people who are concerned with work-related stress but are hesitant to visit psychiatrists (Miyaoka 1999, Matsushita 1997).

CHAPTER FOUR

Pathology of Overwork or Personality Weakness?: The Rise of Neurasthenia in Early-Twentieth-Century Japan

The First Instance of the Medicalization of Everyday Distress

BEFORE WE EXAMINE the history of depression in Japan, I would like to call attention to the fact that, although psychiatry has only recently begun to expand institutionally into the realm of everyday discourse via depression, there was a time when it held a considerable conceptual influence over the way ordinary Japanese talked about their everyday distress in the popular discourse. This was during the alleged "epidemics" of neurasthenia at the turn of the twentieth century, the risk of which was elaborated upon and widely cautioned against by not only medical experts but also influential intellectuals at the time. As this occurred just when lay Japanese were beginning to understand their ailments in biomedical terms, the neurasthenia concept helped familiarize them with psychiatry as a language of everyday experience. In this chapter, I give a brief account of this prewar history and show how both the medical and popular discourses about neurasthenia indirectly provided a conceptual framework for the later theorizing of depression in Japan. I also illustrate how the neurasthenia discourse shared some parallels with the current depression discourse, one of which is the heated debate over its causality—whether or not neurasthenia (like depression a century later) was an illness of overwork or of personality weakness.

Yanagita Kunio, the father of Japanese ethnology and a prominent intellectual of the twentieth-century, commented in *Asahi Shimbun* in 1931 on the effects of modern Westernized medicine. He said that thanks to the new medicine, a number of serious ailments that "have never been heard of" and "would have gone unnoticed" were now being successfully treated. Concurrently, however, Western medicine brought unexpected consequences. While it gave Japanese a radically new knowledge about their bodies, it had made them more anxious than ever. Japanese were now "constantly worried over the slightest changes in [their] health" and had, as a result, become "more vulnerable to illnesses." They were even suffering from something that resided in the gray area between illness and nonillness; the primary example Yanagita had for this was, *shinkeisuijaku* (神経衰弱: literally meaning "nerve weakening" or neurasthenia) (Yanagita 1967:288).[1] The rise of neurasthenia was, indeed, the first instance of the broad-scale medicalization of everyday distress in Japan, preceding the current popularization of depression by a century.

Neurasthenia, an illness category popularized by American neurologist George Beard in 1869, originally referred to a nerve weakness or nervous exhaustion, a condition that was regarded as the ill product of modernity (Gosling 1987, Lutz 1991, Clarke and Jacyna 1987). Epidemics of neurasthenia swept over America and Europe in the late nineteenth century (Oppenheim 1991, Gijswijt-Hofstra and Porter 2001, Rabinbach 1990); Japanese intellectuals began to discuss the notion of neurasthenia by the 1880s. By the 1910s, the Japanese media was calling neurasthenia a "national disease" (Yomiuri, July 8 1917). The media initially depicted it as an inevitable outcome for people at the forefront of the processes of modernization, for whom exhausted nerves even became a mark of distinction. An unprecedented number of cases of neurasthenia among elites—including government officials, company executives, university professors, and artists—began to be reported. Like depression today, neurasthenia was soon linked by medical experts and social commentators with "overwork" (karō)—among other perils of modern life—as well as rising rates of suicide. As newspapers began to feature daily advertisements for various pills to treat it, neurasthenia gradually spread among the general public and became a commonly used idiom of distress by the 1910s (see figure 4.1). Its academic importance for psychiatrists began to decline in the 1910s. In the 1920s, some psychiatrists campaigned against the prevalent "abuse" of the notion of neurasthenia for explaining all sorts of everyday distress. From the late 1930s, the notion slowly began to lose its social significance, as neurasthenia came to signify little more than a weakness of personality. Though neurasthenia continued to be used interchangeably with neurosis for a while, the term faded into obscurity in the postwar period. While neurasthenia had many vicissitudes and conceptual uncertainties, what this notion did for Japanese psychiatry was to help establish its legitimacy as an intimate language for expressing people's everyday distress.[2]

[1] On the rather complex, earlier history of how shinkeisuijaku came to be adopted in the Japanese lexicon, see Watarai (2003).

[2] The sources I use are the following: First, newspaper articles were culled from the databases of *Yomiuri Shimbun* from 1874 to 1945, and *Asahi Shimbun* from 1879 to 2000. Second, popular representations in magazines were examined in an intellectual magazine, *Taiyo*, from 1895 to 1928, as well as in four popular books on neurasthenia published between the 1920s and 1940s. Third, psychiatric discourse regarding neurasthenia was examined in *Shinkeigaku Zasshi* (*Journal of Neurology*) that changed its name in 1935 to *Seishin Shinkeigaku Zasshi* (*Journal of Psychiatry and Neurology*) between 1902 and 1970, and in five psychiatric textbooks published between 1890s and the 1970s.

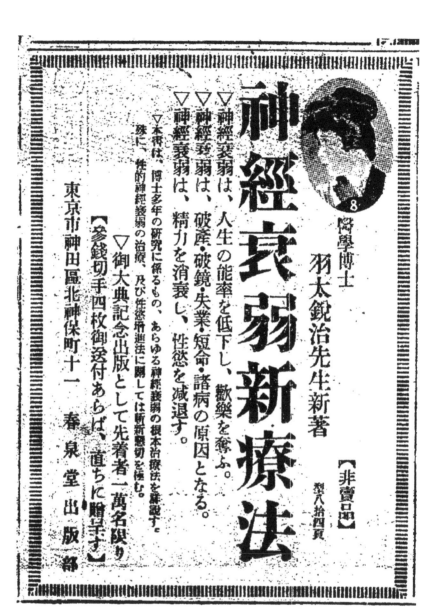

Figure 4.1. An advertisement for a book on how to treat neurasthenia, appearing in Yomiruiri on November 22, 1928 (courtesy of The Yomiuri Newspaper).

The New Language of Experience—"Nerves"

The success of this early medicalization is striking, particularly when we consider the fact that, only a few decades prior, Japanese could not have suffered from neurasthenia at all. This is because, as historians of Japanese medicine have pointed out, Japanese simply did not have "nerves."[3] As Sakai Shizu (1982) writes, within the paradigm of Chinese-derived traditional medicine, there was no concept of nerves, nor was the brain regarded as an important organ. Thus when Sugita Genpaku, the first Japanese doctor to have conducted official dissection, wrote *Kaitai Shinsho* (New Human Anatomy) in 1774, he literally had to create the Japanese word *shinkei* or nerve (also see Kuriyama 1992). "Nerve" remained a highly technical term for the following century; its spread to lay people occurred after Western medicine was officially adopted by the government in 1874 (K. Kawamura 1990). "Nerve" being not at all self-evident to Japanese, experts of Western medicine took care to explain "nerve diseases" in detail. In a 1906 *Yomiuri* newspaper article—titled "The hygiene of nerves"—Tamura Kazaburō commented on how fashionable it was to talk about nerves, but that people had misconceived ideas: "many people seem to think that nerves are invisible; they are in fact tangible, visible things"; nerves are like "white threads" whose normal width was that of "cotton thread," and they function like "electric wires" that "would make a train run." Just as an electric train would not run if the wires were "exhausted beyond use," or if the wires were "cut," the citizens who were the driving force for the advancement of modernity would not function without taking proper care of their nerves (Tamura 1906). In a vision of bioeconomy, psychiatrists talked about nerve diseases as triggered by a deficiency and dysfunction of nerve power (Sakaki 1912). And when it came to the economy of nerve power, Japanese elites, who had launched a national campaign of modernization to join the Western superpowers, had much to worry about.

The media encouraged people to pay attention to their nerves and often provided self-diagnostic tests for the symptoms of neurasthenia. An influential intellectual magazine called *Taiyō* (Sun) featured an article in 1902 with a title that conveyed a sense of national emergency: "Neurasthenia: operators, writers, government officials, and students, read this" (XYZ 1902). The article said that government officials were known to take a leave of absence due to neurasthenia and that "one third of patients who visit hospitals for consultations today" were reportedly suffering from the disease. Such patients were mainly elites engaged in intellectual labor and were thus prone to an excessive use of nerve power.

[3] It is important to remember that, even in the West, "nerves" were not self-evident entities till the nineteenth century; prior to that time, nerves remained mysterious and were often discussed in terms of animal spirits (Clarke and Jacyna 1987).

The symptoms included everything from excitability of the mind (*kandō*), insomnia, lack of concentration, decreased mental capability, oversensitivity, irrational fears and worries, headaches, upset stomach, fatigued eyes, and abnormal sensations in the body such as the feeling that one's head was covered with a heavy pot (a common complaint among depressed patients in contemporary Japan). These symptoms were said to be caused by pathological changes in the nerve cells of the brain. The possibility of heredity was mentioned, but it was emphasized how neurasthenia affects anyone, given certain external life events. The article cited the cases of a businessman suffering a loss in stock trading, a government official humiliated by his colleagues, and a student experiencing heartbreak over love or humiliation for failing an exam. It was also suggested that neurasthenia mostly affected "middle-aged people who are in their primary working years" (again a parallel with the depression discourse in Japan today). Hospitalization was recommended for those who received too much stimulation as a result of work or family interactions. If left untreated, neurasthenia could result in full-blown insanity or suicide (XYZ 1902:134–39, also see Yomiuri July 8, 1917). Commencing in the 1900s, a relentless campaign put out in the media along these lines by medical professionals and intellectuals on the prevention of neurasthenia placed this ailment high on the list of people's health concerns (see figure 4.1);[4] this no doubt created the kind of high anxiety that Yanagita was talking about.

For many Japanese intellectuals, neurasthenia was an ailment of modernity —not just any modernity, but the particular Japanese modernity. Natsume Sōseki, arguably the most important writer in Japanese modern history and also the best-known neurasthenic, asserted that Japanese were suffering from neurasthenia en masse because they were thrown into a modernization that was not of their own choosing. In his legendary speeches, such as "The Enlightenment of Modern Japan" (1911) and "My Individualism" (1914), Sōseki reiterated the theme that Japanese were faced with the task of achieving industrialization and urbanization in less than half the time that it had taken Westerners. The consequence of this "unnaturally" accelerated development, imposed on Japanese by the external threat of colonialism, could be "neurasthenia" from which Japanese would not easily recover (Natsume 1986). Writers at the time were increasingly turning inward to examine the effects of social forces upon themselves, documenting their inner torment by resorting to the idiom of "nerves." Nerves were imagined to be both physical and psychological objects that became fatigued, exhausted, sharpened, overstimulated, or dulled, calmed, and paralyzed. Such images of exhausted nerves bombarded readers of serial-

---

[4] A 1908 book, titled *Eisei Taikan* (Hygiene Encyclopedia), claimed that neurasthenia was due to a wide range of causes, including heredity, mental overwork, sorrow, physical exhaustion, and masturbation. The book suggests that neurasthenia was curable by stabilizing the mind, rubbing and strengthening the body with cold water, taking a cold bath, electrification, or massage.

ized newspaper novels and magazine articles at the time. Concurrently, the media continued to feature advertisements claiming all sorts of "cures" for the damaged nerves, along with graphic pictures of the brain.

By the mid-1900s, the epidemic of neurasthenia was being blamed as the direct cause for the rising rate of suicides. Around the time of the Japan-Russo War (1904—5), with the heightened sense of social unrest, Japanese were experiencing the first suicide boom since the rise of the modern state. Japan's first so-called "modern suicide" in 1903 was reported with much sensationalism in the media. An elite student, Fujimura Misao (a student of Sōseki), jumped over a waterfall in scenic Nikkō north of Tokyo, after inscribing his suicide note on a tree trunk, using a phrase that became famous—"life is incomprehensible." Disputes over the meaning of his act soon erupted among intellectuals. Some intellectuals, particularly artists and writers, attributed social and philosophical meanings to suicide. Tsubouchi Shōyō, a revolutionary literary figure, for instance, wrote a long reflection on suicide and discussed it as a source of freedom for those who must contend with the impossible demands of modernity (Tsubouchi 1903, also see Robertson 1999).

However, some politicians, along with academic psychiatrists (most of whom were trained in German neuropsychiatry and its ideas of degeneration) strongly asserted that individuals who kill themselves do so because they have an "inborn, physical, pathological" nature (such as neurasthenia) that would drive them to "autocide." These individuals, according to this theory, were "unfit" to survive in the highly competitive modern society. Katayama Kuniyoshi, the authority in forensic medicine and a former acting chair of psychiatry at Tokyo Imperial University, wrote in *The Tokyo Asahi* newspaper in 1906 that suicidal individuals were "dispersing poison in society" and that the nation must "strengthen its body and mind so that it can eliminate such pathological molecules" (Katayama 1906, see also Kure 2002 [1894–95], 1917). Ōkuma Shigenobu, a highly influential statesman of the time, was also a central figure in the mental hygiene movement, helping organize "Kyūchikai," a voluntary association for helping the mentally ill. When he was invited to a gathering of psychiatrists and lawyers in 1906, Ōkuma had this to say about the suicidal:

> These days, young students talk about such stuff as the "philosophy of life" [applause from the floor]. They confront important and profound problems of life, are defeated, and develop neurasthenia. Those who jump off of a waterfall or throw themselves in front of a train are weak-minded. They do not have a strong mental constitution and develop mental illness, dying in the end. How useless they are! Such weak-minded people would only cause harm even if they remained alive [applause]. (Ōkuma 1906: 616; note that the whole speech was published in the *Journal of Neurology*)

The surprising fact is that Ōkuma himself later confessed in this speech that his own brother was afflicted with mental illness. The fact that even the family of the mentally ill came to speak of them in such a disparaging tone shows the extent to which the degeneration paradigm permeated the intellectuals' ways of thinking at the time. Kure himself wrote in the *Yomiuri* newspaper in 1917 that the recent increase in the number of suicides among prostitutes (which apparently became a social concern) was the result of mental illness. He wrote that, even though lay people might think that these women were driven to suicide by despair at life's hardships, this would be "amateurish thinking." From an experts' point of view, Kure said, the cause of their suicide was that these women had "inherent, mental abnormalcy" to begin with, which (he said) would also explain why they would turn to such an immoral profession in the first place (Kure 1917:5). Suicide, for the leading medical experts of the time, was thus "self-destruction" of the "pathological molecules" (see Tsubouchi 1903) and neurasthenia a manifestation of abnormal tendencies and even a precursory symptom of suicide (Katayama 1912).

Psychiatric Disputes over Neurasthenia

In the meantime, disputes over the cause of neurasthenia—which paralleled the earlier debates on suicide—began to intensify among psychiatrists by the 1910s.[5] The first group of psychiatrists followed Beard and argued that neurasthenia was indeed an illness of overwork that anyone would experience in the increasingly complex modern world. Matsubara Saburō, who had trained under Adolf Myer for four years in New York, wrote an extensive piece on neurasthenia in 1914 in order to elaborate on the idea that neurasthenia was an illness of "people of culture" (Matsubara 1914). However, most Japanese psychiatrists at the time were trained in German, Kraepelinian neuropsychiatry, and as a result shared a strong adherence to genetics as the cause of mental illness. Kure wrote in a 1913 *Yomiuri* newspaper commentary on neurasthenia that no one could develop mental illness from working too much—if they did, they must have a predisposition to begin with. Kure further preached the importance of recognizing what he described as the "predisposed level of talent," so that people would not push themselves beyond their limit and develop neurasthenia (Kure 1913). As well, Sakaki Yasuzaburō, professor at Kyūshū Imperial University and brother of Sakaki Hajime (the first professor of psychiatry in Japan), stated in his book, *Kawarimono* (the Abnormal), that neurasthenics were "generally born with an inherent weakness in the brain." The neurasthenic, Sakaki wrote, was like a "poor man" who "only has half the mental capacity of a normal person" (Sakaki

---

[5] Note that the ideas about neurasthenia developed differently in different places (see Gijiswijt-Hofstra and Porter, 2001, and Lee 1999).

1912:264). Some psychiatrists began to contend with the issue of the scientific legitimacy of this illness category, which was debated in a symposium on neurasthenia held at the Japanese Society of Neurology in 1913. By this time, Beard's original formulation of neurasthenia as an illness of overwork had been largely refuted in the West (Lutz 1995). Following this conceptual change, Japanese psychiatrists began to introduce the distinction between "true neurasthenia" and *shinkeishitsu*, or nervous temperament/disposition (discussed below). Miyake Kōichi, the successor to Kure at Tokyo Imperial University, had already made these distinctions in a *Journal of Neurology* paper in 1912 and said that about 10 to 20 percent of the so-called neurasthenic patients actually suffered from true neurasthenia, which was the result of external stimuli such as "overwork" (Miyake 1912, 1927).

By the 1920s, psychiatrists were lamenting the fact that too many people were casually using the label of neurasthenia and claiming themselves to be neurasthenic (again the striking parallel with the current depression discourse among psychiatrists). Some began to assert that most of the patients who would come to see a doctor complaining of this ailment were not suffering from neurasthenia at all: it was merely a manifestation of shinkeishitsu. This general sentiment among academic psychiatrists was clearly expressed in a public lecture given by Uematsu Shichikurō, professor at Keio University (who later helped establish the Mental Hygiene Law in 1950) at a "Mental hygiene exhibition" held by the Red Cross in 1929. The Red Cross exhibition opened in the center of Tokyo with the aim of "promoting knowledge of mental illness." Held at a time when Japan was attempting to build up the health of its citizens, the exhibition sought to enlighten people about the horror of mental illness, the danger of passing it on through marriage, and the importance of hygiene of the mind and body in defense of diseases. Mental illness was presented as exotica, its horror conveyed in easy-to-digest graphs and pictures. In a lecture titled "Urban life and neurasthenia," Uematsu pointed out that people once believed that neurasthenia was caused by overwork, but the truth was that these neurasthenics "rarely have apparent causes nor do they seem to improve with rest." This was because, according to Uematsu, these people were shinkeishitsu, and were merely responding to external stimuli in an "abnormal, persistent way," which gave rise to "stimulus fatigue." Addicted to material culture and tormented by deep anxiety about competition, such people had, in other words, a "weak resistance":

> [N]eurasthenia is not a disease but the kind of person. Headaches, dizziness, ringing in the ear, and forgetfulness are all abnormal mental responses and do not themselves constitute a brain disease. Many lay people seem to think that neurasthenia can be cured by injection and medication. What is cured are merely symptoms such as headaches, dizziness, and insomnia. The fundamental disease—that is, the personality itself—can never be cured by medication. (Uematsu 1929:17)

Though Uematsu hastily added that such a pathological personality was something that anyone might have to some extent, he concluded that the only cure
for neurasthenia was a "philosophical attitude or resignation." He reiterated
this position in a series of *Yomiuri* newspaper articles in 1936, titled "Unveiling
neurasthenia," and he denounced this disease category altogether in his widely
used textbook (Uematsu 1948; the textbook went into the ninth printing by
1957). As the concept of neurasthenia dissolved into that of a pathological disposition within psychiatry, and as the national call for cultivating the "spirit"
rose with the impending war, the number of reported neurasthenics rapidly
decreased in the 1930s. Uchimura Yūshi, who as the successor to Miyake chaired
the psychiatric department at Tokyo University both during World War II and
its aftermath, gave a speech at the inaugural ceremony of the Mental Welfare
Association in 1943. In front of two hundred attendees, including the Ministry
of Interior, he said: "The spirit of the citizens is healthy, and this is apparent in
many ways. One example is the decreasing number of neurasthenic patients
since 1937; the number is now half what it was before. However, we have no
time to be complacent, when the various nerve wars (*shinkeisen*) are being
fought" (Uchimura 1943:527). Apparently there was no place for neurasthenics
in wartime Japan, when citizens were constantly being urged to strengthen
both their spirit and body.

After World War II, the notion of neurasthenia was becoming obsolete in
academic psychiatry, almost entirely replaced by the category of neurosis. This
was already suggested in 1942 by Shimoda Mitsuzō, professor at Kyūshū University (and the famous theorist of depression), who wrote in a book for a popular audience called *Seishin Eisei Kōwa* (Lectures on Mental Hygiene), that
"there is no other disease category so widely used and abused as neurasthenia";
"Most of the early phases of mental illness are called neurasthenia; people use it
as an excuse for taking time off work, and even doctors use it when they cannot
find an exact diagnosis" (Shimoda 1942:88). After the war, Nakagawa Shirō of
Tokyo University published a thorough study on neurasthenia, in which he examined 440 patients diagnosed with neurasthenia and shinkeishitsu and found
that 74.9 percent of them had a good prognosis and most would now fall into
the category of neurosis (Nakagawa 1947, Muramatsu 1953, T. Takahashi, 1998:
on the particular history of traumatic neurosis in Japan, see Satō 2009). As
neurasthenia became incorporated into the notion of neurosis, its official usage
quickly declined and the term became a euphemism for insanity. In newspaper
articles of the postwar era, there were scattered references to neurasthenia in
the cases of violent suicide attempts and homicides in the 1950s: for example, a
neurasthenic mother strangled her child (1951), a neurasthenic set himself on
fire (1954), and a neurasthenic craftsman killed his father-in-law with a hatchet
(1960). During the 1960s, the term was seldom used: one of its last appear-
ances in *Asahi* was in 1974 in an article about Lilly the Panda at the Paris zoo,
who developed "neurasthenia" and died during a hunger strike (*Asahi*, April

24, 1974). The word lingers on as the name of a card game (called "Melancholy" in the West), and is still recognized as a term connoting mental illness—albeit with a sense of anachronism.[6]

Up to this point, the story of the fall of neurasthenia from an illness of over-work to a personality weakness deviated little from what had happened earlier in the West. What came after this, however, were two distinct Japanese develop-ments. The first was the way in which neurasthenia became popularized through the rising psychological discourse about shinkeishitsu in the Taishō Era; the sec-ond was a new concept of depression proposed by Shimoda Mitsuzō.

Transformations of Neurasthenia into a Personality Type —Shinkeishitsu

Despite the official dismissal by psychiatrists that neurasthenia no longer con-stituted a disease entity, lay people who had come to think of their distress in terms of nerve disease continued to resort to this category. While they were left uncured, one of the doctors who offered an alternative to biopsychiatry was Morita Masatake, who was beginning to cultivate, in opposition to biology and Western psychoanalysis, his own theory of psychology. Morita had originally entered Tokyo Imperial University with an interest in studying neurosis, and soon emerged as an authority on neurasthenia and neurosis at a time when these notions were becoming increasingly psychologized. Writing in the 1930 *Gendai igaku daijiten* (Contemporary Medical Dictionary), Morita explicitly denied the disease category of neurasthenia, arguing that stimulus-exhaustion was a symptom that accompanied illnesses in general and that it was highly subjective, changing from person to person. Instead, drawing on ideas such as Hippocrates's theory of oversensitive constitution, and Kraepelin's theory of he-reditary neurasthenia, Morita proposed an interpretation of shinkeishitsu as a disposition characterized by "self-reflexivity and intelligence."[7] Morita argued that the key to the cure was to simply encourage patients to "realize" that what they were suffering from was not really a disease but simply the way they were (Morita 1930:83–85, Watanabe 1999). Morita said that 60 percent of his shinkeishitsu patients recovered in less than forty days through this therapy, and his disciples such as Kōra Takehisa were able to claim that the conventional idea that chronic neurasthenia was based upon hereditary predisposition and was incurable had been refuted, as shinkeishitsu patients could return to their normal state by the psychological changes induced by Morita Therapy (Kōra 1938). This marked the birth of a new psychological theory in Japan, in which

[6] As Kleinman demonstrates, interpretations of neurasthenia in China have been subject to shifting paradigms of Chinese psychiatry (such as Pavlovian neurophysiology) that have been inti-mately linked to dominant political theories of the time (Kleinman 1986:22–35, Lee 1999).

[7] Morita contrasted this with the "hyper emotionality" of a hysteric.

the meaning of shinkeishitsu changed from merely a sign of incurable abnormality to an *excess of self-reflexivity*, which was supposedly brought about by the disruptions caused by modernity.

These striking reports of cure by the Morita group went largely ignored by mainstream psychiatrists, who were only interested in the "real" (that is, biological) diseases and moved away from neurasthenia in contempt of its dubious scientific status. However, intellectuals of the time took a keen interest in Morita Therapy and began to form a therapeutic movement, which helped create a kind of psychology boom beginning in the Taishō Era. Morita himself energetically promoted his idea through the publications of his books, *Shinkeishitsu oyobi shinkeisuijakushō no ryōhō* (The Treatment for Shinkeishistu and Neurasthenia) in 1921, and gained a wide audience through his national radio talk on neurasthenia in 1926. At the same time, prominent writers such as Kurata Hyakuzō, known for works like *The Priest and his Disciples*, published accounts of their own recovery from shinkeishitsu through Morita Therapy (Satō et al. 1997:198). Most notably, Nakamura Kokyō, the editor of *Hentai Shinri* (Abnormal Psychology) was an ardent Morita supporter. A former disciple of Natsume Sōseki, Kokyō had lost his brother to mental illness and himself suffered from neurasthenia. Critical of modern medicine from his own experience and arguing that its "materialistic" treatment "disregard[ed] the depth of human psychology," Nakamura became a well-known therapist in his own right, publishing numerous case studies that explained in depth—from his perspective—what overcoming neurasthenia was all about (Nakamura 1930, Oda 2001).

In serial articles Nakamura originally published in the magazine *Shufu no tomo* (Friend of housewives), which was later published in book form (*Shinkeisuijaku wa dō sureba zenchisuruka* [How to fully recover from neurasthenia]) in 1930, he discussed the life stories of neurasthenics who finally found a cure in Morita Therapy after a long quest. In one of Nakamura's articles, for instance, a thirty-seven-year-old graduate of Tokyo Imperial University, who had needed to take a year off from his government work because of his neurasthenia, fully recovered with five sessions of hypnotic suggestive therapy and was now "successfully working as a governor." Another patient was a twenty-six-year-old graduate of a vocational school, who claimed to have suffered from neurasthenia since grade school. He had seen numerous doctors, most of whom simply prescribed medicine and vitamin injections.[8] In desperation, the patient even resorted to a "special medicine" that would make "part of his brain paralyzed" in order to "create changes in the brain encephalon," but it failed

---

[8] His illness history illuminates the range of treatment that was available for neurasthenics at the time: he had received electric therapy, hypnosis, willpower treatment (*kiaijutsu*), the Great Path to Spirit (*daireidō*), and thought-projection therapy (*nensha ryōhō*)—but all in vain. Other kinds of treatment that Nakamura's patients had tried were also far ranging and included massage, self-control therapy, deep-breathing, exercise, abdominal respiration, chiropractic, water therapy, and more ordinary treatments of vitamin shots and hormone therapy by medical doctors.

miserably. Convinced that "it is natural law that the weak must perish," he decided that the "only contribution [he] can make to society" was to "leave this world." Nakamura's advice was that the weak person would only exhaust himself if he wished to be stronger than he was capable of. The cure was to simply recognize who he was: "He has to be resigned to his own weakness, be satisfied and grateful" (Nakamura 1930:42–53). Despite this unflattering fatalism, Morita Therapy won popular appeal, probably because it apparently provided a much-needed cure where biopsychiatry had failed.[9] At the same time, Morita Therapy may have served to de-emphasize the social etiology of neurasthenia by instilling its own distinctive process of psychologization in a Japanese soil that did not accept psychoanalysis.

A New Illness of Overwork: Localizing Depression

In the meantime, as the medical category of neurasthenia was beginning to be dismissed by academic psychiatrists, another illness "resembling neurasthenia" emerged on the horizon of Japanese psychiatry—that was depression. As I will discuss in the next chapter, this notion was formulated by Shimoda Mitsuzō, who noted that a group of patients shared not only neurasthenic symptoms but a certain type of personality. Arguing that they were in fact suffering from depression, Shimoda further illuminated how these patients had the personality traits of those who were diligent, thorough, highly respected members of society. As if to revive the earlier discourse about the overworked neurasthenics, and to save those from the quickly degrading implication of neurasthenia itself, Shimoda's theory of depression established—just when Japan was plunging deeper into the war effort—a new category of illness that was not necessarily of a morally degenerate kind. Yet the moral ambiguity of the neurasthenia concept was also inherited in Shimoda's depression concept. While this later came to aid psychiatrists in discussing the pathology of Japanese social structure, this new notion of depression also left unanswered the question of where the real causality lay—whether the blame should be placed on the society that produced the demand for overwork or on the individuals whose personality drove them to such overwork—a question that Japanese psychiatrists are again having to confront with regard to the rising rates of depression and overwork suicide today.

[9] The idea of neurasthenia and shinkeishitsu penetrated into society by the 1920s, creating diverging interpretations. Compared to the Tokyo-based Nakamura, Usa (1925) from Kyoto, originally a Zen priest who became a disciple of Morita, had a more working-class clientele and showed a strikingly different picture of neurasthenia as being continuously *physical* in nature. His patient population varied remarkably in terms of their occupations—including a potter, famer, chirographer, fisher monger, dye shop worker, oil container seller, goldsmith, as well as photographer—suggesting a spread of neurasthenia in the 1920s well beyond the intellectual circles of the 1900s.

In the next chapter, I examine how Japanese psychiatric notions of depression have evolved in the course of the twentieth century. Notably, Japanese psychiatrists have come to develop localized theories about depression not only by incorporating (and at times questioning) Western knowledge but also by exploring what is meaningful for them at the clinical, therapeutic level. The result is a set of distinctive ideas about depression that are not blind to the forces of society. That is, through their attempts to theorize depression, Japanese psychiatrists have come to grapple with the question of how to understand the interplay between individual biology and society. By tracing these theoretical developments, I show how understandings of the "biology" of depression in Japan have taken a localized form.

CHAPTER FIVE

Socializing the "Biological" in Depression:
Japanese Psychiatric Debates about *Typus Melancholicus*

Unpacking the Meaning of the Biological

As THE CURRENT medicalization of depression has been spurred on by the advent of new antidepressants, North American critics have expressed concern that psychiatry is promoting a form of biological reductionism. By reducing the complex causality of depression to "chemical imbalance" and disseminating the idea of the "neurochemical self" (see Rose 2007), psychiatry—these critics argue—serves to impoverish people's understanding of depression, thereby homogenizing the diverse local resources from which they have dealt with life's hardships (see Elliott and Chambers 2004). During my fieldwork in Japan, however, I found that medicalization does not necessarily promote the same old reductionist biological thinking that critics have warned. Instead, medicalization has gained considerable persuasive power not because of the idea of depression as an isolated neurochemical occurrence, but because Japanese psychiatrists have been able to popularize an alternative—and rather distinctive—language for understanding the "biology" of depression. As I will demonstrate in this chapter, this biological language has effectively captured the Japanese imagination as it seems to speak to their "phenomenological sense of the lived experience of the body-self" (Scheper-Hughes and Lock 1987:7).

I noticed the intriguingly localized ways that "biology" is interpreted immediately after I entered the field of Japanese psychiatry, where I found the dichotomy between the biological and the psychotherapeutic—one that I had become familiar with through my fieldwork in North American psychiatry—soon broke down. When I asked psychiatrists what their theoretical orientation was, some of them—particularly those whom I considered to be more psychotherapeutic in their approach—asked me in return exactly what I meant by "biological psychiatry." These doctors knew full well that such a dichotomy exists and continues to divide North American psychiatry (Luhrmann 2000), and would themselves critique certain forms of biological reductionism. Yet, because they are—like all Japanese psychiatrists—trained first in neuropsychiatry, even those who later adopt psychotherapy regard biological perspectives as an essential foundation for the way they think and operate. The differences did not stop there. While all the Japanese psychiatrists I have met thus confidently state that depression is primarily a neurochemical disease, they also depart in their opinions from their North American counterparts in two important aspects. First, they often depict depression not so much as an illness of emotion (as their North American counterparts do) as an "illness of the (whole) body" (*karada no byōki*)—a physiological problem of fatigue, decreased energy, and inaction—that ultimately affects the "whole person." Second, through what they regard as a *scientific* theory called "Typus Melancholicus," Japanese psychiatrists observe that those who are prone to depression have a set of endogenous personality traits—that is, being serious, diligent, thorough, considerate, and responsible—that tend to drive them to overwork, and in some cases, even to psychiatric breakdown. Using these theories along with the neurochemical account, Japanese psychiatrists have explained the rise of depression in terms of an accumulated sense of fatigue that Japanese have been experiencing in the prolonged recession. By weaving the bio-psycho-social narratives in this way, they have successfully transformed depression from something rarely heard of into a ubiquitous illness that is not only acceptable but also attractive for lay Japanese.

Thus, beneath the surface of the global "biologization" of depression lie rich undercurrents of local discourses about depression. In fact, the current neurochemical discourse seems to even encourage the flourishing of local interpretations because depression explained at the level of neurochemical changes appears, at least for many Japanese, too experience-distant and removed from the realm of lived reality. One may even argue that the neurochemical imagery serves as an *empty symbol* (cf. Barthes 1982) into which rich meanings can be inscribed, making local interpretations ever more diversified, creative, and evocative. Also important is that, while it has become somewhat commonplace to assert the presence of different voices within and across biomedicines (Mol and Berg 1998, Atkinson 1995) and to think of biomedicine as a "collection of regional rationalisms" (Osborne 1998:260),[1] some of these local theories—however exotic they may seem to outsiders—operate not simply as cultural knowledge but as *scientific theories*. Historically, these theories (like ideas about fatigue and Typus Melancholicus in Japan) have emerged at the intersection of diverse theoretical currents within psychiatry (including those imported from Europe and the United States as well as those domestically developed) and local ideas about health and the body, which together make up what Margaret Lock (1993) calls "local biologies." Thus, in order to understand how the particular interpretation of the "biology" of depression has become possible in Japan, we first take a look at the kinds of *scientific* discourses about "depression" during the twentieth century, as well as the ways they have been transformed before and after the advent of the new antidepressants. More specifically, I will focus

---

[1] Osborne asserts that biomedicine can be understood as a "collection of regional rationalisms" with a kind of "spirit" that is ideological not because it is false but because it represents more than just the sum of its local, institutional realities (Osborne 1998:260).

on how Japanese psychiatrists have come to shape their *biological* language of depression via their own struggles with traditional biological reductionism, through different historical phases that I call somatization, existentialization, and politicization.[2]

Somatizing Depression: The Groundwork for Medicalization via Modern Psychiatry

The conceptual seeds for medicalizing depression were sown in Japan in the late nineteenth century, when Japanese psychiatrists imported a German psychiatric concept that defined depression as a heredity-based neurological disease.[3] This idea was more firmly installed as textbook knowledge in the 1900s, when the Kraepelinian nosology, which defined depression as one pole of manic-depression (which, together with schizophrenia, made up the "two major psychoses"), was officially adopted. Generations of Japanese psychiatrists, including the already-retired doctors I interviewed, were trained with this neurological concept of depression, which they sometimes explained to me in terms of so-called "alarm clock theory." This theory asserted that people who were susceptible to depression had a kind of internal, genetically wired alarm clock that operated independently from external environment (Iida 1974:14). This internal clock automatically turned itself on and off, periodically making patients manic or depressive depending on which phase they happened to be in. Because of this fatalistic understanding of depression, early Japanese psychiatrists, who were mainly interested in laboratory investigation of manic depression (particularly anatomical dissection of the brain), showed relatively little interest in clinical exploration of depression per se (Tatsumi 1975). Also, the presumed prognosis for depression, which was, unlike schizophrenia, thought to naturally diminish within three to six months without medical treatment, dissuaded psychiatrists from aggressive intervention. Subsumed under the category of manic depression, depression as such remained a mechanical, experience-distant disease concept, devoid of psychological meaning or social significance.

[2] In order to examine how utsubyō has been discussed in Japanese psychiatry, I checked every article on depression (and suicide) that appeared in the *Japanese Journal of Psychiatry and Neurology* from 1902 to 2003, as well as a number of other psychiatric journals and major psychiatric textbooks published between the 1870s and 2000s. I supplemented the archival research with oral history research, visiting ten university psychiatric departments around the country and a number of private hospitals in the Tokyo area, while conducting interviews with more than fifty psychiatrists.

[3] Originally, for the early Japanese psychiatrists trained with Henry Maudsley's textbook (published in 1872 and translated into Japanese in 1876 [Maudsley 2002]), melancholia served as an all-encompassing category for insanity (Okada 1981:76–78). Melancholia's importance soon waned, however, after Kure instilled the Kraepelinian nosology as the doctrine of Japanese psychiatry. Noting in his clinical lectures the ingenuity of the Kraepelinian notion of manic depression, Kure emphasized how the seemingly unrelated diseases—mania and depression—were in fact two sides of the same coin (Kure 1914, 1915).

Though this biological determinism became firmly entrenched in the thinking of early Japanese psychiatrists, some of them began to engage with other psychiatric intellectual currents of 1920s–1930s Germany, which were developing as critiques of Kraepelin's brand of anatomy-based neuropsychiatry. Drawing upon one such work by Ernest Kretschmer of the Tubingen School, who emphasized the power of clinical observation and the importance of excavating patients' life histories (Ishikawa 1925),[4] Shimoda Mitsuzō, professor of psychiatry at Kyūshū Imperial University, set out to investigate the pathological process of depression in the 1930s. At the time, Shimoda's group (Naka 1932) noticed a considerable number of patients seeking medical care for their neurasthenic symptoms, such as despondency and sleep disturbance, but who did not seem to recover even after a period of rest. Diagnosing them to be suffering from unipolar (presenile) depression, Shimoda's group suggested that these patients were not feeble degenerates as the Kraepelinian conception of the mentally ill might indicate, but rather socially adaptive people ("many from the upper class") who developed depressive symptoms only later in their otherwise successful lives (20 percent of the patients were doctors). Contrasted with Kretschmer's 1921 idea that manic-depressives had a constitution called cyclothymia, Shimoda argued that his own patients possessed what he called immodithymic constitution (*shūchaku kishitsu*). Shimoda explained that patients with this constitution had "abnormal emotional processes," where an emotion would persist with intensity until the patients developed depression at the height of their exhaustion:

> The essence of this constitution is the abnormalcy of its emotional processes. That is, for those with this constitution, an emotion that once occurs does not cool down after a certain period as it would in a normal person and instead persists for a long time at a certain level of intensity, which can even grow stronger. People with this abnormal constitution are enthusiastic about work, meticulous, thorough, honest, punctual, with a strong sense of justice, duty, and responsibility, and unable to cheat or be sloppy. They are the kind of people who gain trust of others by being reliable, who are praised as *model youths, model employee, and model officers.* (Shimoda 1950: 3, emphasis added)

[4] Shimoda's theory of personality was a product of a dialogue with an entirely different strand of German intellectual thought that had been newly introduced to Japan in 1925. Up to that point, German psychiatry meant Kraepelinian neuropsychiatry. What Japanese psychiatrists seemed not to realize was that this kind of biological reductionism was in fact a reaction against the previously dominant Romantic psychiatry in Germany, and that the two currents continued to interact and develop together within Germany itself. Thus when Kretschmer's theory of constitution and mental illness—which was heavily influenced by the Romantic thinking that linked depression with geniuses (such as Goethe and Humboldt)—was introduced to Japan by Ishikawa Sadakichi in *The Journal of Neurology* in 1925, there was considerable excitement among psychiatrists and other intellectual figures (Ishikawa 1925).

At the basic level, Shimoda's theory, like the alarm-clock theory, reiterated the biological theme of the genetic vulnerability of the depressed. People with this constitution pushed themselves beyond their limit because they were unable to sense their own exhaustion. Depression functioned like an internal thermostat built into a machine that, when overheated, shut down the system so as to protect itself. Depression, for Shimoda, is thus a "biological response for self-preservation" that occurs at the height of one's fatigue—a protective mechanism of adaptation (Shimoda 1950:2, 1941).

Notwithstanding its biological determinism, Shimoda's theory also departed from its predecessors in important ways by illuminating the complex relationship between biology, psychology, and the social environment. While the theory illuminated how this pathogenic constitution made people socially successful in their work in the first place, it also accounted for why they tended to break down later in life when their declining physical strength could no longer accommodate their inherent drive to work. By emphasizing how genetics shaped a particular personality, which then gave rise to a pathogenic situation leading to the final collapse, Shimoda's theory opened a path for later conceptualizations of personality cause (*seikaku-in*) and situational cause (*jōkyō-in*). One may even argue that this theory, as it ventured to explain the latent abnormality within seemingly normal, hardworking people, captured the pathology of the militaristic state where such blind, unreflective "hard work" would have been normalized and encouraged rather than problematized.

Though Shimoda's theory set the mold in which Japanese psychiatric understanding of depression was to be later developed, it was largely ignored at the time, as most prewar academic psychiatrists were far more interested in laboratory investigations than clinical explorations; they tended to be dismissive of discoveries made by one of their own colleagues (even by a highly respected scholar like Shimoda) and not by prominent scholars from the "West." It took until the postwar period for the theory to be rediscovered and for a broader medicalization of depression to take off.

Existentializing Depression: The First Attempt at Broad Medicalization

The discovery of antidepressants in the 1950s brought the first serious attempt by psychiatrists to widely medicalize depression.[5] Some of these psychiatrists

---

[5] With regard to depression before the advent of antidepressants, David Healy writes:

> Depressive disorders, at least in Europe, were restricted to the melancholias, with or without delusions, and severe depressive personality disorders that led to admissions to hospital at a rate of approximately 50 per million of the population. These early figures need to be set beside current estimates for depressive disorders which run at 100,000 per million. It fol-

believed that this would cement the triumph of the biological approach to mental illness once and for all. Due to their aggressive promotion of antidepressants from the 1960s on, depression soon became a much-discussed category in the media, which helped psychiatrists and internists to also "discover" a significant number of depressed patients in the community (Hirasawa 1966). This medicalization, though it was of a much smaller scale than what was to come in the 1990s, brought a considerable expansion of psychiatric practice, as doctors nationwide began to report a rapid increase of outpatient depression: Jikei University in Tokyo recorded the rise of depression in its outpatient clinic from 7.1 in 1964 to 18.5 percent in 1971 (Shinfuku et al. 1973); at Kyoto University, from 10.8 (1958) to 19.2 percent (1968), to 29.3 percent (1978) (Kimura 1975).[6] Behind the success of this medicalization lay a series of efforts by psychiatrists to overcome the strong stigma attached to mental illness by reshaping their own representation of the "biological," particularly by shifting their focus from genetic determinism to more flexible forms of somatic representation.

In an attempt to make depression familiar to lay Japanese, psychiatrists first of all found various ways to present depression on par with other physical illnesses. While some psychiatrists stayed with technical, neurochemical terminologies, others with a more clinical orientation began to portray depression by evoking a set of culturally resonant idioms, some of which were suggestive of traditional medical holism. They explained depression as a "disorder in vital rhythm," "stagnation of vital flow," and "lowering of vital emotion" (Iida 1974:6, Shinfuku 1969). They also used other metaphors to naturalize depression, describing it as a phenomenon where "the body enters from a sunny spot into shadow," thereby trying to familiarize depression as if it almost lay within the range of ordinary life experiences (see Okazaki et al. 2006). These attempts also paralleled the advent of a new field in Japan at the time called psychosomatic medicine (*shinryō naika*), which attempted the overcoming of Cartesian dualism built into biomedicine by emphasizing the intimate relationship between mind and body. Though similar attempts were made overseas, what was characteristic about this Japanese psychosomatic medicine was the way in which doctors approached the problem by focusing not on the mind (as psychotherapists would) but rather on the body (as Japanese traditional doctors would), with the belief that inducing changes in the body would also help heal the mind. Further attempts were made to de-stigmatize depression by way of de-psychologizing depression. For example, Shinfuku Naotake (1969), a dis-

---

lows that conditions currently described as primary care depression or community depressions, and thought to be in some way continuous with hospital depression, before 1950 must have been subsumed within the general pool of community nervousness and as such must have been viewed as discontinuous with melancholia. These non-hospital nervous conditions were more likely to attract a diagnosis of anxiety or mixed anxiety depressive disorder or 'nerves.' (Healy 2000:395)

[6] A 1973 questionnaire survey of 200 psychiatrists confirmed the commonly held impression at the time that depression was on the rise (Ōhara 1973).

ciple of Shimoda, used V. Kral's notion of "masked depression" to call attention to the form of depression that showed almost exclusively somatic presentation (such as loss of energy, disturbed sleep, and changed appetite) in the absence of depressed emotion. In these ways, depression as it was widely introduced to lay Japanese for the first time, was a "bodily" entity—de-emotionalized and de-psychologized.

Yet these body-centered approaches gradually showed their limitations, as psychiatrists began to experience therapeutic failures with antidepressants. They observed that a significant number of patients on antidepressants were not getting better, with some experiencing relapses and others turning into chronic patients (Takahashi 1974, Kasahara 1976). Depression experts even began to wonder if the use of antidepressants was inhibiting the natural recovery process, thereby changing the *nature* of depression itself (Kasahara et al. 1992). While some psychiatrists continued with biological/pharmaceutical investigations, other psychiatrists began to explore, beyond the biological fix, alternative approaches to depression. What many of them turned to was not Freudian psychoanalysis (which continued to be criticized by leading academic psychiatrists as pseudoscience) but rather German phenomenological psychopathology, which had begun to develop in the pre–World War II era and yielded significant influence both in Germany and Japan in the postwar period. Japanese psychiatrists found intellectual affinity with this approach partly because they shared the understanding of German neuropsychiatry (upon which psychopathology was built) as the foundation of their own discipline and also because they could identify with the German struggle to overcome the negative legacy of prewar biological determinism. As many depression experts told me, what fundamentally changed their perspective on depression was their encounter with Hubertus Tellenbach's 1961 notion of Typus Melancholicus, a German psychopathological theory of depression developed as an attempt to synthesize prewar biological psychiatry with postwar humanistic/existential psychopathology (Tellenbach 1980[1961]). For these Japanese psychiatrists, Tellenbach concretely showed how the depressed, while manifesting a set of endogenous traits through their personality (such as a love of order and consideration for others), also interacted with the social environment in distinctive ways that would eventually structure their depression. He thus conceptualized the personality of the depressed not only as an inborn, rigid, static entity but something dynamic, with a possibility of agency, and in constant engagement with society. Japanese psychiatrists, who immediately found in Tellenbach's notion striking similarities with Shimoda's immodithymic personality, began to use these theories to critically reexamine their own assumptions about the "biological" nature of depression.[7]

---

[7] Note that German psychiatrists also began to explore situational cause (jōkyō-in), as they faced the question of how to assess the nature of "depression" prevalent not only in returning soldiers but also in Holocaust survivors, many of whom had led a "normal" life before the war. As they investi-

These Japanese psychiatrists' intellectual efforts were crystallized in their debates about Typus Melancholicus as a "social personality." Since the 1950s, the notion of "social personality"—as exemplified by Erich Fromm's 1941 book on the pathology of the German psyche (*Escape from Freedom*, translated in 1951)— was discussed in various symposia of the Japanese Society of Psychiatry and Neurology as a useful concept for reflecting on the pathology of the Japanese war-time mentality. Now faced with the sudden increase of depression from the 1960s on, Japanese psychiatrists were asking why it was especially those with a socially adaptive, normative personality that were falling into depression en masse. They began to explore whether there was something about the Japanese psyche—or society—that was problematic, even pathogenic. Some psychiatrists ventured to explain how social change ("modernization") was affecting individuals' biology as well as their psychology. Doi Takeo, who later wrote the highly reputed *Anatomy of Dependence* (1971), argued that the epidemic of depression was caused by the disintegration of families and traditional communities and the transformation of the work style, factors that were destroying people's "illusionary identification" with the collective (Doi 1966). Drawing on Max Weber's notion of the Protestant ethic (and paralleling social critics such as Norman O. Brown, who discussed how the industrial capitalist order had instilled and rewarded an "anal" personality type in the West [Brown 1959]), Nakai Hisao (1976) traced the historical production of work-obsessed melancholic personality in Japan to the Edo Era, when a certain work ethic of "reconstruction" began to permeate Japanese society. Nakai also suggested how this personality type was no longer rewarded in the emerging economic structure, thereby making Typus Melancholicus maladaptive in today's social order. In the 1972 symposium on manic-depression held by the Society of Psychiatry and Neurology at the height of the antipsychiatry movement, the social themes were reiterated by the panelists, where they discussed how the rise of industrialization and nuclearization of families were causing alienation for melancholics, whose love of order and strong desire for a sense of belonging made them inherently vulnerable at a time of radical social change (e.g., Iida 1973). Iida Shin, a prominent psychopathologist, further elaborated on these themes in 1974:

> Melancholics [or people who have constitutional vulnerability to depression] face crisis at a time of social change, when their particular way of

---

gated the impact of situational causes, German psychiatrists turned to concepts such as "uprooted depression" and "existential depression" in an attempt to do justice to the magnitude of social suffering people had experienced. These psychiatrists were then asked to determine the precise etiology of these people's depression, particularly in legal cases where survivors demanded economic compensation for their suffering. This led to a number of heated—and ultimately unresolved—debates within German psychiatry about whether or not genetic factors were always at work in psychopathology (as their prewar biological determinism would have presupposed) or if a stressful situation alone could serve as a cause for psychopathology (Omata 2002).

being no longer works. . . . (1) Because melancholics rely on stability and order, they lack the ability to change perspective and leap into a new phase of being and are unable to easily adjust to rapid social changes; (2) In today's society where individual values have become diversified, where the location of authority is no longer clearly defined, it is difficult for melancholics, who are inherently pro-establishment and conservative, to find meaning in life; (3) What is important for them is the sense of emotional satisfaction they feel from personal relationships and the real feeling that they are being useful for others and society. Yet, in contemporary society where machine civilization has become highly developed and social institutions enormous, where individuals are mere cogs in the wheel, melancholics are no longer able to obtain such a sense of satisfaction. (Iida 1974:13–14)

Through the discourse of Typus Melancholicus, depression became a symbol of social upheaval (Iida 1974, 1976, Ōhara 1973).[8] What was originally conceptualized as an individual biological defect in Shimoda's discussion, had now become a collective pathology behind the postwar reconstruction of Japanese society and what lay at the core of the "Japanese self."

The Void of the Psychological

However, this highly abstracted and socialized theory of depression, molded in the spirit of the then-popular *Nihonjinron* (theories of *the* Japanese self), posed new challenges to psychotherapeutically oriented psychiatrists. Despite their high-minded, left-wing ideas about how individuals were victims of social forces (from which they could supposedly be emancipated to become agents of their own), these psychiatrists, after years of trial and error, ultimately left individual psychological exploration in a void. Initially, some of them explored ways to combine pharmaceutical and psychotherapeutic approaches. Drawing on the premises of Typus Melancholicus, they would urge recovering depressed patients to reflect upon their own personality—how they themselves might have contributed to structuring a pathogenic situation (e.g.,

---

[8] As Alain Ehrenberg (2010) points out, psychiatric epidemiological research has repeatedly suggested that social stress (including economic disparity or social inequality) in itself does not directly cause depression; instead, whether it translates into depression largely depends on one's interpretation of the stress (if it is thought of as within the range of the expected, for instance). Some researchers have thus argued that depression is not so much an illness of economic disparity or even social inequality per se as it is an *illness of social change*, which creates a discrepancy between what people expect and what they actually experience. In other words, they are most susceptible to depression when their taken-for-granted sense of the world comes crumbing down (Ehrenberg 2010).

Yazaki 1968). However, these attempts were unsystematic and sporadic, without producing definitive results. When these doctors faced therapeutic failures, they tended to discuss them not in terms of their own professional inadequacy or lack of training, or even the inherent difficulty of doing psychotherapy, but rather in terms of patients' inborn traits of Typus Melancholicus. Prominent psychiatrists began to assert that the depressed, given their rigidity and love of order, would feel threatened by reflexive self-transformation (Kasahara 1978, Hirose 1979, Yoshimatsu 1987). Thus, the highly socialized discourse about the Typus Melancholicus—as it defined the depressed as a product of both innate personality and of social environment—created a curious blend of biological and social determinism while leaving little space for conceptualizing individual agency. Consequently, in sharp contrast to the situation in the United States where depression (or neurotic depression) remained the "bread and butter" of psychotherapists for a long period (Healy 1997, Luhrmann 2000), therapeutic approaches other than the pharmaceutical remained largely undeveloped in Japan for decades to come.

Instead, when psychological perspectives were brought in, they were often used as diagnostic—rather than therapeutic—tools for differentiating the depressed from the neurotic. By defining Typus Melancholicus as what lay at the heart of "true" depression (that is, biologically based, endogenous depression), psychiatrists began to classify the people who did not fit into their idea of normative Japaneseness into "new types" of depression (that is, psychologically based, neurotic depression), which were then discussed as synonymous with "treatment-resistance patients." These typologies echoed the neurasthenic discourse of the 1920s–1930s, when psychiatrists were increasingly differentiating the "true neurasthenics" (legitimate patients who fell ill because of overwork) and the "self-claiming neurasthenics" (illegitimate consumers of medicine who fell ill because of their personality weakness). In the same manner, Typus Melancholicus began to serve as a moral, as well as medical, category. For instance, Hirose Tōru argued in 1977 that there was an increasing number of patients with "escaping-type depression," by which he referred to a group of young patients who shared certain characteristics with Typus Melancholicus (such as perfectionism and thoroughness) while deviating from it in that they tended to quickly withdraw when faced with a difficult task and seemed able to enjoy non-work-related activities even when they were on sick leave (Hirose 1977). Miyamoto Tadao also proposed "immature-type depression," referring to patients around age thirty, whose characteristics included: dependence, selfishness, self-centeredness, attention seeking, and quick to lose energy when encountering "trivial" stress (Miyamoto 1978:68). As a result, the theory of Typus Melancholicus produced rather monolithic and fatalistic ideas about the depressed, who were trapped in a timeless universe, reproducing the same "Japanese self" generation after generation without the prospect—or power—for change.

Despite its theoretical inadequacy and the repeated criticisms from biological psychiatrists that the theory lacked scientific validity, Typus Melancholicus has remained textbook knowledge in psychiatry for decades. This is partly because the theory came to acquire—beyond mere clinical folklore—the status of standardized scientific knowledge by being incorporated in Japan's first official diagnostic criteria for manic-depression. In 1975, two leading psychopathologists, Kasahara Yomishi[9] and Kimura Bin, developed a system for diagnosing manic-depression by joining the criteria for symptoms and prognosis as well as premorbid personality and situational cause (Kasahara and Kimura 1975). This attempt preceded the DSM-III by five years with its use of multi-axis criteria, and also reflected the zeal of international psychiatry at the time, when organizations like WHO emphasized the importance of recognizing cultural variations in the manifestations and prognosis of mental illness. Even though its influence began to wane after the introduction of the DSM-III in 1980, this diagnostic system long remained important as the manual for training new generations of Japanese psychiatrists (Makino 1997) and was frequently cited by veteran psychiatrists I interviewed as what shaped their ideas about depression most significantly. Indeed, the establishment of local clinical knowledge in the form of scientific diagnostic system gave Japanese psychiatrists a foundation with which to "resist" and withstand the global hegemony of American psychiatry, while helping create the distinctive local popular discourse about depression that began to be widely disseminated in the media from the 1990s.

Politicizing Depression: The Current Medicalization

Notably, while psychiatrists had, by the mid-1970s, a readily available set of idioms with which to normalize and popularize depression, they did not actively promote a broader medicalization of depression at the time. The most obvious reason for this was the antipsychiatry movement, when psychiatrists themselves became critical of their own discipline's tendency to medicalize social problems. As discussed in chapter 3, the antipsychiatry movement from 1969 was particularly vehement and long-lasting in Japan, where psychiatric institutions, including many academic societies and university departments (especially at elite schools like Tokyo University and Kyoto University), disintegrated and remained chaotic for the decades following. As many psychiatrists I interviewed pointed out, whether they agreed with it or not, they had to confront the argument that was debated daily within their departments and hospitals— that all mental illnesses (including depression) were in some ways socially pro-

---

[9] Note that Kasahara, who introduced R. D. Laing's work through his translations, was also known during the antipsychiatry movement as one of the fierce critics of biopsychiatry.

duced. Biological psychiatrists told me how they were accused of being the most oppressive agents of labeling and social control, how they had to refrain from using terms like "genetics" (which became one of the taboo words), and how their study groups had the feel of secret sect meetings. Psychotherapeutically oriented doctors also insisted that they were even more harshly condemned for being "insidious tool[s] for managing and manipulating individuals," and were urged to reflect on how they had "intruded into" and "emptied out" patients' interiority. Even the socially oriented psychiatrists I met lamented the fact that, during the 1970s and 1980s, their work in community mental health was significantly hindered as their interventions were critically scrutinized as potential invasions of human rights. Any attempts at psychiatric epidemiological survey became an impossibility, which meant that they had little means of grasping how many people suffered "depression" or any mental illness in the community during these decades.

Despite all these radical self-criticisms, psychiatric reforms lagged behind in Japan, impeded by the institutional, structural problems of Japanese psychiatry that continued to rely heavily on private mental hospitals, whose main source of income came from institutionalizing patients on a long-term basis (see chapter 3). Judging from my interviews with psychiatrists and research in the popular literature of the 1970s–1980s, perhaps the most productive aspect of psychiatric practice in this era was its vigorous cultural critique of "social pathology"—including depression that was said to be born of an alienating society (see Lock 1986, 1987). In the media, psychiatrists began to elaborate on various forms of depression, such as "relocation depression" (*hikkoshi utsubyō*), "promotion depression," "apartment-complex depression"—suggesting that social event and environment could become causes for depression. In the way that it served to familiarize Japanese with the psychiatric rhetoric for conceptualizing social ills, the antipsychiatry movement may have provided the groundwork for the later medicalization of depression.

Thus, when the new generation of antidepressants was introduced in the 1990s, psychiatrists, rather than creating a whole new set of idioms, simply recycled the same themes and rhetoric from the 1970s to 1980s to elaborate upon a new language of depression. For instance, their attempts to normalize depression via local somatic idioms only intensified. Unlike in the United States, where the idea of depression as a "chemical imbalance" of the brain has risen as a popular metaphor, Japanese psychiatrists have continued to combine the technical, neurochemical imageries of depression with familiar cultural idioms that present depression as a *generalized* illness of both mind and body, as something that anyone can be afflicted with when placed under too much stress. They are again using similar explanations of depression such as a "temporary decline of vital energy" and "generalized illness of the whole body . . . and the whole person" (Okazaki et al. 2006). This holistic theme is most clearly expressed in the phrase that became widely popularized (both by psychiatrists and pharmaceutical companies) in the early 2000s: depression as a "cold of the heart," for which antidepressants are again pitched as an effective cure. What is new is the extent to which lay people have absorbed this language and begun—beyond simply following doctors' recommendation for antidepressants—to explore how to treat depression themselves by watching their diet, getting regular exercise, developing good sleep habits, and generally trying to lead more healthy lives.

What has again helped make depression a persuasive category for lay Japanese is the same rhetoric of Typus Melancholicus. While the patients' Typus Melancholicus of the 1970s were said to be alienated by the forces of modernity, the patients' Typus Melancholicus of the 2000s are portrayed as the victims of globalization, made vulnerable by the new merit-based system of competition and the collapse of lifetime employment. What has radically changed is the way this discourse of the Typus Melancholicus has gone beyond mere rhetoric and acquired political, institutional power, as it has been employed to give credibility to grassroots medicalization. That is, using the theory to represent the depressed as mainly hardworking people, workers and lawyers have successfully argued for the social causality of depression, holding corporations and the government liable for workers' psychiatric breakdowns (to be discussed in chapter 9). As both biological and social psychiatrists have come together to create a powerful narrative about how depression can be understood as both a biological and social disease, they are creating new understandings about local forms of oppression. In these ways, the social themes developed in the antipsychiatry era seem to have fully bloomed.

At the same time, however, this bottom-up medicalization poses its own problematic in the way that its assertion of social causality is based upon implicitly moralized local understandings of what counts as "social." Through her works on the medicalization of everyday life in Japan, Lock (1988, 1993) has demonstrated the ill effects of the "social" component in popular medical discourse in Japan, which serves to homogenize and overdetermine the meaning of people's affliction. In a similar manner, the discourse around Typus Melancholicus has served to conceal the complexity and diversity of the depressed by creating a static, timeless, homogenized image of Japaneseness. As psychiatrists are employing this theory to differentiate those who deviate from their ideas about the "truly depressed," they may be reproducing the same moral codes they did in the 1970s in determining who counts as legitimate sufferers and who do not. Consequently, people who resort to the depression diagnosis as a way of claiming legitimacy for their distress are subjected to shifting and politicized interpretations about the nature of depression. So far, these individuals have little recourse to talk back and officially rewrite the "scientific" discourse, even if they are aware that the "biological" is morally infused, culturally negotiable, and political malleable.

Beyond Local Knowledge

Rather than erasing and emptying out preexisting cultural resources, the global medicalization of depression has given rise to hybrid discourses about what depression means in the local context, a phenomenon that is happening concurrently in other parts of the world (to be discussed in chapter 11). Such local heterogeneity often remains undiscussed in biomedicine partly because of the dual structure of psychiatric practices. As Allan Young (1995) has shown, psychiatry continues to be characterized by the division between medical science and clinical practice. Medical science retains a largely stable core of knowledge—or a "style of reasoning" (Hacking 1982, 2002)—with its set of ideologies regarding objectivity and universality, while clinical medicine works at the level of local knowledge and remains multiple, implicit, and unstable. Psychiatric practitioners themselves often see these two as different orders of knowledge, and are not troubled by their own conflicting voices or about maintaining hierarchical order between the two (Gilbert and Mulkay 1984). The scientific style of reasoning tells them that not all scientific facts are to be invested with the same "truth" value, and thereby provides them with a sense of order and coherence (Young 1995). As an important actor in this medicalization, the pharmaceutical industry certainly understands this and seems to have capitalized on this dual structure by strategically mixing the scientific discourse with local discourses, using whatever rhetoric (such as Typus Melancholicus in the case of Japan) best suits the marketing of antidepressants in each locale (Petryna, Lakoff and Kleinman 2006).

What further complicates this power relationship between the two orders of knowledge is the fact that scientific psychiatry still comes from a few power centers—most of them in the West—and travels to the more "peripheral" regions, while clinical psychiatry is often made to remain "local" as it rarely travels back to the sites where scientific psychiatric knowledge is produced. Thus, while Japanese practitioners are content to use their local theories such as Typus Melancholicus in everyday clinical practice, and often express criticisms of the DSMs for what seems to them as culturally bound understandings of psychopathology, they are far more ambivalent about seriously exploring or articulating such difference in international psychiatry. For Japanese psychiatrists who derive their expert authority from a commitment to the universal biological language—and who are also aware of their own marginality in the global production of medical science—local differences can be sources of epistemological tension as they try to establish their international legitimacy. Thus, in front of their international colleagues, they either go out of their way to erase such differences, or in cases where they do speak about it, do so "less through any engagement with clinical reality but primarily through the oppositional dialogics of international legitimacy" (Cohen 1995:330). Thus, the wealth of local knowledge is often lost, silenced and buried beneath the official scientific discourse.

Given that this dual structure has served to solidify and reproduce the familiar hierarchy between global medical science and local clinical practice, anthropologists concerned with the place of local knowledge should not content themselves with simply articulating heterogeneity or celebrating local diversity. The dual structure makes it easy for both global psychiatry and local psychiatries to proceed with business-as-usual even in the face of growing gaps and contradictions between scientific representations and clinical realities (which I will demonstrate in the following ethnography). The lack of dialogue becomes an even more serious problem when medical science further moves the data away from the realm of local, clinical practices, replacing patients' narratives (which leave the possibility for raising contradictions) with fragments of voiceless material bodies in the laboratory. In this last phase of biopsychiatrization, local subjectivity may no longer matter, when the dislocation of the ownership of self-knowledge becomes complete (Young 1995). Ultimately, this may have the unfortunate effect of keeping psychiatry from living up to its professed standard of scientific falsifiability (Young 1995). As I see it, therefore, my job as an anthropologist is to illuminate what lies in these borderlands between scientific psychiatry and clinical psychiatry, with the hope that the anthropological articulation of local knowledge and local differences might help create a new dialogue with rapidly globalizing scientific psychiatry. We need to ask how local knowledge is (re)produced and made to remain "local," what possibility exists for dialogue between local knowledge and globalizing psychiatry, and in what forms local knowledge can begin to influence the knowledge production of global psychiatric science—questions I will examine in the remainder of the book.

PART TWO

Depression in Clinical Practice

IN PART II, I examine how depression is actually talked about by psychiatrists and patients in local clinical practice. Nakai Hisao, one of the most influential contemporary scholars of Japanese psychiatry, once asked why Japanese psychiatric accounts of depression seemed so obsessed with work (Nakai 1976)—a tendency that seems to have only been reinforced since the 1990s. As I have shown through historical investigations, work as a cause of fatigue—and subsequent depression—has been an important theme in Japanese psychiatry, perhaps even a singular aspect of its theorization of depression. Notably, work stress and fatigue of all kinds—including physical hardships suffered by manual laborers, mental pressures by office workers, and emotional strains by housewives—are featured in this theorization, leaving the border between physiological fatigue and psychological fatigue blurred and ambiguous. Especially in the debates surrounding overwork depression, the presence of physiological overwork alone is often used (by lawyers) to argue for the assumed existence of psychological fatigue, thereby leaving the role of individual psychology, subjectivity, and agency in the making of depression largely unexplored.

While psychiatrists have made fatigue from work stress an evocative theme through which Japanese have come to understand depression, psychiatrists certainly do not think that this is the single cause of depression and neither is it the only object of their professional concern. While depression is often represented as an ailment of virtuous, hardworking victims, depressed patients in clinical practice are a highly heterogeneous group, whose life histories, reasons for breakdown, and types of "depression" vary significantly. Given the complexity of depression, What kind of language do psychiatrists actually use to persuade patients of the pathological nature of their "depression"?; How do they succeed in mediating the disruptions in these people's lives?; and How do patients respond to such medicalization? Based on two years of ethnographic fieldwork I conducted at three psychiatric institutions (a university hospital, a private mental hospital, and a small clinic specializing in psychosomatic medicine), I examine how psychiatrists and patients actually deal with depression in everyday clinical encounters. By illuminating the Japanese psychiatrists' explicit focus on the biological nature of depression, I explore in what ways psychiatric persuasion may be liberating for patients, and where—and particularly for whom—it becomes subjugating as it begins to overdetermine the meaning of people's experience.

In chapter 6, I first demonstrate how psychiatrists *successfully persuade* patients of the pathological nature of their depression via a certain kind of biological persuasion. This begins with the question of why it is that many Japanese psychiatrists—even those who are critical of biological reductionism—regard (psychoanalytically oriented) psychotherapy as taboo for treating depression. Describing diagnostic interviews, hospitalization, and case conferences, I elucidate how psychiatrists try to contain patients' reflexivity and avoid intruding into the realm of the psychological, in order to protect patients' already fragile sense of self. Defining depression as an alienation from one's own body, psychiatrists instead urge patients to focus on their bodily changes and social distress. What emerges is a surprisingly uniform set of narratives about depression, designed to create a sense of social legitimacy for patients' suffering. Psychiatrists here employ biological language as a means of partial persuasion, a symbolic "lid" used to contain the potential contradictions that lurk beneath the official representation of the depressed. In so doing, these psychiatrists, notwithstanding their clinical sensibilities, leave unexamined the important issue of how the depressed can act—beyond merely passive recipients of biological cure—as agents of self-transformation.

In chapter 7, I explore where psychiatrists *fail to persuade* patients of the biological nature of their "depression." The limit of this biological persuasion— particularly its failure to address the question of individual agency—becomes a focal point in psychiatrists' confrontations with suicidal patients. Although what is most notable in the current medicalization is that psychiatrists are having some effect in persuading Japanese that suicide—traditionally depicted as an act of free will—is caused by depression, clinical encounters show that this effort is fraught with conceptual tension. In chapter 7 I analyze the ways in which psychiatrists try to persuade patients of the pathological nature of their suicidal intentions, and how patients respond to such medicalization. I also explore psychiatrists' ambivalent attitudes toward pathologizing suicide and how they limit their biomedical jurisdiction by treating only what they regard as biological anomaly, while carefully avoiding the psychological realm. One ironic consequence of this medicalization may be that psychiatrists reinforce the dichotomy between normal and pathological, "pure" and "trivial," suicides, despite their clinical knowledge of the tenuousness of such distinctions and the ephemerality of human intentionality. Thus, while the medicalization of suicide is cultivating a conceptual space for Japanese to debate the location of the border between normality and abnormality and how to bring the suicidal back onto the side of life, it scarcely seems potent enough to supplant the cultural discourse on suicide that has elevated it to a moral act of self-determination.

In chapter 8, I examine how psychiatric persuasion actually works in structuring *patients'* own understandings and experiences of depression by calling attention to the peculiar "gendering" of depression in Japan. Despite the fact that depression is often depicted in the West as a "female malady," in Japan, men have been represented as likely to suffer depression as women. Behind this gender anomaly lies, I suggest, selective medical and social recognition of pain. Through the narratives of those who have recovered from depression, I show how men, on the one hand, are provided with a public narrative of depression that highlights their sense of fatigue and overwork as well as the injustice of economic and social systems. On the other hand, women, while reflecting on their sense of hopelessness, rarely seem to link their suffering to the recognized structural causes of depression. While men recover when submitting themselves to the protective, if paternalistic, relationship with a psychiatrist, women often express resistance to the way psychiatrists try to cure them by fostering dependency and instead seek to gain control through a quest for the right doctor. Thus, the experience of depression takes on different forms according to gender—not because Japanese women suffer more than Japanese men or vice versa but because the nature of their social suffering is structured differently. While suggesting that this politics of gender is rapidly changing in the current medicalization, I also argue that the Japanese approach to recovery by way of "relinquishing control" is at odds with new demands and expectations in the age of neoliberalism, where Japanese are increasingly encouraged—even pressured—to take control of their lives.

CHAPTER SIX

Containing Reflexivity:
The Interdiction against Psychotherapy for Depression

> [T]he body is the locus of *all that threatens our attempts at control.* . . . For, as Plato says, "Nature orders the soul to rule and govern and the body to obey and serve."
> —Susan Bordo on the Western thought on the body,
> *Unbearable Weight* (1993:145, emphasis original)

> [P]sychoanalysis helps promote in the minds of those who engage in it the *precious illusion of control* over fate, that is, the sense of autonomy.
> —Doi, "The Cultural Assumptions of Psychoanalysis"
> (1990: 269, emphasis mine)

Against Psychotherapy?

I CHOSE TO DO MY FIELDWORK in the psychiatric department at JP Medical School[1] because of its emphasis on psychopathology (*seishin byōrigaku*). Psychopathology, a subfield of clinical psychiatry, developed by scholars who drew upon phenomenology and psychoanalysis, might be hard to grasp for those who are used to the American opposition between biopsychiatry and psychoanalysis. Based on German neuropsychiatry, psychopathology is not opposed

[1] The discussion below mainly draws upon the narratives I heard within clinical settings: i.e., the data from 40 individual consultations, 128 case conferences, and 14 group therapy sessions that I observed at JP Medical School. It also incorporates a series of interviews I conducted with patients in a hospital consultation room (which usually lasted between 30 and 90 minutes). I also did follow-up interviews with some patients over the period of a few months, and in one case, nearly two years. To explore possible counterdiscourses to these "clinical narratives," I also participated in a patient self-help group (which took place in a commercial building in Tokyo) and conducted interviews with patients at a clinic specializing in psychosomatic medicine and different hospitals (which lasted between 1 and 6 hours). Some of these interviews took place in a consultation room, others in public spaces (cafes and restaurants). Although I had been initially concerned that the nature of clinical settings would seriously limit the kinds of narratives I would hear from patients in my interviews, most of the patients seemed relaxed enough to be quite blunt and at times critical of the doctors or medical treatment they were receiving (a point I explore in chapter 8). In fact, the university hospital's ethics committee made sure that I incorporated a statement in the informed consent form to assure patients that whatever they said—or whether they collaborated in my research or not—would have no bearing whatsoever on the clinical treatment they received. I understood that the changes in their narratives had more to do with the stage of the course of their illness and medical treatment: how long these patients had suffered "depression."

to the use of biology in psychiatry but rather regards it as an integral part of it. It involves a particular way of performing clinical observation and a diagnostic method that emphasizes phenomenological approaches in an attempt to understand the "lifeworld of the psychotics." Psychopathologists have thus critiqued biopsychiatrists' disregard for the subjective meanings of mental illness and have provided the main objection to the predominance of the neurobiological perspective in Japanese psychiatry since the 1960s. They have also promoted distinctive theories about melancholic premorbid personalities (see chapter 5) and established many of the commonsensical ideas about depression in both professional and popular discourses in Japan. As inheritors of this tradition, the psychiatrists at JP pride themselves on the close attention they pay not only to biology but also to the subjective experience of the mentally ill, as well as the situational causes that together make up the experience of mental illness. Yet, these psychiatrists are also aware of how marginalized their field has become in the increasingly DSM-ized Japanese psychiatry of the last two decades, and are actively seeking ways to establish and re-energize this perspective.

Most psychiatrists at JP say they deliberately sought employment in this department because they wanted to learn something other than straightforward biological psychiatry. The department is headed by Professor Higashi, a psychopathologist who is also the grandson of a pioneering social psychiatrist. He was trained in France and has extensive knowledge of both French and German philosophies. Other senior psychiatrists are scholars who share a deep interest in philosophy, art, and creativity. The department has regularly sent its staff for training in Germany, France, and England; many departmental members have good linguistic skills in various European languages. Both the professor himself and other senior staff conduct a number of weekly seminars with residents after a day's busy clinical work. In these seminars, they together read such authors as Immanuel Kant and Jacques Lacan in the respective German and French original, in an attempt to relativize and reflect upon their own clinical practice from a different perspective. Though they use the DSM-IV and ICD-10 alongside more conventional nosology, the psychopathologists maintain a skeptical attitude toward American psychiatry and occasionally critique it when articulating their own clinical perspectives. JP's psychopathology group maintains a surprisingly peaceful coexistence with their biologically oriented colleagues, who formed a smaller group headed by an associate professor, a gentle man in his forties well respected for his works in neurobiology.

The department's congenial balance between the more dominant, European-trained psychopathologists and its subordinate, American-trained biopsychiatrists also creates an intellectually vibrant atmosphere. This is reflected in the wide range of interests discussed in the weekly departmental seminars. While I was doing fieldwork, the presentations included, for instance, a lab report on serotonin syndrome by a neurobiologist, a linguistic analysis of schizophrenic delusion with reference to Wittgenstein, and the exploration of anorexic narratives in light of the philosophy of Simone Weil. However, the department's apparent interest in the *meanings* of mental illness seems curiously confined to backstage, intellectual discussion. In their daily clinical practices, the psychiatrists at JP emphasize a straightforward pragmatic, biological approach, which seems to differ little from that of the few other, more biologically oriented psychiatric institutions where I had done observational research. Contrary to their interest in narrative-based perspectives, they remain particularly "biological" with regards to the treatment of depression, and they even proclaimed to me: "Psychotherapy is taboo when it comes to depression."

This seemed puzzling not only because of the doctors' intellectual disposition but also because psychotherapy has long been regarded as an effective cure in North America even after the advent of Prozac. In fact, the increasing dominance of the biological cure has attracted much criticism there, where intellectuals have been concerned that such a simple cure may impoverish people's ability for self-reflection (for a review of this debate, see Kramer 1993, 2005). Politically conscious critics have even worried that biologization of depression may serve to numb people's critical insights and impose conformity (see Elliott and Chambers 2004); thus, the fact that in Japan it is the psychological cure for depression—and not the rise of antidepressants—that seems to have created discomfort, even explicit prohibition, among psychiatrists, is an intriguing difference.

When I asked these Japanese psychiatrists why they would go so far as to disclaim psychotherapy for depression, the responses varied.[2] Generally they pointed out the overall unpopularity of psychoanalytically oriented psychotherapy, and the lack of institutional and economic support for it. Under the current system, the reimbursement for "psychotherapy" remained a set fee, which meant that psychiatrists would receive the same amount for doing fifteen minutes of so-called therapy as they would for an hour.[3] Yet the lack of eco-

---

[2] Note that this situation is gradually changing with the rise of cognitive behavioral therapy in Japan over the last decade.

[3] Anyone who observes the practices of Japanese psychiatrists at university hospitals and many other large hospitals would immediately recognize that most of the doctors work on incredibly tight schedules. At JP Hospital, the outpatient unit is flooded with patients every morning. Because it operated on a "first come first served" basis at the time of my initial fieldwork (this has since changed), patients would wait for a long time, sometimes for hours, before they were seen by their doctors. Psychiatrists, many of whom saw patients both in outpatient and inpatient units (as well as juggling administrative work, conducting research, writing textbooks and journal articles, organizing conferences, and medical school teaching simultaneously) would see patients all day at least a few days a week. I would often see them coming back to the departmental lounge around 4:00 P.M. exhausted. They would report having seen more than forty, at times even sixty, patients per day, telling me how they were "near collapse towards the end." Given the tight schedule, as well as the structure of national health insurance that pays little for psychotherapy, in-depth psychotherapy was seen as a luxury, saved only for patients whose illness demanded that kind of approach or whose illness happened to intrigue doctors intellectually. In these cases, doctors would make a point of using what little spare time they had for the treatment. Thus they would sometimes tell me how envious they were of me, who, as an anthropologist conducting research on the experience of depressed patients, was able to spend as much time as I wished talking to patients. The problem of

nomic incentive alone did not explain why some of these psychiatrists occasionally engaged in extensive talking cures for other types of patients (such as anorexics) but rarely for the depressed. When specifically asked about depression, they emphasized that this was a biological disease, for which antidepressants should be the primary therapeutic tool. Then they would point me to Kasahara Yomishi, an authority in psychopathology who also established, together with Kimura Bin, the first comprehensive nosology for mania and depression in 1975 (see chapter 5). In his widely read papers, Kasahara has asserted that depression be treated first and foremost with medication and rest. He suggests supportive listening and giving advice on practical matters but strictly warns against the kind of psychotherapies that seek to promote psychological insight in depressed patients (see also Hirose 1979, Yoshimatsu 1987). He also writes that the Japanese approach—which attends to both bodily and psychological recovery—is more "holistic" than the cognitive approach coming from America, which, he says, is too "partial" in its primary focus on the mind (Kasahara 2003). Should the Japanese interdiction against psychotherapy be understood, then, not as just a matter of biologization but as a cultural articulation of holism of some sort (cf. White 1982, Kirmayer et al. 1998)?

Drawing on anthropological analyses of psychiatric encounters, I want to examine how these Japanese psychiatrists provide the depressed with a language with which to express and mediate the disruption in their lives (Lock 1988, Young 1995, Corin 1998a, 1998b, Kirmayer 1992). My aim is to examine how they construe the biological understanding of depression in lieu of psychotherapy. Does their psychiatric language, as some critics of biopsychiatry have argued, serve to silence patients, suppressing their reflexivity? Or as Kasahara seems to insinuate, is it an attempt to promote a culturally "holistic" reflection upon the nature of their alienation? Alternatively, do these psychiatrists have another way of construing the reflexivity over the biological—and psychological—nature of depression? Japanese resistance to psychotherapy has long been noted (Lock 1980, 1982, Ohnuki-Tierney 1984, Ozawa 1996, Ozawa-de Silva 2002, Doi 1990), yet there have been few ethnographic investigations into how Japanese psychiatrists, particularly more psychotherapeutically oriented ones, actually treat their patients in everyday clinical practice (except for Breslau 1999). This chapter attempts to fill this gap.

Diagnostic Interview

JP Medical School, located in a city outside of Tokyo, attracts patients from across the demographic spectrum. The waiting room fills up quickly in the

---

time constraints seemed common in the ten university hospitals I visited for my fieldwork. Clearly, the Japanese institutional system of psychiatry does not foster a psychotherapeutic atmosphere for treating depression.

morning, and each psychiatrist sees anywhere from between thirty to sixty patients per day. There is a general animation in the air as doctors, nurses, a few psychologists, and a social worker busily move around in white coats. Consultation rooms are minimally furnished, containing an examination bed, a desk, and a couple of chairs. From the outside, the psychiatric unit differs little in appearance from other units in the university. Yet its waiting room—which is segregated from the corridor by a closed door—has an atmosphere that is always a touch more tense than other units. When I looked at the anxious faces of the patients, and later heard them talk about how they took pains to avoid a chance encounter with an acquaintance, I realized that the media campaign for depression that has increasingly brought more patients to this university had yet to fundamentally diminish the stigma associated with psychiatry.

What seemed to most strongly characterize the patients' initial encounter with a psychiatrist was their heightened feeling of uncertainty. This is partly because, unlike in internal medicine where patients have basic familiarity with the kinds of diagnostic questions asked, psychiatry is alien territory for most patients. The questionnaires they have to fill out before the consultation—Zung's depression scale and the department's own set of questions—might add to this sense of unfamiliarity. The latter includes the usual medical questions, such as the patients' demographic data, illness history, and current symptoms. It also includes, however, apparently *psychiatric* items such as an extensive list of personality traits to choose from, and a family tree (suggesting hereditary factors) in which patients are supposed to fill in the illness histories of close relatives. Such pre-diagnostic questions indicate that psychiatrists are concerned not just with the physiological symptoms but also with what kind of person a patient is. Patients' unfamiliarity with the psychiatric framework was evident in the pre-diagnostic interviews that I observed conducted by less-experienced resident psychiatrists, with whom some patients seemed confused about where to start their narratives or exactly what constituted "psychiatric" symptoms. I was occasionally surprised to see how their narratives changed quite drastically when later interviewed by a senior psychiatrist. It is against this uncertainty among patients—and the malleability of their narratives—that psychiatrists attempted to first establish a solid framework for understanding the distress via a biological model of depression.

Victor Turner has demonstrated how a therapeutic ritual serves to contain chaos by providing a name for the affliction (Turner 1967). The diagnostic interviews I saw certainly strived for this goal, where psychiatrists approached the patients' emotional chaos with the calm assurance of a medical authority. For instance, one morning in the outpatient clinic, Dr. Oda and I were looking over the questionnaire, and called in a man whose ailment Dr. Oda suspected to be depression. Takayama-san, a well-dressed, fifty-six-year-old businessman, came into the consultation room looking haggard, restless, and preoccupied. After Dr. Oda introduced me as a research student (Takayama-san nodded to me) and asked him what seemed to be the problem, he began to pour out the stories about the recent incidents at work that had been distressing him. Ever since he had been promoted to Sales Director, he had felt both over-whelmed and isolated in the office. He thought about work all night and could not sleep. And he was deeply resentful about the treatment he was receiving under the new position: "I think the company is dumping more work on me than I deserve, and my colleagues are not taking any responsibility." As he talked on, he seemed to grapple with his own anger, whose intensity I could feel as it seemed to fill the room. After he talked on for a few minutes, Dr. Oda, who had been quietly writing down the details, looked up and said: "You have gone through a hard time" (*taihen deshita ne*).

At this moment, Takayama-san's shoulders fell, his face visibly relieved. As I have since witnessed many times, psychiatrists' simple words of recognition seem to produce in patients an effect that is reminiscent of religious or psycho-therapeutic affirmation: "You have suffered" (cf. Levi-Strauss 1963b). As pa-tients revealed in my later interviews, a surprising number of them had had their worries dismissed by their families, even by other doctors. They thus found great relief in meeting someone who had even an inkling of what they were going through. Perhaps it was because of this that patients talked about the acknowledgment from a psychiatrist to be a defining, transformative mo-ment. As one woman said to me: "I knew, at that moment, that he understood, that I could entrust myself to him." Establishing this moment of connection was, for doctors as well, important for ensuring diagnostic accuracy and thera-peutic efficacy. Psychiatrists pointed out to me how some patients go home without saying what was really troubling them because they were afraid of being labeled as mentally ill or because they could not trust the doctor enough to reveal themselves. Beneath the verbal exchanges, there was much that went on, as the patients were deciding whether or not to disclose their deepest fears and yield themselves to the power of psychiatrists.

This psychological, cathartic moment of connection was kept brief, however, as the psychiatrist swiftly moved onto the diagnostic questions. Changing the tone and the pace, Dr. Oda began with the basic symptoms: "You said you have been losing sleep. What about appetite?" Takayama-san: "Come to think of it, I have not been eating much. I've lost some weight." Asked about the sleeping patterns, Takayama-san told us how he had been waking up regularly at two or three A.M. and laid awake for the rest of the night. Dr. Oda asked about the level of concentration, energy, and changes in the mood. Takayama-san pointed out how he felt intensely depressed in the morning but that this would recede in the afternoon (a distinctive sign of depression that psychiatrists call diurnal varia-tion). Robert Barrett (1996), in his ethnography of Australian psychiatric prac-tices, demonstrates how psychiatrists make patients understand the biological nature of their experience not through overt persuasion but through a subtle process of repetitive questioning and evading what they regard as irrelevant information (also see Atkinson 1995, Osborne 1994). This is also what was happening here to an extent, as the psychiatrist began to translate the patient's highly emotional, psychological torment into a set of biological signs that were beginning to form a pattern and then into the definite shape of a *disease*. The psychiatrist's focus on the bodily aspects of depression here is not really an expression of cultural holism (a way of engaging with the patient's emotions through somatic symptoms); rather, it appears, at this initial stage, to be simply an expression of their biological reductionism, whereby psychiatrists treat the bodily symptoms merely as the indices of the underlying biological disease.

Only after the psychiatrist has clearly extracted the biological contours of depression does he move onto situating the patient's distress in the social and psychological context of his life. Dr. Oda began to ask Takayama-san about his daily routines, particularly around the time of the onset of depression, in order to determine how the biological symptoms appeared independent of other factors (social and psychological). Inquiring of Takayama-san about his family situation and seeing no problem there, Dr. Oda then asked how his life changed before and after the promotion. Takayama-san reflected how, under the increased workload of the new position, he had recently begun to get up early and come home late at night and how he had felt chronically tired. Then Dr. Oda moved on to ask about his longer life history to see if he had experienced anything like this before. Takayama-san recalled that ten years ago he had barely survived a critical case of an ulcer, when his boss fell ill before a major project deadline and he was put in charge. Previous episodes of physical collapse (particularly ulcers), such as this, were not uncommon among the depressed patients I met. These histories of illness served for the psychiatrists as a way of understanding patients' patterns of response to a socially stressful situation.[4] Lastly, Dr. Oda asked him about his personality, to which Takayama-san said he was probably a "serious" (*majime*) type. Dr. Oda, content with this further indication of underlying depression (based on the theory of Typus Melancholicus discussed in chapter 5), seemed certain that what Takayama-san suffered from was endogenous depression.

The inquiry about biological changes, when done effectively, serves to symbolically disconnect the patients' (normal) self from the disease (Estroff 1981, Luhrmann 2000). As Takayama-san concentrated on mapping out all the physiological symptoms that he had suffered, he appeared as if momentarily lifted out of the uncontrolled emotions that had seized him. This must have had the effect of making him recognize anew the serious changes that were occurring both in his mind *and* his body, which he might have been too preoccupied to notice or too frightened to admit to himself. Notably, after he had been bitterly expressing his resentment towards his colleagues, he suddenly broke down and said: "I don't know what is happening to me. I can't show gratitude to the people I'm

---

[4] In a society where psychiatrists also practice under the banner of (much-less stigmatized) psychosomatic medicine (shinryō naika), psychiatrists and patients seem to naturally share the assumption that stress can be manifested differently—both over the mind and the body—at different times.

close to. I can't even say hi to the people who have been good to me." This burst of self-confession illuminated how genuinely scared he was of the mysterious changes that were occurring, and of the intense emotions that were spinning out of control. Assuring him that this was a "disease," Dr. Oda told Takayama-san that taking medication—as well as an immediate leave of absence from work— would ensure recovery. By the time Takayama-san left the room with a return appointment in two weeks' time, he seemed calm, liberated, at least momentarily, from the alarming sense of the incongruities he was experiencing. Dr. Oda believed that Takashima-san's emotional confusion would eventually dissipate as the biological depression itself lifted. He would not deny that certain events might have occurred or psychological conflicts existed and might even have served as pathogenic factors. But his plan was to first test the medication out to see if the patient might change his *interpretation* of such events and recover his innate power to cope with life's difficulties. It is for this reason, first of all, that psychiatrists place the priority on the bodily aspects of depression.

The power of such biological language lies in its ability to temporarily suspend patients' search for social meanings for their emotional confusions, and place them firmly under biological management. On another morning, Dr. Satō and I met a thirty-year-old housewife, Yamanaka-san, who complained of experiencing dejection and strong anger. She thought her emotional torments were initially caused by her husband's infidelity, but said they had since grown much more intense. Sobbing nonstop in the consultation room, Yamanaka-san recounted how she felt a surge of rage every morning and wondered aloud why she could not control her emotions. She emphasized that she was "no longer [her]self" and asked Dr. Satō if she was suffering from a "personality disorder or something." Listening quietly to her account, Dr. Satō, as he told me later, was focusing on two alarming signs of depression: First, the intensity of the emotion that she was exhibiting, which even the patient herself seemed to think was disproportionate to the stressful event (her husband's affair); and, second, the time lag between the stressful event and the onset of her depression, as she said it began months after her reconciliation with her husband. Suspecting that her depression was more endogenous (a biologically rooted anomaly) than psychogenic (a reasonable response to a stressful event), Dr. Satō gave her a set of diagnostic questions in order to ascertain its endogeneity. He asked, for instance, when the anger was likely to occur ("always in the morning") and if it stopped at a certain time ("it usually lasts till about ten o'clock"). Continuing with this line of inquiry, Dr. Satō elicited the intensity, durability, and periodicity of her "anger," which began to appear as if it had a life of its own. By shifting her attention from the psychological *content* of her anger to the biological *form* it took, Dr. Satō seemed to successfully persuade the patient that she was a victim of forces beyond herself.[5]

These cases illustrate how the biological model of depression prevails in ini-

---

[5] For alternative interpretations of "anger," see Hochschild 1983, Boddy 1989, Holmes 2004.

tial psychiatric encounters as it is used to temporarily suspend patients' uncertainty. Professor Higashi often emphasizes that depression lies at the "limit of language." That is to say, depression in its core represents a psychotic experience, which creates a fundamental disruption in the sense of self. The psychiatrists' sensibility about the psychotic aspect of depression also means that they implicitly placed mere psychological torments lower in their moral hierarchy of mental illness. They carefully differentiated endogenous depression—which is presumed to have biological etiology—from neurosis, and often referred to the latter in a dismissive tone. They even called the first "true depression," to distinguish it from the DSM-IV's concept of major depression, which they think has carelessly expanded the boundary of depression to include neurosis and is thus quite useless in clinical practice. This implicit moral hierarchy means that patients who are judged to be suffering from psychological problems are at times told that there is nothing medically wrong with them and that there is not much doctors can do (except to refer them to a smaller clinic).[6] Still, there were ambiguous cases in evidence that call this simplistic version of the biological model into question.

Hospitalization

While the biological model of depression predominates throughout clinical encounters, psychiatrists often carefully introduce approaches beyond the purely biological perspective as well (including what one may even call "holistic" approaches), particularly after patients come out of the initial, acute phase of depression. This was evident in the ways in which these psychiatrists treat those who are hospitalized. In a society where long-term hospitalization is often used as an opportunity for rest, particularly for salarymen who tend to be provided with generously paid sick leave, this is a preferred method of treatment for depressed patients who do not promptly respond to medication. Psychiatrists structure hospitalization for these treatment-resistant patients in a way that allows them to explore what factors are inhibiting their recovery—if the matter is purely at the level of the biological (the mismatch between the symptoms and the antidepressants), or alternatively rests more on psychological and social factors (such as stressful family/work situations). In terms of the biological inquiry, hospitalization undoubtedly provides an ideal, quasi-laboratory setting for the psychiatrists, who closely monitor the patients at three levels. First, they give patients a battery of tests to scan their *physiological* condition,[7] while checking the daily reports (kept by the nurses) on the patients' temperature, weight

---

[6] In such cases, patients are often told not to worry about it, or referred to a smaller clinic. Psychiatrists themselves were split on the issue of what to do with "neurotic" patients but they clearly saw them as outside of their main responsibility and only dealt with them when time allowed.

[7] These tests may include X-rays, electrocardiogram, echocardiogram, head CT, MRI, electroencephalogram.

changes, blood pressure, sleeping and eating patterns, and urination and bowel movements. Secondly, they observe patients' *behavioral* changes, examining the level of energy and what kinds of activities they engage in. Third, psychiatrists monitor *affective/cognitive* changes in patients through individual consultation and note their facial expressions, tone of voice, and other signs of angst, agitation, anxiety, or dejection. The way these psychiatrists commonly talk about patients as "going up" (meaning "turning manic") or "going down" (turning depressed) on varying doses of antidepressants does illuminate the extent to which they rely upon the biological model of depression. Listening to them talk in this way, I initially wondered if the psychiatrists saw patients as little more than passive vehicles upon which depression left its mark.

However, the psychiatrists never let patients hear them talk in these technical terms, and instead use another kind of language when they interact with them—what we may call *a language of the body*. Here they try to construe a common understanding by urging patients to reflect—phenomenologically— upon how depression is experienced as a "physical disease" *(karada no byōki)*. At the initial stage of hospitalization, they encourage patients to leave aside their emotional, psychological torments and instead to focus on recovering through rest. And it is through bodily changes that patients begin to recognize how thoroughly fatigued they had been and how unaware they were of the dysfunctions happening inside their bodies. I was often surprised at how much psychological meaning patients attributed to the physiological symptoms, as they talked about burdens of responsibility they suffered (such as heavy workloads, family obligations, and discord in human relationships: to be elaborated on in chapter 8)—referring often to stiff shoulders *(kata ga koru)*, heaviness of the head *(atama ga omoi)*, and lead in the chest *(mune no namari)* (cf. Kirmayer 1999). Perhaps it is here that the kind of holism that Kasahara discussed as the strength of the Japanese approach is most evident, where psychiatrists try to get patients to see the link between the psychological torments and their bodily changes. Through such phenomenological talks, patients began to share the idea that—as Dr. Kanda put it—depression creates profound "alienation of the mind from the body," and that the recovery is a matter of restoring this connection. Without delving into the question of which is the cause and the effect— the body or the mind—psychiatrists usually succeed in persuading patients how depression affects their whole being, for which the biological treatment presents one path to recovery.[8]

Thus it is important to note that these psychiatrists do not use biological

[8] Compare this with the more explicitly biological, Kraepelinian approach, which introduces a sharp division between the subjective and objective (or behavioral). Radden characterizes this approach as follows: "The subjective captures what is able to be introspected, that which we alone know directly from our privileged and exclusive access to our own mental and psychological states. The behavioral is that which may be known from the detached perspective of third-person observation, without the subject's cooperation or verbal report" (Radden 2000:29).

language in a totalizing way. That is to say, they do not lead patients to think that depression occurs in the absence of other, psychological or social factors. In fact, they emphasize that such simplistic models of depression belong to the past, when traditional psychiatrists believed in genetic determinism and assumed that depression happened "for no good reason." Instead, they emphasize the interplay among biology, personality, and environment and create ample opportunities for exploring nonbiological aspects of depression. For instance, as patients begin to recover at the physiological level, the doctors usually encourage them to join one or two of the many weekly group therapies that the department offers, which include undirected discussion, painting, collage-making, pottery, calligraphy, and music. Psychiatrists use their observations of these activities for understanding the aspects of depression patients might not (or cannot) readily talk about. For instance, I observed that they would compare the same patient's artworks from different weeks and discuss the changes in the themes, colors, overall moods, and levels of energy that these works exhibited; the more psychotherapeutically oriented staff would even venture to make comments on patients' unconscious desires. Sometimes they would exhibit these artworks in case conferences (discussed below) and analyze the patients' personality structures, hidden psychological themes, and conflicts. It was unclear to what extent they used these artworks in their individual consultations (I had the impression that very few did) but many of the psychiatrists regarded art therapies as a distinctive strength of their psychopathological tradition and pointed out their value as nonverbal, nonintrusive therapeutic tools.

Patients seemed to find making art therapeutic and talked about themselves as they performed these activities. And because of the way hospitalization was structured, away from families and work, some patients came to reflect intensively upon themselves in a way they said they had never done before. The patients often shared such insights with psychiatrists (who mostly simply listened) and their fellow patients. Thus, psychiatric hospitalization undoubtedly provided a *refuge* from the outside world, where patients experienced an unusual level of introspection. This, no doubt, contributed to creating a special environment, where the biological remained the most prioritized, official language, but where other, diverse languages of depression were also actively cultivated and coexisted at different levels.

Case Conferences

(Referring to what Kretschmer said) "A depressed person is essentially like a river with a dangerously low level of water. Because the water (= energy) is so low, the rocky river bottom becomes exposed. The psychiatrists' job is

> not to try to remove these rocks (= personality flaws) but
> simply to let the water level return to normal."
> —Dr. Kondō Kyōichi, a depression expert;
> for Kretschmer's citation, see Tolle 1991

Given that I observed how the hospitalization period was rife with psychological talk, it was interesting to see how psychiatrists and patients came together at
the end to create the official narrative of depression through the discharge case
conferences. Professor Higashi, who interviewed each incoming and departing
patient in front of thirty or so staff members, regarded this as an important
function and required all the doctors to attend. After the resident-in-charge
handed out a summary of the patient's illness history and held a brief presentation and a discussion, they called in the patient.[9] Most patients, after being
greeted by Professor Higashi, seemed to gradually overcome their initial nervousness and recount their story (which usually lasted from fifteen minutes to
half an hour). At one level, the case conferences served as a means of quality
control, whereby they ensured the departmental standard of diagnostic validity
and therapeutic efficacy. More importantly, however, the conferences—particularly the discharge conferences that are the focus of this section—provided a
platform from which patients could tell their stories. Because the structure of
the interview paralleled that of diagnostic interviews, I often found it striking
how patients were able to provide a psychiatrically coherent narrative, which
suggested the extent to which they had mastered—if not necessarily internalized—the language of psychiatry (cf. Saris 1995).

Here, psychiatrists strived to help patients reach what they called "narrative
integration" (*katari no tōgō*). The interview often began with the professor leading the patient to demarcate the chronology of their depression in terms of its
attendant etiology, course, and prognosis. Patients described the physical
symptoms they suffered and reflected upon when and how they began to feel
not quite themselves. Then they were urged to narrate the social circumstances
that led to their gradual breakdown. Usually the last question—in which Professor Higashi asked what kind of personality patients thought they had—was
given to not only validate the theory of melancholic premorbid personality but
also to legitimize their depression as an illness that was born out of their hard
work and their consideration for others. Professor Higashi referred to these
encounters as a place where psychiatrists could serve as secretaries for record-

---

[9] The case conference serves many purposes at once. It is a system of training residents (who
usually report the cases as doctors-in-charge), of negotiating and coordinating different viewpoints
among the psychiatrists, and of establishing the agreed-upon professional standards within the
department. Thus there is a bit of lively discussion after the resident-in-charge hands out a case
summary of the patient in question and goes over the symptoms, illness history, test results, treatment outcome, final diagnosis (one according to DSM-IV or ICD-10 criteria plus the one based
upon the Japanese "conventional diagnosis"), and future treatment plans.

ing patients' testimonies of suffering. Though this view downplayed the power that psychiatrists wielded by determining the order and the length of the interview, it does suggest how psychiatrists saw this as an opportunity for acknowledging how patients had overcome their difficulties. In these ways case conferences served as a place where psychiatrists tried to bring a symbolic sense of closure and returned the authorship of their narrative to the patients themselves (cf. Kleinman 1988a, Kirmayer 1994, 2000).

The point of the case conference was thus not to gruelingly scrutinize the patient or even to establish a solid consensus about the nature of depression (cf. Light 1980). Patients offered their interpretation, and at times said things that contested psychiatrists' understanding of the illness. Psychiatrists would not dispute patients' versions at such times, however, as long as the basic facts about biological symptoms largely remained in place. This was evident in a conference with a fifty-five-year-old businessman, Sakata-san, who had been hospitalized for the second time for depression. Prompted by Professor Higashi's questions, Sakata-san recounted a number of physiological symptoms with utmost fluency—apparently, he remembered what kinds of questions would be asked from his previous hospitalization. He then elaborated on his long commutes, difficult work situation, and frequent business-related drinking, as well as his "serious" personality, all of which he presented as contributing factors for his depression. It was notable how he particularly stressed that his depression began "for no good reason." This was not necessarily unusual (some patients found no apparent stressful circumstances behind their depression) but the firm, determined tone in which he relayed his answers implied that he would rather end this inquiry sooner than later. After Sakata-san left the room, psychiatrists began to examine what it was that triggered his second depression, which they suspected might have nonbiological causes that needed examining in order to prevent a further relapse. Dr. Kanda, a veteran psychiatrist in charge of Sakata-san, said that his patient was facing complex family problems that he did not seem to wish to discuss. Psychiatrists then halted further exploration in this direction and left the patient in the care of Dr. Kanda. It was obvious in this case how the patient used the biological language of depression to construe a public narrative, which left the potentially threatening, psychological problems in the realm of the private.

On other occasions, psychiatrists themselves explicitly drew on biological language to keep from having to deal with underlying psychological issues that patients insisted on. In one instance, a forty-two-year-old civil servant, Miyao-san, had protracted depression, which seemed to have improved but again became suddenly worse before his scheduled discharge. Miyao-san himself told Professor Higashi that he did not want to go back to work (where he faced demotion) and dwelled on how thinking about work made him depressed. Professor Higashi, however, impressed upon him that what was beneath all this was *depression*, that he had a "hardworking" personality, and assured him that he would feel differently once medication began to kick in. After Miyao-san left the room, however, some psychiatrists pointed out that Miyao-san's workload seemed not necessarily heavier than that of his colleagues and that there might be certain vulnerability in his "personality structure." As they began to discuss how psychology—more than biology—might be at work, Dr. Satō, who was in charge of him, instead emphasized how utterly bureaucratic and unsupportive Miyao-san's boss had been, and how difficult it was to intervene in his work situation. The discussion then shifted to solving the practical issues of how to support Miyao-san's return to work, how to help improve his relationship with his boss, and how to monitor his changes carefully as the level of his exposure to (social) stress would gradually increase. As was usually the case, psychiatrists did not hesitate to intervene in the social aspects of patients' depression, giving their families and supervisors advice about how best to treat the patient, even inviting the company people to the hospital for consultation, if necessary. When the biological model alone failed to work, they mostly concentrated on adjusting social relations rather than examining possible psychological reasons behind protracted depression.

Though in-depth psychological excavation in front of the patient was apparently off-limits, in the case of a young depressed patient, an enthusiastic young resident explicitly went against the general interdiction. Shima-san was a twenty-six-year-old businessman, who was hospitalized with what appeared to be a straightforward case of a salaryman's *overwork depression*. He had been working long hours and on weekends for months, routinely coming home at two or three in the morning. After his request to be transferred to a different section was turned down, Shima-san became severely depressed and suicidal. It was apparent that his work conditions were to blame. His own boss had already become depressed from the heavy burden and was seeing a psychiatrist himself. Despite a situation that was typical among depressed inpatients, what made Shima-san stand out was his persistence with the "big questions" of life. He kept asking why he had become depressed, what the meaning of his life was, and why he should continue living at all.

Other psychiatrists would have waited to see such psychological conflicts pass with the biological recovery. They would, as a senior psychiatrist told me jokingly, rather "impose the biological explanation on the neurotic and provide a generic narrative" than let the psychological take hold. Dr. Mori, however, who seemed to generally have a good reputation among the patients because of his devotion and sincerity, reciprocated Shima-san's existential ponderings by spending many hours listening to him. Under this doctor's care, Shima-san made a brisk recovery, while elaborating on the meaning of his collapse and understanding the patterns of his relationships at school and at work. All seemed to be going well, until Shima-san, with a prospect of soon returning to work, began to again suffer severely from various physical symptoms. At the same time, he began to express strong emotions—particularly anger against his company—which he started to redirect at Dr. Mori himself, who was, in Shima-san's eyes, now failing to resolve his problems. Though Dr. Mori and his supervisor tried desperately to set the treatment course straight, Shima-san's "aggression" became more intensified.

His anger seemed to affect other inpatients, as it soon came to transform one therapy group that had been tranquil (if rather uneventful), into a highly emotional, explosive outlet for dissenting patients. Some of them began to raise doubts about the effect of medication, demand more psychotherapy, and express their concern that they "needed to be taking more control" of their own illnesses. This turbulent situation, which lasted for weeks, ended abruptly when Shima-san—who seemed to have mostly recovered on the physiological level by then—decided to transfer to another hospital. The subsequent case conference, held without the patient himself, had the feel of soul-searching for the psychiatrists involved. They labored to determine exactly what the patient's biological depression was and how the psychological problems ("neurotic components") had begun to take over. Professor Higashi pointed out how the doctor must have become, for Shima-san, an omnipotent being, whom he expected would be able to provide the ultimate meaning for the magnitude of the suffering he endured. Yet, as the professor said, such a grand expectation for a unifying meaning would be hard to fulfill (also see Kleinman 1995). While one psychiatrist raised the issue of Shima-san's vulnerability and suggested "personality disorder," Professor Higashi immediately cautioned against the use of this notion. He pointed out how this diagnosis would label him with the ominous implication of being incurable and implicitly place the blame on the patient. Without resorting to the notion of personality disorder, senior psychiatrists discussed how those with melancholic premorbid personality had embedded within them such "hidden aggression" (Kasahara 1976, 1978, see also Yokoyama and Iida 1998). They had pointed out, in discussing this among themselves, how *essentially endogenous* depression could *turn neurotic* through such (genuine but misguided) psychotherapeutic intervention.

As it became clear from their discussions over the weeks, what lay behind their interdiction against psychotherapy seemed to be their particularly localized, historically situated, understanding of depression. The senior psychiatrists brought out the examples of the 1970s and 1980s, which they nostalgically talked about as the time when their supervisors were engaged in intensive psychotherapeutic endeavors—when some would "spend all night in a locked room with an acutely psychotic patient." This was the height of the psychotherapeutic zeal among psychopathologists, who began to regard depression as a kind of cultural alienation, caused by the breakdown of the old Japanese values (Iida 1978). As discussed in chapter 5, these psychiatrists illuminated how the people with a melancholic premorbid personality—who were taught selfless devotion to the collective good—were most prone to depression in the emergent social order. While some psychiatrists emphasized at the time the importance of changing their value system (Yazaki 1968), what others began to reveal was how threatening such psychological probing turned out to be for these patients. The literature from this era notes how depressive patients reacted strongly when their internalized social norms or their identification with the collective became questioned (Kasahara 1978, Hirose 1979, Yoshimatsu 1987). Such probing could also lead to expand and diffuse the nature of their depression, furthering their sense of vulnerability, producing dependency. Psychopathologists such as Kasahara (1978) instead emphasized that the depressed were well-adapted people to begin with, and the aim of the treatment should not be to question or change their way of being but rather to help them return to the way they were.[10]

Containing Reflexivity

Thus psychiatrists' reliance on biological language stemmed not from their belief in some timeless, cultural holism (although their practice certainly has an aspect of this [cf. Ozawa-de Silva 2002]) but rather, was a historically situated sensibility about the potential danger of their own power. Psychiatrists at other institutions also told me that the only thing still standing after the vehement antipsychiatry movement was neurobiological psychiatry, as all the others—including psychotherapy and psychopathology—were thoroughly criticized as intrusive, even insidious tools for colonizing thought, which might even end up "emptying out the patient." Thus some psychiatrists talked about the importance of letting the patient determine the terms and the extent of their psychological reflexivity. Even if patients engaged in extensive psychological reflection over the meaning of their depression—and even if such depth intrigued psychiatrists intellectually—psychiatrists believed that it was important, therapeutically, to try to "place a lid on it" (keep it contained) (Yokoyama and Iida 1998). This also meant that even for the patients whose depression had a dubious biological basis, psychiatrists maintained a policy of minimum intervention. For instance, I observed a case conference for a twenty-four-year-old hairdresser, who was, as psychiatrists came to conclude, hospitalized with a mistaken diagnosis of depression when in fact he only had neurosis. After the interview in the case conference, the doctors agreed that this patient's biological symptoms never really "deepened" or attained the clear shape of depression, and his com-

---

[10] The aim was to provide a secure sense of order, even if this meant on the part of the psychiatrist to consciously reproduce the hierarchical work relationship by playing the role of the superior (Suzuki 1997).

plaints—low energy, sleep disturbance, and despondency—were only an extension of the way he had lived his life. Judging that his problems were of the kind that lay beyond psychiatrists' control, these psychiatrists agreed that it was better to immediately discharge him rather than let him develop "hospital dependency." Their general sentiment was summed up by Dr. Kawano, who said at the end of the conference that it would be better "not to psychiatrize him" (*seishin-iryōka shinai*). This sentiment was also repeated in a training seminar, when another senior psychiatrist made an explicit warning to the residents about the danger involved in the intricate power relationships of psychiatry: "Do not turn the patient into an object of your own desire. A mere human being cannot change another, and such a desire would only produce a perverted relationship." Such an act, he declared, "belongs to the realm of magic." For these psychiatrists, the distinction between the "biological" and the "psychological" served to demarcate the boundaries of not only what was "true depression" but also where they saw their jurisdiction and their responsibility end.

What emerged from these practices was also a different vision of what recovery meant. Emphasizing the danger of colonizing the patient, these psychiatrists defined clinical encounters more in terms of a crisis management than inward exploration for self-enlightenment (they may have thought that such a self, construed through psychiatric encounters, may have risked fostering an "illusion of control," as Doi put it). Some psychiatrists were explicit about the differences between their ideal model of the therapeutic and the American psychoanalytic model. As Dr. Eguchi Shigeyuki put it, North American psychotherapy adheres to a *dialectic* model of recovery, where an increased awareness of the accumulating contradictions in one's life inevitably leads to a confrontation that allows the patient to reach a new self-awareness "in a moment of epiphany." In the Japanese clinical practices I observed, patients' claims for having made such a dramatic transformation—particularly via psychological insight—were received by psychiatrists with concern, even skepticism, in terms of the genuineness of their recovery. Instead, they urged patients to reflect upon their bodily changes, thereby implicitly demonstrating the historical continuity between traditional medicine and current practices in terms of the belief in the interconnectedness of mind and body (see chapter 2; also see Lock 1980, 1981, 1982). Their attempts to downplay patients' excessive psychological reflexivity was thus based not on a simplistic belief in the power of the biological but rather on their concern about deflecting patients' deeply internalized sense of self-responsibility and protecting patients' fragile sense of the self.

At the same time, however, these psychiatrists' actual clinical practices might come to resemble, ironically, those of the biological reductionists, who bracket out social and existential questions about depression. In fact, the seeming predominance of the "biological approach" of Japanese psychiatry is a source of frustration for some patients—particularly female patients, as we will see in the patient narratives explored in chapter 8. Psychiatrists' emphasis on the body and the near absence of psychotherpy also created a major problem with the rise of depression during the 2000s, when over-reliance on psychopharmacology began to perpetuate an overuse (and abuse) of antidepressants (these more recent changes are discussed and analyzed in chapter 10). Before we tackle these issues, however, I first turn to suicide in the next chapter as a problematic issue in Japanese psychiatry, where confrontations between psychiatrists and patients who insist on the existential nature of their ailment become most intense.

CHAPTER SEVEN

Diagnosing Suicides of Resolve

> Suicide . . . the act of intentionally destroying one's own
> life. . . . Its existence is looked upon, in Western
> civilization, as a sign of the presence of maladies in the
> body politic which, whether remediable or not, deserve
> careful examination. It is, of course, impossible to
> compare Western civilization in this respect with, say,
> Japan, where suicide in certain circumstances is part of a
> distinct moral creed.
>
> —*Encyclopedia Britannica*, 11th edition (1910–1911:50)

> Suicide cannot be comprehended as merely a "psychiatric
> problem," yet it is central to a psychiatry that asks questions.
> —Lifton, *The Broken Connection* (1979:239)

The Boundary between Pathological Suicides and Suicides of Resolve

UNDER THE EXPANDING power of psychiatry in Japan, few subjects have so thoroughly resisted medicalization as that of suicide. Early-twentieth-century Japanese psychiatrists adopted the biological view of suicide then dominant in the West, and proposed that it should be understood as a matter of a diseased brain or a genetic predisposition (Kure 1900, Miyake 1900). This biological determinism provoked a heated debate in Japan for a few decades, but since has had little persuasive power over lay people beyond the narrow circles of biological psychiatry. This may be because Japanese, according to Maurice Pinguet (1993) in *La mort volontaire au Japon*, have rarely criminalized suicide as a matter of principle, and have even granted suicide an aura of legitimacy (also see Takahashi 1994, Morris 1975, cf. Gates 1988, MacDonald and Murphy 1990). This cultural logic dictates that, far from being pathologically driven, those who chose to take their own lives are in full possession of their senses and act with intentionality (Takahashi 2003).[1] This image of suicide prevailed in the postwar period, and has been reinforced in the media and in various art forms, such as the annual broadcasting of the legendary drama of Chūshingura (a suicide pact

---

[1] Partly because of this cultural valuation of suicide, Japanese psychiatrists—unlike their Western counterparts who were able to emerge as "liberating" agents by asserting that suicide is not a religious sin or crime but the product of an illness to be treated—have largely failed to have a similarly significant influence on Japanese thinking about suicide.

of samurais) and school-recommended modern novels featuring suicide, like Natsume Sōseki's *Kokoro*. The endurance of this cultural logic was recently demonstrated in the way Japanese responded to the suicide of the postwar literary giant Etō Jun, in 1999, who left a note stating, "I've decided to do away with what remains of me" (*Asahi*, July 23, 1999). Admiration from fellow intellectuals flourished in the media, with some proclaiming that Etō's death embodied "first-class aesthetics." Few commentators questioned the normality of Etō's state of mind at the time of death or the intentionality of his suicide, and the voices of a few psychiatrists who dared to suggest that his suicide might have been caused by depression went largely ignored. Etō's suicide, for many Japanese, seemed to embody the continuation of the cultural logic that defines suicide as the ultimate expression of personal will, or what Japanese often refer to as *kakugo no jisatsu*, or "suicide of resolve."[2]

The cultural legitimacy of this idea is, however, being challenged today by some psychiatrists, and their influence is being felt on an unprecedented scale. Amid public concern about rising rates of suicide in Japan—hitting historical highs of more than 30,000 per year for twelve consecutive years—psychiatrists are increasingly appearing in the media to stress the link between suicide and depression. A series of lawsuits concerning overwork suicide has also given psychiatrists a public platform from which they argue that those who take their own lives under tremendous social pressure might also be victims of depression. Following these lawsuits, the Ministry of Health, Welfare, and Labor has adopted new criteria for diagnosing suicide, which has had the effect of significantly expanding the domain of what falls within "pathological" suicide. Under the new system, the kind of suicide that would have been automatically labeled suicide of resolve—such as the death of someone who left a note stating his or her intention to die—can now be regarded as caused primarily by "major depression." Furthermore, the government has established the Basic Law on Suicide Countermeasures in 2006, which includes plans for psychiatric intervention in workplaces and schools. These changes have increasingly brought the subject of suicide under wider psychiatric scrutiny. The current medicalization of suicide is helping create an important conceptual shift in the way Japanese think about the normalcy and intentionality of those who take their own lives.

However, for those who question the medicalization of suicide in Japan, the cultural logic of suicide of resolve apparently serves as a powerful point of reference, as the term continues to appear in popular writings on suicide, government records about overwork suicide, and everyday conversations in the clinical practices that I observed. Notably, such resistance to medicalization is not totally absent in the psychiatric community. On the one hand, there are cer-

---

[2] While the Japanese have recognized different degrees of intentionality in those who commit the act—from a reckless desire for escape from an unbearable reality to a fully premeditated act—suicide of resolve represents the ultimate expression of intentionality.

tainly many Japanese psychiatrists who are enthusiastic about diagnosing and treating a wider range of suicidal cases. They genuinely believe in what they think of as their own humanitarian attempts to intervene, and many of them also cast doubt on the notion of "suicide of resolve." As a forty-eight-year-old suicide expert said in an interview with me, "I know some people bring up the issue of free will [when discussing suicide]. But our job is to save lives, and not to be bogged down in a philosophical debate." Some of them go so far as to claim—echoing the early-twentieth-century Japanese psychiatrists—that most suicides are caused by mental pathology.[3] On the other hand, there are Japanese psychiatrists who express ambivalence about the underpinnings of increasing medicalization and wonder where that kind of pathologization might lead. When I began asking the then-current director of the National Institute of Mental Health about "depression and suicide," he frowned in visible disapproval and poured out his criticism of the "new idea" that directly links suicide and depression. His stance originated in the suicide boom of the late 1950s, he told me, when he became a psychiatrist in order to investigate why so many of his own friends had killed themselves in a time of peace, especially puzzling because they had only recently survived World War II. He implied that explaining away their suicides in terms of "depression"—which, to him (and to most Japanese psychiatrists, who are steeped in Kraepelinian neuropsychiatry) was a matter of biological pathology—was to dismiss their existential angst and the determination with which they took their own lives. His strong reservations about the expanding power of psychiatry in dealing with suicide was shared by many of the younger psychiatrists I interviewed, and also seems to remain strong in Japanese society in general (Kayama 1999, Okajima 2005, Ozawa-de Silva 2008).

Given these opposing views, one may wonder how Japanese psychiatrists actually medicalize suicide in everyday clinical practice. How do they persuade patients of the "truth" of the psychiatric account of suicide, when its fundamental premise goes against the cultural logic of suicide? Anthropologists have repeatedly demonstrated the tension-laden ways in which psychiatry becomes localized in the process of becoming a persuasive force. The current medicalization of suicide in Japan needs to be examined similarly, if we are to understand how psychiatry is overcoming Japanese resistance to framing everyday distress in psychiatric terms. Until relatively recently, psychiatry in Japan was able to maintain its authority not because its knowledge was accepted as cultural common sense, but because it was able to monopolize medical knowledge and exercise its jurisdiction for treating those diagnosed as mentally ill even without their consent. In practicing such institutional power, there was no need

[3] However, this idea is far from being shared beyond psychiatry. For example, the suicide statistics compiled by the Police Agency classify the reasons for suicide into the following categories: family problems, sickness, economic hardship, work-related problems, relationship problems, problems in school, alcoholism or mental disorder, other, and unclassifiable.

for psychiatrists to persuade patients of the naturalness of the psychiatric worldview or expect them to accept it—let alone internalize it. Today, particularly through the medicalization of depression and suicide, psychiatry is beginning to seek to operate at the conceptual level, turning its language into an "internally persuasive discourse" that requires individuals' voluntarily acceptance as psychiatric subjects. Yet this change is fraught with tension because of the nature of psychiatric encounters, which, as anthropologists have repeatedly demonstrated, often remain sites of contestation rather than total conversion (Corin 1998a, Estroff 1981, Kirmayer 2000, Saris 1995).

Given the strong and persistent cultural resistance against medicalizing suicide in Japan, how do psychiatrists try to persuade patients, and how do they deal with the potential criticism that they might be trivializing patients' existential angst and social suffering? In examining these questions, I draw on my two years of fieldwork at the psychiatric department of the JP Medical School. At JP, I was allowed to participate in almost every aspect of the daily clinical practice. I talked to suicidal patients, discussed these cases with psychiatrists, and observed how the suicidal are treated. Here, I draw on data from 48 case conferences that I observed, where patients' attempted suicides were discussed and their suicidal ideation was explicitly an object of medical intervention (of 48 cases, 37 patients were diagnosed with depression, 3 with schizophrenia, and 8 with other categories such as eating disorder and neurosis). I also draw on my interviews about suicide with 25 patients with depression and 35 psychiatrists, both at JP and at other psychiatric institutions. First, I show how psychiatrists diagnose the potentially suicidal and how they determine which patients should come under their care. Second, I demonstrate how psychiatrists medicalize suicide through a process in which they attempt to persuade patients to see their suicidal acts as pathological in nature. Third, I examine psychiatrists' own reflections on suicide and examine how they respond when they are confronted with patients who resist their efforts at persuasion and insist that their failed suicide attempts be understood, instead, as attempts at suicide of resolve.

Determining the Objects of Psychiatric Intervention

Given the prevailing concern about the abuse of medicalization in Japan, the first thing that struck me upon entering the field was how the psychiatrists at JP Medical School carefully limited the object of psychiatric intervention with regard to suicide. This is, first of all, because the psychiatrists think that suicide in itself is not a pathology and that their task is to treat only those who are suffering from a mental illness (i.e., depression, schizophrenia, or personality disorder). In this regard, they are certainly not descendents of J.E.D. Esquirol, who once declared: "I think I have proved that no man takes his own life unless he is in delirium, and that all suicides are deranged" (cited in Pinguet 1993:23; on Esquirol's theory of suicide, see Goldstein 1987). Pressed further, these Japanese psychiatrists even go so far as to state that the decision to die, for people without mental pathology, belongs to the realm of free will (*jiyū ishi*), where psychiatrists have no right to intrude. However, this seemingly clear-cut principle—which appears to support the cultural notion of suicide of resolve in certain circumstances—easily breaks down in the reality of the clinic. Unlike the idealized notion of suicide of resolve, people's intention to die is notoriously difficult to determine, and varies significantly in degree. What psychiatrists soon learn in their practice is the malleability of people's intentionality and the uncertainty of determining agency in a suicidal act.

At JP, psychiatrists are now becoming more involved in suicide intervention. Previously, unless patients exhibited apparent signs of mental disturbance, they would have been let go without a psychiatric examination (see Igarashi and Ishii 2000, Sakurai et al. 1998, Suzuki 2000). Recently, the hospital installed a new system in which psychiatrists are requested to examine all patients brought to the emergency unit after a failed suicide attempt. Thus, after emergency medical treatments are provided, psychiatrists are called in to determine the cause of the suicide attempt and decide what psychiatric intervention, if any, is necessary. If the patient is still in critical condition, psychiatrists first gather information from the family and/or the police. There are a number of questions they ask first in order to determine whether the attempt was fully intentional and, if so, whether the patient's mind was influenced by mental pathology. First, they ask about the presence or absence of a suicide note. Second, they inquire about the method employed and its lethality; for example, what kind of knife was used, how deep the cut was, or how many pills were taken.[4] Sometimes patients choose a deadly method, such as swallowing hundreds of pills with alcohol or slashing their own throats; in such cases, their suicidal intentions appear unquestionable.[5] Other times patients may have swallowed (only) ten pills or made several minor cuts on the wrist, leaving the degree of seriousness of their intention to die rather ambiguous. The third question psychiatrists ask is the situation in which the patient was discovered. For instance, was a patient found at 2:00 A.M. on a wooded mountain having taken an overdose of sleeping pills, where no one would likely pass by, or was he discovered having hanged himself at home around 8:00 P.M., when his family was expected to arrive at any minute? Finally, psychiatrists try to gather information on the possible reason(s) why the person attempted suicide. From this circumstantial evidence, psychiatrists make a tentative diagnosis. Such a diagnosis is only an early interpreta-

---

[4] Common suicide methods are by overdose, cutting the wrists, cutting the throat, evisceration, and jumping from a building, etcetera, as well as hanging, poison, and drowning.

[5] Information on how to kill oneself is disseminated through websites on suicide, which have been mushrooming of late, and best-sellers such as *The Complete Manual of Suicide* (Tsurumi 1993), which has sold more than a million copies.

tion, however, which psychiatrists know can be easily contradicted later by patients' own subjective accounts.

According to the psychiatrists who have worked at the emergency unit, a considerable number—about half—of the patients who have attempted suicide are released directly after being given a brief psychiatric consultation. This is because these patients are deemed to be more or less in control of themselves— that is, they can logically explain the act, show repentance, and are judged to be in no immediate danger of repeating a suicidal attempt. Some patients say that they really meant to die—suggesting that their attempt was more in line with a suicide of resolve than an impulsive act—but somehow taking the action "cleared away" their deadly intention. Others say that they had no lethal intention and only acted in the heat of the moment, and they now regret what they did. While interviewing these patients, psychiatrists carefully look for any signs of gaps, strangeness, or breakdown in the coherence of their narratives, and any disconnection between the given reasons and the act committed. If psychiatrists are satisfied that there are no signs of mental illness (that is, if the patients' accounts fall within the realm of culturally comprehensible reasons for a suicidal attempt), patients are discharged (though often with a referral to outpatient psychiatry). As psychiatrists admit, this leaves open the possibility that some are so determined to die that they would successfully hide their intention and convince psychiatrists that they should be let go (as discussed below). What is important to recognize is that, for the time being, the medicalization of suicide in Japan remains selectively targeted to a small portion of the potentially suicidal, almost all of whom are suspected by psychiatrists as suffering psychopathology.

Among those who are judged to be requiring immediate psychiatric care, there are two types of patients. The first group is the patients who still remain suicidal after the first attempt; most of them (but not all) are immediately given a diagnosis of a mental illness. Some of them appear to be totally "out of control"—that is, restless, agitated, and possessed by an urge to die. These patients are kept under close watch, even tranquilized, for fear that they might wander out into the corridor and jump from a window. As a man who checked himself into the hospital aptly described this state of mind: "It isn't that I wanted to die; it was more that I didn't know what I would do if I were all by myself." This split between the self—or *intention* identified by the self—and the pathology clearly places these patients outside the realm of the cultural notion of suicide of resolve. (This is also one of the key pieces of psychiatric knowledge that these doctors learn before entering emergency psychiatry.) The second group is the patients who appear to be under control and now regret the act, but whose suicidal behavior leaves some mystery to be accounted for. That is, neither the patients themselves nor the psychiatrists can fully explain why suicide was attempted. Fearing the possible risk that these patients will make another impulsive suicide attempt—without a clear intention to do so—psychiatrists try to place them under close monitoring to attempt to discover and treat what they suspect is an underlying pathology.

Treating Pathological Suicide

The dialogues between psychiatrists and patients provide us with a glimpse of how psychiatrists try to persuade patients of the pathological—particularly biological—nature of their suicidal acts, and how patients respond to such medicalization. The dialogues we see here between inpatients and Professor Higashi took place at a weekly case conference held both at the time of patients' admission and at their discharge from the hospital. I must note that these dialogues occurred in the early 2000s, when Japanese were just beginning to be exposed to the public campaign by doctors and the state promoting the idea that suicide is a psychiatric problem. Thus, few of the patients that I saw during the two years seemed to have voluntarily decided that their suicidal urges might have been a product of depression or any other psychiatric illness. Even those who seemed puzzled about why they were feeling like killing themselves, apparently "needed" psychiatric persuasion to begin to regard their suicidal urge as something that lay beyond the realm of normality. Thus, for instance, Professor Higashi invited into the admission conference room a patient in an acute phase of depression, a sixty-year-old retired worker, Kimura-san, who appeared visibly agitated and restless. Soon after sitting down Kimura-san told Professor Higashi: "I can't describe it in words. I feel like I'm being driven to die." Professor Higashi, in an attempt to determine exactly what was generating this urge, asked him:

H: The feeling that you are driven to die, is it stronger in the morning?

K: I feel it more in the morning.

H: How does your head feel when you wake up? Do you feel like you've slept well?

The priority in the diagnostic interview is given to discerning the presence of an endogenous depression that has taken over the patient's body and mind. Here, the psychiatrist began to translate the patient's psychological torment into a set of biological signs, finding a pattern and, eventually, the definite shape of a *disease* (see chapter 6). Having detected in Kimura-san the typical signs of endogenous depression—such as diurnal variation (with which depressive mood moves with regularity) and disrupted sleeping patterns—Professor Higashi moved on to examining his life history. Kimura-san seemed to calm down a little as he began to discuss his gardening hobby. Shifting to the subject of his future concerns, however, he again became agitated and too preoccupied with his suicidal thoughts to talk of anything else. Seeing that his urge seemed to be welling up from inside, Professor. Higashi assured him:

> **H:** For now, leave it to your doctor. If you try to think, your thoughts will only be circular.
>
> **K:** I can't prevent these thoughts from coming into my mind. I try to tell myself that I shouldn't think about death but the thoughts keep coming back to me.
>
> **H:** . . . We will make sure to treat your anxiety. Your doctor will see to it.

Here the psychiatrist tried to tame Kimura-san's suicidal thoughts by translating them into "anxiety," a de-existentialized, pathological condition (and a symptom of depression) that can easily be controlled by medication. (Professor Higashi later instructed the resident in charge of Kimura-san to "reduce his anxiety level.") Since his suicidal urge is considered a mere symptom of depression, it is expected to dissipate as the depression "lifts." Based on this belief, psychiatrists caution patients not to dwell on their suicidal ideation because they feel that too much introspection while in a depressive state will only exhaust the patients (and no doubt the psychiatrists as well). I remember a morning round in which a petite elderly woman with "delusional depression" suddenly grabbed the sleeve of Professor Higashi's white coat and insisted that she was going to die anyway and that there was nothing they could do (she later wondered aloud in the case conference how she could have believed that). Perhaps because they constantly treat patients in such severe conditions, these psychiatrists emphasize how patients' thinking under the influence of depression will likely be circular, repetitive, making it impossible for them to understand their situation based on calm reasoning. As patients themselves are initiated into this way of thinking, they begin to talk about the uncontrollable impulse, as a force external to their sense of "self." "I always try to watch a movie around four o'clock because I know that the suicidal urge always happens around then," said a forty-five-year-old businessman, who had taken a long sick leave from work. For many psychiatrists, then, the biological impulse for self-destruction lies at the core of the suicides they deal with and, as such, leaves little room for psychological exploration.

At times, even when patients dwell on the external reasons and psychological motives that drove them to attempt suicide, psychiatrists retain their focus strictly on the internal, biological mechanisms. This has an effect of conceptually shifting the agency—the locus of control—away from the suicidal patient. For instance, a thirty-three-year-old factory worker both slashed his stomach and attempted to hang himself in one night, only to survive these deadly acts. In the case conference, he talked about how he had recently been promoted in the labor union but that he felt he was not meeting other people's expectations. Failing to manage the workload and despairing about his lack of ability, he came to believe that he was better off dead. As he talked on, however, the psychiatrists were puzzled by the light-hearted and even sometimes humorous manner in which he discussed what he had done to himself. The only time the psychiatrists saw this patient become grave and emotional during the interview was when he was asked if he had "hesitated" before the suicide attempt: "I did, and that is why I didn't succeed." Also, the magnitude of the violence seemed like an aberration in his life history and personality (described by him as "serious and responsible"). Rather than seeing his act as a failed attempt of suicide of resolve, psychiatrists concluded that the patient had suffered depression, which, they speculated, had turned into a milder form of mania after the rescue. Some psychiatrists suggested that depression would explain his emotional disconnection from his suicidal acts and the way he behaved during the interview, while others still worried about the possibilities of undetected organic disturbances in the brain, which could trigger further impulsive, dangerous behavior. In such ways, these psychiatrists saw their job primarily as the managers of biological anomalies, finding cues for the latent structure of a disease, which would otherwise remain hidden to suicidal patients themselves.

At the hospital where I carried out my fieldwork, such biological concerns were thus always given priority over other possible explanations, and psychiatrists often deliberately stayed away from the realm of the psychological. Though psychiatrists would occasionally mention hidden intentions and unconscious desires behind such an act, they would rarely elaborate on them, nor would they ever hint at them to patients. In another case, a thirty-nine-year-old office worker was rescued while trying to hang herself. Seeing that she had no memory of the incident or what had happened prior to it, Professor Higashi tried to determine if she had committed the act in a state of dissociation or if it was a retrograde loss of memory. She said she did it after one of the usual quarrels with her husband; she discussed the ongoing conflicts that she had with him because of his lack of consideration for her work, and her desperate attempts to balance marriage and work. She also expressed her fury at the psychiatrist for the fact that she was the one, not the husband, to be given medication "for [her] anxiety." Apparently, there were long-standing psychological issues that went into her thinking as she was driven to the suicidal act, and at one point she even muttered, seemingly more to herself than to the doctors: "I wonder if I'm better off if I do not recover my memory." After she left the room, Professor Higashi mentioned how this particular case made him "want to think about her psychological background." But the discussion that followed hardly touched on such issues, while the psychiatrists examined in depth the level of her agitation, signs of psychomotor retardation, and precise nature of her dissociation. One of the reasons for this omission was the heightened sense of risk of, and uncertainty about, her possibly being seized by another suicidal urge. Especially in the early phase of treatment, psychiatrists give stronger emphasis to impulsive and biological forces than to the deliberate, intentional aspects of suicide.

In the final step of treatment, when patients are clearly out of danger, psychiatrists allow themselves to venture into what might be loosely called a "psychological" intervention. Before these patients are discharged, psychiatrists make sure that patients can reflect on their suicidal acts and integrate them into their life history. They refer to this process as "narrative integration." (Even this remains consciously and cautiously framed in a kind of biological narrative, which might seem, particularly to a psychoanalytically oriented observer, surprisingly "limited" in terms of psychological depth.) The main structure of this narrative is the one in which patients are encouraged to distance themselves from their formerly suicidal selves so that they can recognize it as an aberration from their normal self. In one case conference, a forty-four-year-old businessman explained how he had been so driven to the edge by accumulating debt and the fear of being prosecuted that he became determined to pay the debt off with his own life insurance.[6] Asked if he had made the decision calmly, he denied it firmly and said: "No, I was exhausted and I wasn't myself. I kept thinking how my life was not what it should have been." When Professor Higashi asked him if he was happy to be alive, he nodded and said: "I didn't imagine that I would be feeling better like this again. I'm truly thankful for what you've done."

Such psychiatric persuasion—and the patient's adoption of psychiatric thinking—is at times so thorough that it seems to suppress all other possible interpretations of patients' suffering and behavior. I once witnessed a humorous exchange between Professor Higashi and a forty-one-year-old patient who had taken a massive overdose of antipsychotic drugs after being "ordered by divine forces" to kill herself. Schizophrenia was first suspected but in the end this patient was diagnosed with hypothyroidism, which had caused the psychotic symptoms. After listening to her discuss the spectacular visions she saw of the struggles between God and death, Professor Higashi, who has written extensively on creativity and religious themes in psychotic experiences, appeared impressed and asked what she would call that experience: "Doesn't it sound like a mystical experience?" he said. The patient's response was blunt:

P: No, I do not think it is. It's simply a disease. [Laughter from the attending staff.] Well, the doctors told me that it was.

H: [with an amused, embarrassed smile] Well, I think that you had a rich experience, very religious, I'd say.

[6] As the economic recession has dragged on, many men have taken their own lives for the sake of leaving the life insurance money for their families. This has become a social problem.

Other times, however, the existential pondering that went into the suicidal act seems too painful to reflect on—the suicidal urge so apparently frightening for the patient that psychiatrists try to tame the experience by biologizing it. In fact the belief in the power of taming the existential angst by way of biologization is one of the main reasons why these psychiatrists make the biological persuasion so central in their practice, a stance that seems to be appreciated by some patients. When Professor Higashi asked an eighty-one-year-old woman about the time leading up to her suicidal attempt, she began to describe the incident in detail, only to soon fall silent—as if she was re-experiencing the dreadful moment before the act—and to tell the professor that she could not go on: "My son and I agreed that it would be best to forget it and never speak of it again." Seeing how disquieting such reflection can be for some patients, psychiatrists maintain the principle of nonintrusion, listening attentively to what patients say voluntarily while carefully suspending any questions that would impose further psychological introspection. In its place, they try to provide a generic framework for a recovery narrative by stressing the discontinuity between the diseased, suicidal self and the recovered, normal self. Another patient, a seventy-year-old retired worker, discussed how he had thought that he would be better off dead, as his memory was fading in his old age, and how he, serving as the chair of a local community meeting, felt "ashamed" of what he perceived to be his poor command of things. Indeed, even after being hospitalized, the patient was insisting on his intentionality to die for a while. In the final, discharge case conference, Professor Higashi asked him:

H: You said before that it was no use being here.

P: I wanted to die. I thought it would be of no use receiving any treatment.

H: You no longer feel that way?

P: It must have been a disease. . . . I kept thinking about jumping in front of a train or being hit by a car then.

H: [empathetically] You couldn't sleep then.

P: No, I couldn't sleep.

In such ways psychiatrists empathize with the patients' struggles, highlighting how natural it might have once seemed—from the patients' point of view—to take their own lives. Professor Higashi often uses expressions such as, "For you, it was a calm decision" and "There's no denying that you went through a lot," as a way of acknowledging patients' suffering and existential concerns that cannot simply be reduced to mere effects of biology. He then gradually shifts the agency to the pathology by reminding patients how they were driven to the edge by a force they had no control over. In the end, patients are induced to regard their act not as a product of personal will and they are more willing to accept it as a result of mind-affecting psychopathology. In highlighting this point, Professor Higashi frequently poses the question more dramatically, drawing a contrast with the culturally pervasive idea of suicide by asking: "Was it a suicide of resolve?" Patients' flat-out denials—as usually is the case—allow psychiatrists to ascertain that the treatment is now complete.

Resistance Stemming from the Cultural Logic of Suicide of Resolve

Psychiatrists' Own Ambivalence and Doubts

In contrast to the centrality of the biological perspective in their everyday practice, these psychiatrists revealed, in their extraclinical discussions, that they are also products of local cultures; indeed, in interviews many of them talked about suicide with a certain sense of romanticism. Some discussed suicides of their friends and the influence these acts had on their decisions to become doctors, and others evoked the suicides of their favorite writers, citing passages about suicide that had left an impression on them. Most of them explicitly stated that they had chosen psychiatry as a profession expecting to have a glimpse into the depths of the human mind. It is probably because of this initial expectation and romanticism, however, that many of them also stated somewhat cynically that it was rare to encounter a suicide of resolve in the "true sense of the term." In a widely read text on this topic, suicide expert Inamura Hiroshi drew on the work of German psychiatrist P. Feudell to express similar disillusionment: "Relatively speaking, I find it surprising how petty people's reasons for suicide tend to be and how casually they considered it. We often approach the bedside with an initial feeling of intense expectation, only to be betrayed. Instead of encountering depth, what we find is the vulgar imperfection of the human mentality" (Feudell cited in Inamura 1977:61).[7] As Dr. Oda said, "Most of the time I cannot help but wonder why the patient has attempted suicide for such trivial reasons. I have rarely encountered anyone who has carefully contemplated the act beforehand." (Though the question remains as to how much patients would allow that kind of self-revelation in a medical setting.) As psychiatrists repeatedly witness patients' minds altered simply through medication accompanied by rest, they become used to the ubiquity of what they call "petty" suicide attempts and grow weary of the patients who phone the doctors on-call at night to talk persistently about their plans to kill themselves. Learning to dispense with their

---

[7] Translated from the Japanese translation of Feudell's text cited by Inamura (1977:61).

initial romanticism, some psychiatrists even come to wonder if there really is such a thing as suicide of resolve.[8]

Suicide of Resolve by a "Psychotic" Patient

Yet, there are moments in clinical practice when psychiatrists are compelled to reexamine their biological model of suicide. During my entire two years of fieldwork at JP Medical School, there were at least three cases where psychiatrists debated whether these patients' acts constituted (attempted) suicides of resolve. One of them was an attempted suicide by a schizophrenic, whose suicidal intention the psychiatrists failed to—in fact chose not to—explicitly medicalize. This forty-three-year-old worker, who had been previously treated for hallucinations but had long lived a seemingly stable life, was brought to the emergency unit after drinking insecticide. The life history he relayed in the discharge conference illuminated an increasing deterioration in his relationship with his family (his wife had left him, taking the children with her) and his difficulties in holding a steady job because of the illness. Despite the long-term remission of schizophrenia, he had apparently had persistent fear of a possible relapse and its devastating effect. Assuming that his suicide attempt was nonetheless a product of schizophrenia, Professor Higashi asked what the reason was for his attempt:

P: I was at a dead end. I knew my existence was causing my family trouble. Taking my life was the best choice for everyone. I would leave the insurance money and the house to my wife and kids. It would be the best thing to do; that was the conclusion I came to.

H: So you had given much thought to it.

P: Yes, I had.

Later, Professor Higashi came back to the same question, this time asking explicitly if the patient was "being induced by a voice." The patient lifted up his face, looked at him squarely and declared: "No, doctor. It was a suicide of resolve." Here, by inserting this cultural expression, the patient was bluntly resisting the psychiatric framing of his act, thereby insisting on the personal will with which he tried to determine his own end. Though I doubt that he implied any criticism of the doctors, his utterance also attested to the psychiatrists' own failure to cure his illness, a factor in his increasing desperation. Professor Higashi fell into a respectful silence and did not further pursue other questions on this point.

---

[8] Though their own idea about what counts as a "true" and "pure" suicide of resolve is not a biomedical category in any sense but is, instead, a product of their cultural assumptions about what is an honorable, meaningful way to die (cf. Lock 2002).

Existentializing Suicide

Here might lie a troubling question posed by the patient's assertion of a suicide of resolve: What if it appears "reasonable enough" that one should want to choose death? Indeed, it was over the question of how to conceptualize the suicides of psychotics that brought about an important shift in Japanese psychiatric perspectives. The previously prevailing biological model of suicide—which began to be contested from within psychiatry in the 1950s (Katō 1953, 1976, Ōhara 1975)—became the object of critique during the antipsychiatry era. Moriyama Kimio, who was to become an influential leader of the antipsychiatry movement from the late 1960s, told me in an interview that his starting point for questioning the established knowledge of biological psychiatry was, indeed, his encounters with attempted suicides of resolve among psychotic patients. In his dissertation, he described how these patients had tried to take their lives after contemplating the gravity of their own illnesses, and argued that to dismiss such patients' acts as impulsively driven biological symptoms is not only to fail to recognize the existential nature of their suicide attempts but also to do further harm to their human dignity. Following this line of thought, Takemura and Shimura (1977) conducted a survey of suicides among institutionalized psychiatric patients. They concluded that in a significant number of these cases (about one-third) there were "comprehensible reasons" behind patients' suicidal acts (Takemura and Shimura 1977, 1987).

What characterized the psychiatric approach of this era was the psychiatrists' passionate commitment to the patients' own subjective accounts, and efforts to bring agency back to patients by granting the possibility of normality and intentionality in their suicide attempts. Yet this debate did not help establish a drastically new psychiatric model of suicide in Japanese psychiatry. Some psychiatrists I talked to pointed out institutional and economic factors that kept a new system of suicide prevention from emerging, while a few others discussed a "muddle" in which psychiatrists found themselves whenever they tried to engage with the suicidal at an existential level. As a cautionary tale, they all brought up the case of Ellen West, the famous patient of the existential psychiatrist Ludwig Binswanger. They discussed how, faced with the possibility of her committing suicide, Binswanger nonetheless discharged her, believing that "in the death chosen with freedom, she was able to break the vicious circle" and "came to the true realization of herself" (cited in Ishikawa 1962:954).[9] They used this example to underline Binswanger's possible therapeutic negligence and the ethical questions involved in taking the sort of philosophical approach that would glorify a patient's death. This kind of existential, humanistic argument, as my archival research revealed, also came to be used, in an ironic way, to pro-

---

[9] Translated from the Japanese translation of Binswanger's *Schizophrenie*.

tect psychiatrists from being held legally responsible for patients' suicides. In one highly controversial lawsuit in the late 1970s, when the family of a mentally ill patient sued psychiatrists for failing to prevent the patient's suicide, the judge acquitted the doctors in charge by suggesting that psychiatrists were only responsible for irrational suicides of those in a pathological state, and that psychiatrists' humanistic care that respected patients' own will and autonomy, may well be incompatible with suicide prevention (e.g., Fukuoka Chihō Saibansho 1982, Nishizono 1986). The irony of this verdict must have been evident to psychiatrists (see Okada 1989), most of whom seem to have since withdrawn from explicitly discussing existential approaches to suicides or how to conceptualize agency in such acts.

Learning the Consequences of Therapeutic Failure

Psychiatrists, also from their everyday practice, seem to quickly learn the danger of existentializing suicide because of the devastation they experience from losing patients to suicide. A patient's suicide apparently leaves a strong mark even on experienced psychiatrists and is certainly something that they "never get used to," as a sixty-nine-year-old depression expert stated. During my fieldwork, I got to know a few psychiatrists who have repeatedly gone back to the files of the first patient they lost to suicide during their residency in an attempt to think over what they could have done differently. And I met a number of veteran psychiatrists who recite the minute details of letters they had received from patients who later committed suicide. A well-known personality disorder specialist, who talked in depth of the three patients he had lost during the decades of his practice, still uses the appointment organizer file that a patient's father gave him as a keepsake after the patient's suicide; he said that he keeps it as a reminder to himself. Young doctors are known to have quit psychiatry, or seriously contemplated quitting, over such intense experiences (for research on American psychiatrists' reactions to the suicides of their patients, see Hendin et al. 2000). Discussing such a time in his life, a thirty-three-year-old psychiatrist talked about having lost three patients in one week—one in a murder and the other two to suicide: "It was like going through a massacre—I was too busy and had too many responsibilities by then to stop and absorb what had happened." A thirty-seven-year old psychiatrist became tearful as she recalled the first patient she lost, a young man who was referred to her by a colleague with the warning that he had "more of a personality problem" (than depression). Seeing that he was steadily getting better under her care, she gave him permission to stay at his home one night, only to find the following morning that he had hanged himself there. Dazed and devastated, she hardly remembered how she spent the following days, only that she had lost her wedding ring amid the confusion that morning. "I still wonder if he committed suicide of resolve or if it was depression and I made a misjudgment. Since then, I never forget the equation: 'Depression Equals Suicide.'"

Suspending Uncertainty

Thus psychiatrists at times intentionally medicalize suicide not because they cannot see beyond pathology but precisely because they know how easily the boundary between pure biology and existential angst can begin to blur. They would stress, as Dr. Oda told me, how suicidal ideation, "unlike delusions and hallucinations," from which they remain detached, is so "easy to imagine and get emotionally drawn into." Persuasion thus can go *both ways*: as some psychiatrists stated, "the more you listen, the more you begin to see the logic that the person has for wanting to die." Psychiatrists certainly meet many patients who have unusually difficult life histories, some for whom, as a suicide expert pointed out, "[s]uicide would even begin to seem as if it were a natural conclusion to their life"—an extremely dangerous mindset for a psychiatrist to hold. Thus the aforementioned expert in personality disorder emphasized how treating the suicidal was a constant struggle in which it was important to stand firm. He said that he had "no doubt" about the rightness of medicalizing suicide, and added: "That's what we are here for. If they try to bring you onto [their] existential ground, you might get swallowed up in it. And if you begin to have any doubts yourself, I think you'll lose." The consequences of being drawn into considering patients' "reasons" and having any doubts about the legitimacy of their medical treatment can be dire. Thus, despite their initial ambivalence early on in their careers, psychiatrists grow accustomed to suspending the uncertainty they once held about treating suicide. By limiting their object of intervention to what they understand as mental illness, Japanese psychiatrists seem to effectively transform suicide into a product of biology. In place of psychological intervention, psychiatrists at JP Medical School do an extensive amount of social work by talking to patients' families, trying to bring about changes in workplace conditions, and creating a rehabilitation plan for patients' return to work. And hospitalization serving as a refuge from society does seem to work as a temporary shield for suicidal patients, nourishing their desire to live and, at times, bringing about quite dramatic transformations.

The Limit of Biological Persuasion

Drawing the Boundary between the Biological and the Existential

Psychiatrists thus come to operate mainly with the biological model of the suicidal mind, assuming a sharp dichotomy between the normal and the pathological. Yet the emerging forces for medicalizing suicide may be reawakening some of the old debates about the tenuousness of the biological model of suicide, particularly in cases where patients insist on their right to refuse medical treatment.[10] At JP, another case where a patient insisted on a suicide of resolve involved a sixty-four-year-old former civil servant, Furuta-san, who was brought to the emergency unit after taking an overdose and was found unconscious by his family. His life story suggested a series of tragedies; born into a landlord family whose history dated back a couple of hundred years, he faced bankruptcy of the family business as well as discontinuation of the family itself. He had had a difficult relationship with his father, who was a powerful local politician; he had become estranged from his oldest daughter and had lost his second daughter to suicide. His third daughter denounced any intention of marriage for fear of handing down the "tainted blood." Exhausted and despairing, Furuta-san insisted that his act was an attempted suicide of resolve, and continued to plead to doctors that he be discharged so that he could realize his "aesthetics of death." Being an intellectually vibrant person, Furuta-san had a ready cultural vocabulary for expressing his wish to die by drawing on historical figures whose suicides were praised as honorable acts of self-determination. Psychiatrists were further shocked and gravely worried when, a few months into hospitalization, Furuta-san was found trying to sneak out of the hospital for another suicide attempt.[11]

Importantly, when patients explicitly resist medicalization in such ways, these psychiatrists respond not by attempting to biologize the existential—that is, reducing existential angst to mere signs of biological anomaly as medicalization critics might assume—but by simply leaving intentionality aside. Instead of directly engaging with his persistent assertion of the suicide of resolve, these psychiatrists kept emphasizing to Furuta-san that they were only treating his clinical depression and that they had no desire or right to intrude into the irresolvable aspects of his life. Professor Higashi made this clear to the attending staff in one of the early case conferences for Furuta-san: "It is our responsibility to cure his depression. Once his mental illness is treated, the remaining decision will lie with him."[12] Though Furuta-san's hospitalization dragged on for an unusual length of time, with little change in his insistence on suicide of resolve, psychiatrists continued to hold this stance. While they did listen to his existential angst, they would try to call his attention to the minute bodily changes that would occur under treatment. Even when Furuta-san finally began to come out of his depression after receiving unexpected news of his third daughter's marriage, psychiatrists continued to discuss his suicidal ideation with him in terms of biological depression, which they said had no doubt become intensi-

[10] For instance, psychiatrists are increasingly requested to consult with other medical units, to help determine to what extent a terminally ill patient's wish to discontinue a certain treatment is a product of free will rather than an underlying depression.

[11] Note that there is no locked ward at this psychiatric department, as a matter of therapeutic principle.

[12] Of course what allowed him to say this initially was the confidence that their biological cure would eventually lift his suicidal ideation.

fied when coupled with life's difficulties. By the time he left the hospital after eighteen months, Furuta-san expressed in my interviews his own ambivalence toward the nature of what he once believed was his attempted suicide of resolve, and seemed to find some comfort in the psychiatric perspective as a plausible account for the dreadful despair he once felt.

The therapeutic approach that these psychiatrists took should thus be differentiated from biological reductionism—or what can be called "biologism"—whereby psychiatrists commonly reduce the patient's existential angst to a localized chemical imbalance in the brain. Instead, without delving into the question of the cause of Furuta-san's depression, the doctors in charge stressed that depression affected his whole being, and that the biological treatment would present one path to recovery. This therapeutic approach resonates with the strands of traditional medical ideas that anthropologists have repeatedly found in contemporary Japanese medical practices, whereby mental distress is often explained—both by medical professionals and lay people—as deeply interrelated to somatic disturbances (Lock 1980, 1982, Marsella 1980, Ohnuki-Tierney 1984, Ozawa-de Silva 2002). In this regard, what these doctors are engaged in is not the overwhelmingly biological approach that they have often been criticized for, but rather what can be glossed as "somatism," a therapeutic principle that does not set out from a mind-body dualism but one in which the body becomes the central medium through which the mind can be cured (see chapter 6). Importantly, however, somatism is not a therapeutic principle that is clearly articulated or consciously theorized by psychiatrists themselves. Without such awareness, the exclusive focus on the body in actual clinical practice may risk slipping into biologism (to be further discussed in chapter 10 with regards to the rapid pharmaceuticalization of everyday distress during the 2000s).

When Psychiatrists Accept a Suicide of Resolve

Despite the surface confidence in biological persuasion these psychiatrists exhibited to Furuta-san, behind the scenes they actually debated among themselves how to truly differentiate the biological from the existential. In the numerous case conferences they held for Furuta-san's case, some psychiatrists even brought up the possibility that his suicidal ideation might well be a product of free will, as Furuta-san insisted, and asked on what grounds they even had the right to treat suicidal patients against their own will.[13] In the end, the consensus that emerged was, as Dr. Satō put it: "We have no philosophical grounds upon which to justify why we should stop suicidal patients from tak-

[13] Note that Japanese psychiatrists are granted the legal power to confine those who are deemed a danger to others and to themselves. While psychiatrists do not hesitate to forcefully institutionalize the first group, in the case of the latter, they can be highly indecisive about taking the same measure if being a danger to oneself means being (simply) suicidal.

ing their own lives. Only, we believe, the fact that the patients are telling their intention to a psychiatrist—who has the medical and ethical responsibility to save lives—already suggests their implicit desire to live."

Psychiatrists hung onto the thin thread of Furuta-san's desire to stay under their care of his own "free will" as the justification to keep treating a determinedly suicidal patient like him. This suggests that the only time that psychiatrists grant the cultural logic of "suicide of resolve" is when patients successfully hide any desire to die while in their care, thereby suggesting their implicit refusal to engage in further dialogues with psychiatrists. The fate of Terada-san, a sixty-four-year-old woman hospitalized around the same time as Furuta-san, was in sharp contrast to his. On the one-year anniversary of her husband's death, she took an overdose of antidepressants and was found unconscious the next morning. She surprised the psychiatrist at the emergency unit when she begged him to assist her in dying, literally suggesting euthanasia. In my interviews with her after her recovery, Terada-san told me about the hardships she had gone through; divorcing after her first husband's infidelity, she brought up two sons on her own by working as a medical clerk, a job she kept for thirty years. Meeting her second husband gave her happiness and comfort, until they were thrown into an uphill battle with the cancer he developed. The memories of the numerous trips they made to mountain shrines to pray for his recovery were still fresh in her mind, and she was proud of having done everything she could to ease his pain, nursing him at home until the very end. Soon after his death, she began to experience mysterious symptoms—including being drained of energy, shivering, rashes, and high blood pressure—that none of the doctors she visited were able to diagnose. Even after she finally met a psychiatrist who prescribed antidepressants for her, she spent many nights sleepless, worrying about gradually turning into an "invalid." Once hospitalized in the psychiatric unit, however, she was amazed by her own brisk and dramatic recovery and soon regained her cheerful former self. She told me repeatedly how the doctor had saved her life, and how she had complete trust in him. The only concern she still had at the time of her discharge, it seemed, was whether her married son would live with her to keep an eye on her fragile health. Before the hospitalization, he had offered to do this himself, but she was indecisive, possibly because she was under the influence of depression but also because she worried incessantly about becoming a "burden" on others.

A few months later, I was told by the doctor in charge of Terada-san that she had taken her own life on the morning she was supposed to enter a nursing home. The doctor was visibly distressed. He said he could not comprehend what had driven her to it and fell silent. As I sat there, thoughts rushed through my mind: Could it be that her depression was not fully cured, as doctors had assumed? Could it be that she chose death because she did not wish to be a burden on her sons? She emphasized that she felt satisfied with her life, and proud of having taken care of her sons and her late husband. Did she want to end it with a sense of pride as a caregiver while she could, rather than becoming an "invalid"—an existence that she had so feared? Or did she die in resignation, possibly even protest, feeling abandoned by her family and by medical professionals? As I tried to recall my conversations with her to search for any signs that I might have missed, the doctor said that he had not predicted this outcome at all. Though it was apparently a planned act, Terada-san had shown no signs of suicidal intention that the psychiatrist could detect in the last few times he had seen her at the outpatient unit. Then he added: "This must have been a suicide of resolve."

Partial Persuasion

The rise of the psychiatric discourse on suicide represents a transformation in the nature of psychiatric power in Japan, from a mode of oppression and coercion to one of persuasion and incorporation, whereby psychiatrists encourage people to share and speak in their own terms (Foucault 1973). However, as the clinical vignettes discussed above illuminate, this transformation is fraught with tensions, as psychiatrists are confronted with patients who bring competing moral views on the nature of their distress (cf. Good 1994, Kirmayer 1994, Kleinman 1995, Young 1995). Despite the routine success of the biological model of suicide, psychiatrists are made to face their own deep-seated ambivalence about medicalization by patients who insist that they had attempted suicide of resolve. These patients thereby (implicitly) question how psychiatrists' expanding jurisdiction might pathologize—and trivialize—the existential dimensions of their suicidal intention. The cultural discourse about suicide that these patients draw on serves to expose the inadequacy of the psychiatric model of suicide, while raising disturbing ethical questions involved in the psychiatric work of treating people against their own will. And psychiatrists' own failures to provide a cure in the end—as in the case of Terada-san, for whom medication was apparently successful in changing her outlook, but only while she remained within the hospital walls—serve to remind them that there is a vast domain of social suffering to which their biologically oriented treatment does not extend. As we have seen, this kind of dilemma has led in the past to heated debates within psychiatry about the nature of psychiatric intervention in the realm of the existential; again today, the rising forces of medicalization seem to be rekindling similar concerns.

One way in which psychiatrists try to solve their dilemma is to knowingly limit their jurisdiction to the familiar domain of biology, where they know they can exercise control and achieve a certain level of therapeutic efficacy. Without aiming for the kind of holistic conceptual transformation that psychiatry's hegemony might seem to require, psychiatrists instead strive for the minimum of shared understanding with patients about the biological nature of the "mental illness," while deliberately avoiding the realm of the existential—and psychological—meanings associated with patients' distress. They try to achieve their persuasion in three steps: First, they "extract" the underlying psychopathology and urge patients to objectify their own body, cultivating an awareness of how fatigued and even alien their body has become; second, they de-existentialize suicidal urges by showing suicidal patients how not only their bodies but also their minds change through biological interventions. They encourage patients to regard their suicidal intention as a departure from their "normal" selves, thereby shifting the locus of agency to the realm of biological pathology (cf. Barrett 1996, Estroff 1993); and, third, as they tame patients' suicidal urges, psychiatrists also call attention to the social pressures driving the breakdown, thereby suggesting patients' victimhood. In this final step, psychiatrists effectively merge the biological and the social in their particular construction of psychopathology, which culminates in a generic framework that at times effectively translates individual misery into a sign of social suffering (cf. Kleinman 1986, Kleinman et al. 1997).

Through this process, psychiatrists are able to get patients to reproduce narratives about suicide with surprising uniformity and consistency, not necessarily because they have thoroughly persuaded patients and transformed their consciousness, but because they deliberately leave much unexplored. Knowing their own powerlessness in altering the social conditions that have contributed to patients' psychological desperation, psychiatrists avoid explicitly intervening in patients' own reasons and intentions for attempting suicide. Thus, the triumph of instrumental rationality discussed by Byron Good (1994) seems to prevail here, as moral and existential questions that cannot be easily answered by routine biomedical practice are bracketed off and left unexamined (also see Lock and Gordon 1988). At one level, psychiatrists' silence over the existential and the psychological aspects of suicide suggests their own critical reflexivity about the potentially insidious—even abusive—power of medicalization (as seen in Japanese psychiatrists' debates between the late 1960s and early 1980s about the suicides of psychotics). At another level, however, psychiatrists' silence also makes psychiatric discourse—particularly for patients who wish to find ways of changing their lives other than merely through biological intervention—fall short of becoming an internally persuasive language with which to explore suicidal ideation in meaningful terms. Thus in the end, psychiatrists, despite their cultural and clinical sensibilities, appear constrained from fully participating in dialogue with patients asserting that their behavior and intention be understood in terms of suicide of resolve.

Furthermore, instead of fundamentally destabilizing the cultural discourse, Japanese psychiatrists may well be complicit in reproducing the cultural assumptions about suicide even when their clinical experiences tell them otherwise. This is most evident in their use of the sharply drawn dichotomy between pathological suicide and suicide of resolve. On the one hand, by upholding suicide of resolve as a kind of "ideal" against which all other (i.e., pathological) suicides are to be judged, psychiatrists often successfully persuade patients to reflect on the fragile nature of their own intentionality and to accept the psychiatric explanation that it was pathologically induced. On the other hand, however, their use of the dichotomy also seems to reproduce and reinforce the implicit moral hierarchy embedded in the cultural discourse, whereby some deaths are aestheticized as courageous acts of *pure* and *true* suicides of resolve, while others are relegated to the rank of "trivial," "petty," and what are now increasingly labeled "*pathological*" suicides. Psychiatrists themselves point out that such a dichotomy breaks down easily in actual clinical practice, and that the boundary between biology and existential angst is often blurred. Even with all their sensibility in this regard, they seem to lack a language with which to convey to nonpsychiatrist audiences the complexities of the suicidal mind or the ephemeral nature of human intentionality. One of the ironic consequences of their cultural sensibilities may thus be that Japanese psychiatrists, despite their therapeutic commitment, scarcely seem poised to challenge and supplant the cultural discourse that, traditionally, has aestheticized the voluntary taking of one's own life as an acceptable expression of free will but has also provided so few clues as to how to bring the suicidal person back onto the side of life.

Up to this point, we have examined how doctors and patients engage in clinical dialogue in everyday psychiatric practice. The relatively seamless transformation of patients' narratives largely owes to the fact that it takes place through systematic clinical intervention over a limited time span, targeted at the acute phase of depression. It is important to remember that, even after patients leave the hospital, their narratives continue to evolve as they grapple with the meaning of their breakdowns in the context of their lives. It is here that we find how psychiatric persuasion works at the level of "internally persuasive discourse," and what long-term effects it has on individuals. In the next chapter, I thus turn to patients' narratives in order to explore how psychiatric persuasion comes to structure their own understandings of illness and in what ways—and particularly for whom—it may be liberating, by focusing on striking gender differences.

CHAPTER EIGHT

The Gendering of Depression and the Selective Recognition of Pain

The Peculiar Gendering of Depression in Japan

DEPRESSION HAS LONG BEEN represented in the West as a quintessential female malady, where women are said to be twice as likely as men to become depressed. This gender ratio has been cited by some feminists to argue that depression epitomizes women's suffering (Jack 1991, cf. Showalter 1985). Japan poses a challenge to this characterization, however, because until recently rates of male depression have been as high as—sometimes even higher than—those of women. Throughout the twentieth century, numerous Japanese psychiatrists have commented on this statistical anomaly (e.g., Hirasawa 1966, Naka 1932, Matsumura 1937, Shinfuku et al. 1973, Nakane et al. 2004).[1] As Margaret Lock called to our attention in 1993, Japan was the only one out of the twelve countries that participated in the 1973 WHO crossnational survey on depression, where slightly more men than women suffered depression (Lock 1993, Nakane et al. 1994). While this data was recently challenged by the epidemiological community survey on depression, which indicated a gender ratio akin to that suggested by the Western data (Kawakami et al. 2002, 2005),[2] and there has certainly been an increase of women with depression during the 2000s, there have been few empirical investigations into what created this peculiar gendering at the epidemiological level.[3]

---

[1] On gender and mental illness, also see Suzuki Akihito's historical analysis of the asylums in the early twentieth-century Japan (Suzuki 2005). On the politics of gender representation in psychiatry, see Micale 1995, 2008, Showalter 1985.

[2] In one recent epidemiological study—conducted for the first time in a long while in Japan—Kawakami et al. (2002, 2005) showed that depression rates may not be so different in Japan from those in the United States. These statistics urge us to seriously examine whether or not the long-held Japanese psychiatrists' clinical observations about gender were indeed just a matter of social accessibility to psychiatry and of experts' selective attention, or if the number of depressed people has itself changed rapidly of late. (As Lock [1993] has suggested, there is a possibility that Japanese women may have had cultural resources that have long protected them from social isolation and a sense of alienation—and perhaps from the experience of depression itself.) Experts also ask if increased rates of depression are merely the result of a new "operational diagnosis" (i.e., the DSM), which gives the false impression of there being an actual biological entity when in fact the definition of depression itself has been significantly changed to include a wide variety of subjective complaints (this has left many Japanese psychiatrists debating the validity of such a diagnosis).

[3] Note that one way in which biological standardization of depression is being quickly estab-

Depression has also been gendered at the level of popular representation, and here, the Japanese difference is even more striking. While the statistical data have repeatedly shown almost an equal number by gender, the popular discourse has represented depression more as a male malady. Particularly since depression has emerged in the 1990s (with record-high rates of suicide) as a "national disease," the media has frequently depicted depression's victims as working men. In the mushrooming number of publications and TV programs on depression, male depression has been featured centrally—so much so that in 2006 NHK (the National Broadcasting Service, which is the Japanese equivalent of the BBC) aired a series of programs proclaiming that "women also become depressed." These programs emphasized that women are much more likely to become afflicted with depression, even if "the image of depression remains that of a working man." Though this representation is also changing rapidly, in contrast to the prevailing image of the depressed person in the West as a melancholic housewife, in Japan, depression's victim has been overwhelmingly represented as a burned-out salaryman.

How do we account for this gender anomaly? Some earlier Japanese psychiatrists used to suggest that men were more likely to become depressed because they simply suffered more. Their reasoning was that, given men's higher social standing, they were exposed to more social stress, while women, with their lower social responsibility, remained more protected. Other psychiatrists have suggested, however, that women's lack of social standing, and their economically dependent status, resulted in inadequate attention to their depression. In other words, women have suffered as much as, if not more than, men, but their suffering has remained largely unrecognized. If so, then this would parallel the ironic situation that had surrounded menopause until recently in Japan—as analyzed by Lock (1993)—whereby "menopausal" women largely escaped medicalization because of the relative lack of Japanese recognition of their distress. While this kept women out of doctors' offices and encouraged them to seek out other cultural resources, even prevented them from pathologizing their experiences, it also had the unfortunate result of making them believe in the hegemonic discourse that de-legitimized their distress even against, at times, their own subjective experience. Drawing upon this interplay between medical representations and subjective experiences, I examined the narratives of 25 Japanese who were recovering from depression (12 males and 13 females). I also participated for a year in a depression support group, the only one in existence in Japan that I could find in 2001, which happened to be exclusively male. These data are analyzed in light of the ethnographic fieldwork I conducted at three

---

lished is through the psychiatrists' use of statistics (Hacking 1990). Lock (1993) has shown how statistics in biomedicine take on peculiar universality, where research findings in the West are too often assumed to be the norm, with little serious investigation into possible local variations. Depression—particularly its gender ratio—seems to be an obvious starting point for such an investigation (Sartorius and WHO 1983, Nakane et al. 1994, Lepine et al. 1997).

psychiatric institutions in and around Tokyo between 2000 and 2003, where I did participant-observation of everyday clinical practice for two years. What emerged from these investigations was that men and women suffer differently because of the particular gendering of depression in Japan.

Male Depression: Overwork as the Cause for Depression?

> Job security, recognition for long service, a system of re-
> wards, company accommodation, social backup: under
> Japanese capitalism the firm neglects no measure which
> can further the integration of its employees, and assumes
> a large part of the welfare role which in the West was once
> played by the Church, and now devolves on the state. Em-
> ployer and employee are bound not by a precise and dis-
> soluble contract for the sake of working capacity, but by a
> personal commitment involving total participation in the
> life of the company.
> —Maurice Pinguet, *Voluntary Death in Japan* (1993:30)

Social and Medical Recognition and Trust in Doctors

The depressed, Japanese psychiatrists say, are the most normative Japanese. With their self-sacrificing devotion, discipline, and sense of responsibility, they are, in the well-known dictum of Shimoda, "model (male) youths, model employees, model officers" (see chapter 5). True to these words, the male patients the psychiatrists introduced me to as "typical patients of depression," were always hard-working men. They first and foremost discussed work stress as the cause of their "depression," and their narratives were remarkably uniform in structure, indicating an increasing amount of work, fatigue beyond limit, eventual collapse, and recovery through simple rest. Men's narratives also characterized a relatively smooth recognition of their depression by their family and by medical professionals, followed by a congenial relationship with their psychiatrist, who helped shape their understanding of depression as a product of overwork.

This was evidently the case with Kobayashi-san, a fifty-year-old civil servant working for the central government, and one of the first people I was introduced to by psychiatrists as embodying Shimoda's notion of melancholic premorbid personality. Kobayashi-san's narrative gives a glimpse into what might go through the minds of some Japanese men, who risk literally working themselves to death. In a small consultation room of a private mental hospital where we met, Kobayashi-san and I exchanged business cards and I explained my research to him. He then began to recount his experience chronologically, recalling what he thought was the initial episode of depression. Ten years previously,

he had been working in Kasumigaseki (the part of Tokyo where most governmental offices are located), and was engaged in an intense negotiation with the
Ministry of Finance over the annual budget for his ministry. A new computer
system for budget management had been introduced, but not wanting to hurt
his computer-illiterate boss's feeling, Kobayashi-san did everything manually
and brought back extra work to do at home every night. Sleeping for only three
hours each night and working on weekends, Kobayashi-san suddenly found
himself one day feeling suicidal.

> I was in the office on a Sunday, when my mind went blank: then the
> thought occurred to me that I might throw myself out of the window. I
> had heard about people jumping (from high rise buildings) in Kasumi-
> gaseki. I wondered if I might just do the same. . . . I simply wanted to es-
> cape from it all.

In the early 1990s, mental health was still not something people talked about in
his office: "We would habitually exceed 100 extra hours of overtime per month.
If someone happened to drop dead, then superiors would consider providing
the deceased's family with workers' compensation, but that was it." Kobayashi-
san said he did not think his problem was depression and thought that he was
simply "weak," lacking the ability to carry out the job. Similar to the illness histories recounted to me by other depressed patients, he was soon hospitalized,
not for depression, but for a duodenal ulcer he had developed.

His initial encounter with a psychiatrist began when he experienced what
Japanese psychiatrists commonly refer to as "promotion depression." At the
time, Kobayashi-san had been transferred to the southern part of Japan as a
stepping-stone to his next promotion. The job proved to be highly stressful,
however, as he had to constantly negotiate with the strong labor union there.
Kobayashi-san recounted with apparent chagrin that he was yelled at by the
union people during an important lecture he was giving to young trainees.
Feeling humiliated but still trying to smooth things out by going out drinking
with union leaders every night (despite his dislike of alcohol), Kobayashi-san
felt thoroughly exhausted after eight months and simply could not go to work
anymore. His worried wife took him to an internist, who then referred him to
a psychiatrist. The psychiatrist, who diagnosed him with depression, seemed to
know exactly what to say to convince Kobayashi-san to take sick leave: "The
doctor said that even a departmental chief from the local government [higher
ranked than Kobayashi-san] was coming to the clinic. I was surprised to learn
that it happened to my superiors as well." The hospital hid the fact that their
diagnosis was depression and kept out all visitors. He "slept as much as [he]
wanted for the first time in a long time" and found himself recovered in two
weeks' time. For Kobayashi-san, depression was apparently a case of work-

related exhaustion or "burn-out," for which a cure (with generous, paid sick leave) was readily provided.

In such ways, the psychiatric master narrative of work-induced depression was the unifying theme of the men's narratives I heard. The uniformity of patients' narratives was intriguing, considering how utterly confused and confusing most patients' narratives were, coming from people who were visiting psychiatrists for the first time. The uniformity seemed to emerge by the time they had gone through psychiatric treatment, which suggests that patients' narratives are coproducts of their own reflection and psychiatric persuasion. As demonstrated in previous chapters, in the everyday psychiatric practices I observed, I often saw patients provided with an assuring narrative from psychiatrists about an inevitable breakdown from stress. Psychiatrists did this by first systematically cultivating an awareness in patients of how fatigued and alienated their bodies had become, thereby shifting patients' attention away from their psychological torments. They reminded patients of their normative personality as well as the social predicaments that had driven them to the edge, thereby illuminating patients' victimhood. In so doing, psychiatrists seemed to achieve what biomedicine has always done best—distancing the afflicted from the self-blame and moral responsibility that they might otherwise be subjected to (Sontag 1978).

Indeed, Kobayashi-san's narrative is typical of men's accounts of overwork-induced depression. This is the basic form of depression that Shimoda had already illuminated in the 1930s, and the mold in which Japanese psychiatric understandings of depression have been cast. As with cases that lawyers involved in overwork suicide litigations have successfully argued, there was little doubt that work stress was a crucial factor for the depression of almost all the men I interviewed. For instance, Narita-san, a thirty-seven-year-old computer engineer, explained to me how he became depressed right after being promoted to section chief. He was exhausted from the added responsibility of managing employees and keeping up with the ever-accelerating pace of the computer industry. As his boss had suffered depression himself, Narita-san was urged to take sick leave and rest, which led to recovery after a few weeks. Another fifty-five-year-old entrepreneur, Watabe-san talked about how he was driven to a suicide attempt after his once-successful chain stores began to fail in the bursting of the bubble economy. Watabe-san said he was driven to the edge while scrambling for funds, worrying about the imminent risk of bankruptcy, and spending many nights sleepless. Such narratives attest to the increasingly difficult working conditions under which Japanese men are placed in the long recession, and suggest how depression may be understood as a work hazard.

While straightforward "overwork depression" dominated the male narratives I heard, some men did, however, deeply reflect on the nature of their illness—particularly after they had suffered chronic or repeated forms of depression—and elaborate on how their work stress came to be closely entangled with problems beyond the workplace. Kobayashi-san was one of them, who had come—over the years of his struggles—to regard depression as not only a temporary sign of work stress but an embodiment of the growing contradictions in his life. He said that at the time he became depressed, he had just found out that his wife had joined the Jehovah's Witnesses. "I hadn't realized how distressed she had been about everything, especially about how to bring up children. I was far too busy with my work to notice her distress, and when I found out, I was thrown into a panic." His wife insisted on new ideas about child rearing, and refused to tend to his family grave (regarded as an important act for preserving the continuation of the family). As his life began to crumble both at work and at home, Kobayashi-san was forced to confront the fact that his personal aspirations were causing strain in his life. He recounted how as a young man, his family had been too poor to send him to college, but that he got his B.A. through night school after joining the Ministry. While this placed him in a higher position than he might have hoped for, he still had to work as an intermediary between the top elites in the central Ministry and the (equally proud) directors of local governments. His reliability at work and unfailing consideration for others had certainly won him many supporters, but Kobayashi-san felt he was always "trying to cover up [his] lack of ability" by maintaining smooth relationships on all sides, for instance, by writing five hundred New Year's cards every year. He realized how this way of being had thoroughly exhausted him. What went through his mind when he imagined himself jumping out of a window, he said, was the fear that he would make an irreversible mistake on the job and would be "destroyed" (*tsubusareru*).

> When I was hospitalized, I really wanted to talk to my father. I went back to see him at the end of the year, and he said: "I understand." He wasn't at all surprised that I had become depressed. My father was only a farmer but had also served on a village council so he knew [what it was like]. . . . He told me not to worry about getting ahead of others and to take it at a slow pace. I was so relieved. . . . He never told me to try harder (*ganbare*). To tell someone to try harder often means driving him to take his own life.

For Kobayashi-san, recovering from depression meant critically reexamining the way he had lived. Through his struggles, he came to feel gratitude towards his wife, who kept telling him not to worry about promotions, saying that was not what she married him for. Watching her do volunteer work every week and bringing up their children with care, Kobayashi-san became reconciled with her religious belief: "I came to realize how she also needed a purpose in life (*ikigai*)." While he still debated taking the exam for the next promotion, he was now also trying not to spend his days worrying about "what [he] could otherwise do tomorrow." Kobayashi-san's dream was to quit work after staying with

the Ministry for another decade and go back to his hometown to take up farm-
ing: "I want to do another budget compilation as my last service, and leave [the
Ministry]. . . . I don't think I would have become depressed if I had been a
farmer all along."

Like other male patients, Kobayashi-san gradually recovered with the help of
his family and the protective relationship that the psychiatrist offered him. Doctors often consciously reproduced the work relationship for these depressed
men, taking up the role of their superiors, ordering them rest, and determining
when they should return to work (Yoshimatsu 1987, Suzuki 1997). Kobayashi-
san seemed to fully trust the doctor's decisions and said, "Dr. Koyama listens to
me well. When I have three days off and I don't feel like going back to work, he
says: 'I feel just the same.' That kind of thing makes me feel so much better." The
men I interviewed seemed to find a sense of comfort and security in such a relationship, as they recovered by readily yielding themselves to the power of
psychiatrists, whose benign shelter helped them nurture their impaired sense
of self.

Meanings of Depression

Should "work" then be seen as a kind of a "cover story" that some men used to
simplify the cause of their depression? Though the psychiatric master narrative
that emphasized overwork certainly functioned as what a veteran psychiatrist
called "a generic narrative" of depression, the men I met seemed to genuinely
regard work as the overarching theme and the deep root of their problems.
Their narratives suggested that because they had become so united with their
work, and work occupied most of their waking hours, the slightest discord
within the workplace could open up an abyss that could destabilize their sense
of self, even threaten their existence.

No one else symbolized this sense of impasse as eloquently as Takashima-
san, a forty-nine-year-old banker with a courteous, gentle manner. Discussing
with me a book on the history of English industrial revolution that he happened to be carrying, Takashima-san began to talk about his depression first as
a product of alienation in the workplace. He graduated from a prestigious university in the residue of the student movement of the 1970s, where he studied
Marxist economics. Instead of pursuing his dream of becoming a lawyer to
fight for the needs of the socially weak, Takashima-san followed his parent's
wish and began working for a local bank. This was the time, he said, when Japanese industry was going through a fundamental restructuring after the oil
shock, and Toyota's strict production control was acclaimed as the model for
the new era. He was put in charge of loans in an area known as a publishing
hub, where tiny factories were in turn controlled by a few megapublishers. Each
shop specialized in a single process of book production, such as binding or

page trimming, and their livelihoods were entirely dependent upon the whims of the big corporations.

> As I took charge of these small firms, I started reading more books on economics than I ever did in college. You know how much these small companies get paid for binding? It's a matter of sen (a smaller unit than a yen, now obsolete), for thousands of books they do. Big companies demand a rebate on top of that! . . . I felt I was seeing real life exploitation.

Through making rounds to these small factories and building trusting relationships with his customers, Takashima-san began to find meaning in his work. He had a promising career ahead of him (as a graduate of an elite university), but remained uncomfortable with the culture of the bank, he said, where turning down a loan request was regarded as a sign of manhood: "I cared too much about my customers. That's why I became depressed. I chose the wrong vocation."

Takashima-san became depressed at what seemed like the height of his career, when he was transferred to help establish a foreign exchange division. Working under a new boss sent from a powerful bank known for its Spartan culture, Takashima-san began to routinely leave home at 6:30 A.M. and work till 2 A.M. in order to keep up with the new work demands. The boss did not take to Takashima-san's style, however. He would often criticize him in front of others; he would hit the desk with the document Takashima-san had prepared and, disparaging him, toss the paper into the air. "I can't forget that sound of the paper hitting the desk, 'bang, bang.' That's when I began to go wrong. He imposed his own style on me. . . . I totally lost confidence and began to wonder what I was doing." Tears would come and he could no longer get up for work in the morning. He soon began to see Dr. Nakata, whom he had been seeing for almost ten years.

Up to this point, Takashima-san's narratives sounded "typical" of the other depressed men I interviewed. Yet, just when I thought I had grasped the cause of his depression to be work stress, Takashima-san suddenly said, "[his] wife was another reason" for his depression. They never got along because their ideas about child rearing were incompatible. His wife having to live with his mother (an arrangement that is becoming less common and is regarded as a source of domestic tension in Japan) led to a constant war between the two women. As his wife refused to divorce him and was living upstairs and he downstairs in the same house, he found himself in limbo: "I love my children. I can't stand it when my wife yells hysterically at them. My mother and my wife fight all the time. I can't stand it." Feeling cornered both at work and at home, he said that the only time he felt tranquility was when he would contemplate on the intricate details of how to commit suicide. Discussing a number of failed suicide attempts he had made, he told me how he wanted to achieve peace of mind by "finding the absolute meaning for [him] self." Talking feelingly about an old woman he saw on the train, a peddler carrying an enormous bundle on her bent back, and wondering how she could persevere in life despite the apparent hardship, he said:

> I can think of the reasons and solutions [for my depression] but I can't actually carry them out. I'm forever analyzing my plight. You know the hardest working people are not necessarily the most rewarded. . . . There were many folks who went through tough times in the rise of the agricultural revolution or the industrial revolution. How did they find the strength to survive that?

Takashima-san's dream was to enter graduate school after retirement to study the history of the English working class, to understand how the underdogs persisted despite the social hardships. "I'm just hoping that I can hang on for the rest of my life—thirteen years and six months before retirement."

As these men's agonies were so much determined by work, one might wonder why they would not simply quit the job and find something else. As Thomas Rohlen once described the life of Japanese bankers, however, quitting work in a society where life employment is still the norm is an anomaly that people frown upon (Rohlen 1974). Though this way of thinking seems to be changing since the recession of the 1990s, losing lifetime employment had long been comparable to social death. This deep fear was evident in the depression support group that I attended over the course of a year. The discussions these men engaged in more than half the time centered around their worries over how to hold onto their job. Veteran members would caution new members on sick leave, who expressed their desperation to get back to work, that a rushed return would likely result in poor performance, which could further damage their employability and exacerbate their depression. To other newcomers who talked angrily about their treatment at work and fantasized about quitting in protest, veterans spoke from their own bitter experiences: "We have to drop the illusion that the [company] will be begging us to come back. Hang onto the job even if they try to make you feel like quitting." While dreaming of a full recovery by finding an alternative self elsewhere (as in postretirement life), few men dared to leave that system and the security it provided. And those on long-term sick leave often expressed their constant anxiety (and accompanying risk of shame) of being spotted by their neighbors in broad daylight, when "decent men" are supposed to be at the office, working. Their being bound to the workplace was, it seemed, both a blessing and a curse for these men, as they seemed unable to envision a life outside the system in which they had long been complicit, even if it was now destroying their health.

Letting Go

Depression thus represented a liminal space, where excessive self-questioning of causes and meanings could lead these men out of the orbit of well-ordered company life. Some of the men, however, seemed to reach—through their struggles—what could only be described as a philosophical resignation. This was the case with Machida-san, a sixty-three-year-old man of few words, who appeared somewhat beaten by years of hardship. He was a former managing director of a construction company, who was—at the time of my interview—cleaning toilets for a living. Until a few years before, he had been running his company with his three brothers. He reminisced about the time of hardship in building the company from scratch, and the eventual success they enjoyed as the business steadily expanded. All this changed with the bursting of the bubble economy. The number of contracts began to decrease, and the fee for each project got smaller and smaller. Soon enough, the parent company started dumping nonprofitable jobs on its small subsidiaries like Machida-san's, threatening them with otherwise discontinuing future business: "We could not afford to turn down any offers of contracts, even if we knew that it was a project no one else wanted because it was sure to produce losses, not profit." Machida-san became uncharacteristically eloquent as he began to criticize the government, whose generous shield of protection for big corporations that were failing (under the Prime Minister Koizumi's banner of collectively "sharing the pain") barely covered little firms like his. As the company struggled to survive, gradually letting go of the trucks and other construction machinery, Machida-san's elder brother died from a cerebral infarction. His younger brother, who took over the management of the company, soon sank into alcoholism, dying from liver damage. Scrambling for funds and worrying about being able to pay salaries to employees at the end of each month, Machida-san hardly realized the changes happening to him, but he was losing energy, concentration, and sleep. By the time he filed for bankruptcy, he was drinking heavily and was severely depressed.

After losing everything—his company, employees, his savings, and his house—Machida-san was, he said, "satisfied" with his simple life now. He spoke with feeling about how his family supported him throughout the hardship, and how that kept him from committing suicide. Working for the cleaning company without worrying about managing funds, he emphasized, was such an easy way to live (he particularly appreciated his coworkers, who all had a "past" like Machida-san—one was formerly a banker, a few others former presidents—who did not hesitate to help and cover for each other). He was "thankful that [he] had a job [he] could do every day," and said that, since the job was something that no one else wanted to do, he found it meaningful to be able to engage in the work of "cleaning and removing the taint." Then, almost as if he were delivering a Buddhist sermon, Machida-san intoned how "human beings become tainted from daily living, how life is constant suffering." His words are intriguing in light of the fact that Shimoda originally termed the melancholic premorbid personality, "shūchaku kishitsu." Shūchaku is etymologically a Buddhist term, translation of a Sanskrit term (*abhi-niveśa*), which refers to obsession, adherence, tenacity, and delusional attachment (Hirasawa 1966:49–52).[4] Though Shimoda himself did not moralize the nature of the melancholic or promote psychotherapy to change the way patients were, except to draw attention to their tenacious attachment to work, his use of the Buddhist term to describe the underlying pathology of the depressed seems to implicitly point to a certain path toward recovery—that is, the idea that letting go of worldly obsessions and desires would bring one to inner tranquility.

This indigenous philosophy of recovery also resonated with what I heard from other depressed men I met in the depression support group. These men articulated how they came to realize, after years of battling with depression, that they could not do anything but "relinquish control."[5] Indeed, the mantra that had naturally emerged from the group was: "Focus on your depression here and now.... Immerse yourself in depression (*utsu ni doppuri tsukaru*)." True to this spirit, one member gladly reported his recovery and added: "But I'm trying to remain modest. And I'm *trying hard not to try hard*." The apparent contradiction in his remark made everyone laugh, as this struggle was something that they all seemed to recognize in themselves. The group shared the understanding that the depressed tended to be the ones who "borrowed trouble" by worrying about things over which they had no control (see Kondō 1999). Depression, they said, forced them to confront their own weakness and abandon the desire to be in control, a point I repeatedly heard from other men I interviewed (see also Ozawa-de Silva 2006).

Recognizing their own limitations also made them realize, most of them pointed out, how embedded they were in social relationships. Watabe-san, the aforementioned entrepreneur, said that the cause of his depression was his own personality: "I used to be egoistic and would easily get upset when things got in my way.... But I've changed since then. I've come to realize that I do not live alone and that I have been supported by many people all along." He was now trying to do the same by helping others in need. (Most of my interviewees cited this to be the reason for sharing their experiences with me—so that people who were suffering from depression now could learn from their hardships.) Emphasizing the importance of rebuilding their relationships, a retired science professor talked about having started an "*Ikigai* (Purpose of life) Club" in his neighborhood, where retired residents got together to give talks on their respective

---

[4] The character "*shū*" is made up of the figure of a person whose hands are bounded in a shackle, thereby symbolizing a criminal, captured in this sense, in delusional attachment.

[5] The support group was originally established by a Morita-oriented psychiatrist and his patients. Though they rarely discussed Morita Therapy and its ideas, some of the philosophy that emerged from the group had affinity with them.

areas of expertise in an effort to remind them of the purpose of life (cf. Plath 1980). Depression for these men was certainly a disruption in their life, but it also provided an opportunity—albeit a difficult and bitter one—to reach a philosophical height that brought them a kind of inner freedom, and helped them establish new forms of social relationships beyond work.

Women's Depression: The Psychiatric Encounter as a Site of Power Struggle

> [I]n the larger context of Japanese culture, women's narrative productions of identity in work are not part of the central story. Their narratives are not the subjects of cultural celebration; indeed, their lives cannot be arranged into a teleological sequence of increasing mastery in work.
> —Dorinne Kondo, *Crafting Selves* (1990:259)

In sharp contrast to the culturally evocative, sympathetic portrayal of overworked salarymen in the popular discourse, until recently no clear master narrative had existed for female depression. And to an extent, this seemed also to be the case in medical discourse. While psychiatrists certainly pointed out the depression of housewives and the increasing number of young female patients, they remained much less eloquent about the plight of these women, as if they could not quite grasp or explicate the nature of their suffering. As some veteran psychiatrists I interviewed claimed, because women's symptoms "lacked clarity of shape" and took "heterogeneous forms," their depression "defied easy classification"—remaining more of an aberration in their model of depression. Perhaps reflecting the lack of a psychiatric master narrative, the women's narratives usually lacked a straightforward and uniform storyline that men's narratives often had. Instead, women's narratives were characterized by three types of "lacks": a *lack* of social and medical recognition, a *lack* of trust in medical professionals in general, and a *lack* of certainty in the meaning of their depression.

Lack of Recognition

Many of the women I interviewed began their narratives by describing their desperate search to have their pain recognized by others. This was the case with Endo-san, a fifty-nine-year-old director of a nursery, whose gentle yet restrained manner seemed to accentuate the quiet agony she suffered. The nursery she directed was originally founded by her father, a social work professor who, in the aftermath of World War II, opened his own home for the children of working parents in the poverty-stricken area in which they lived. Endo-san took over the nursery and expanded it successfully, to now accommodate ninety children and thirty staff members. Asked how her illness started, Endo-san recalled that she began to experience menopausal symptoms in her forties ("It's hard because menopause hits you when you are in the prime years of your work"), which also came to affect her mental state after she turned fifty. She lost interest in everything, did not want to see anyone, and felt too dull to get up in the morning to go to work. The lack of understanding on the part of her family further intensified her desperation: "Their innocent words hurt me, when they say things like why don't I go for a walk [to cheer herself up]. I guess it's no use expecting them to understand since they have never experienced it themselves. . . . I wish there were a barometer for the pain I feel . . . my husband, for one, is very healthy and thinks that I am just being lazy." She sought out various doctors and had numerous tests for the "heavy lead in the chest," but, despite these seemingly typical symptoms of depression, none of the doctors could help mitigate her pain. By the time she was referred to a neurologist, she had been driven to believe, like many of the women I met, that her ailment was incurable and suicide might be the only option to get away from it: "The pain was so bad that I scratched the tatami mattress in agony. . . . I grabbed the sleeve of the doctor's white coat and begged him to do something about it, to please let me be hospitalized."

Such a persistent failure of recognition—not only from families but also from medical professionals—was a theme that predominated in the narratives of the women I interviewed (cf. Lock 1987, 1991, 1993, Boddy 1989, Borovoy 1995, Martin 1987, Todeschini 1999a and b). I remember being taken aback by the harsh tone of a seemingly docile woman I met at a small clinic, who said: "My doctor listens to me all right but to what extent he really understands I have my doubts. I wish he could experience this pain himself so he would know how awful it is." Many women described how their symptoms were treated dismissively by various doctors as either "undiagnosable," and therefore not "real," or more commonly diagnosed as a "disorder of the autonomic nervous system" (*jiritsu shinkei shicchōshō*)—a taxonomic category often used as a "catch-all" diagnosis for what is labeled as nonspecific symptomatology (Rosenberger 1992).[6] Asked why female depression seemed so difficult to diagnose, some psychiatrists suggested that these doctors' failures to spot the underlying depression (or at least give a referral to a psychiatrist) might have to do with the way women often give complex, heterogeneous somatic complaints. Yet, this alone does not seem to explain the failure of medical diagnosis when, as doctors pointed out to me, some Japanese men complained of complex somatic symptoms as well.

---

[6] Note its similarity with the ICD-10's notion of autonomic dysfunction (a somatoform disorder not included in DSM-IV, but common in many other parts of the world because it includes many common somatic symptoms related to anxiety and depression or physiological dysregulation).

This leads me to the second explanation, which has to do with women's style of symptom presentation and causal attribution, whereby, instead of framing their depression as a straightforward product of overwork, women almost always raised multiple possible causes for depression up front. When asked what she thought was the cause of her depression, Endo-san began to explain how, at the time of her depression, she was being swept away by a series of hardships. In the nursery, cooking staff and nursery staff had a major conflict, in which Endo-san had to intervene as an intermediary. At home, her sister moved in with her after her daughter's husband's business went bankrupt. Endo-san, who was the guarantor for his business, suddenly found herself with a huge debt. While she seemed to shoulder all the burden without much help from her husband, her son—who had been the source of her support—married and moved out of her house, which intensified her feelings of loneliness: "I was so exhausted every day that I couldn't shake off the feeling of tiredness at the end of the day." Such narratives reflected the way women's lives were segmented into different roles with competing demands. Yet, their emphasis on the complex domestic and emotional problems may have made their depression appear more psychological in origin, which I suspect had led doctors to treat them with less urgency and concern. That is probably why, even in apparent cases of stress and "overwork"—accumulated both at work and at home—women's complaints lacked, in the eyes of the family and general practitioners, the clear shape of work-induced depression that a burned-out salaryman would be able to present, for instance, simply by stating his hours of overwork. In other words, what might have been at play here were not only cultural constructions of gender and the differential values placed on business (*public*) versus domestic (*private*) work but also *biological* disease versus *psychological* distress.

While this lack of recognition was most striking among the internists that women first sought for help, psychiatrists also seemed to hold moral—and implicitly gendered—orderings of different kinds of "depressions," which might have influenced the way they treated female depression. In the clinical practices I observed, psychiatrists certainly acknowledged women's stress in domestic spheres and rarely played down the significance of their emotional labor. They broadly interpreted the notion of overwork to include women's hardships and kept telling women how they overstretched themselves in demanding situations. Yet, psychiatrists also emphasized among themselves the traditional distinctions between what they considered a biological form of depression (called endogenous depression) and a psychologically caused depression (called neurotic depression) and treated the latter more dismissively.

This psychiatric ordering of soma over psyche seemed to clearly underline the experience of Nagano-san, a forty-nine-year-old librarian with the city library system. Her depression began five years ago, she said, when she was about to be promoted to a managerial position in the administration. As the nature of her work changed drastically, Nagano-san began to get "the shakes" at work, lose concentration, and spend many nights sleepless. Wondering if it was an early sign of menopause, she sought out an authority in psychosomatic medicine (a near branch of psychiatry in Japan), only to be diagnosed with the disorder of autonomic nervous system. The doctor must have treated her dismissively, she thought, because she first told him about her (psychological) problem with her husband that their "personalities were incompatible." Nagano-san was confounded when the doctor immediately scolded her: "You shouldn't be saying things like that," and began preaching and moralizing. She continued to suffer the same symptoms under his care, while people around her assumed that her ailment was nothing serious. The second doctor she met was a psychotherapist, who bluntly declared: "Your problem is a marital problem" ("as if that was all there was to it," Nagano-san said). Because her condition had deteriorated, she knew that the problem could not be that simple. The third doctor, a psychiatrist, "fluctuated in his decisions according to [her] mood." He would prescribe whatever increased amount of medication she requested, and she ended up suffering terribly from side effects of the heavy doses. Nagano-san had no idea how long it would take to be cured, or what goals she should be striving for.

Lack of Trust in Doctors and Quest for a Cure

The lack of medical recognition inevitably led to another lack among women, that is, a general lack of trust in doctors. Many women—while maintaining a congenial relationship with the current psychiatrist, who introduced the women to me—were nonetheless explicitly critical of medical professionals. These women's criticisms seemed to stem in part from their (high) expectations of doctors and their strong ambivalence toward what they perceived as dependency-fostering medical paternalism. Doi Takeo, in his highly acclaimed *The Anatomy of Dependency* (1973), argued for the positive values attached to dependency (*amae*) in Japanese relationships and suggested that the desire for mutual dependency and interrelatedness constitute the core of the "Japanese self." Given this reputed importance, it is interesting how these women (who persisted until finding the right psychiatrist) often explicitly resented such dependency. A number of women recounted how they were encouraged by their psychologically minded, seemingly empathic doctors to become dependent (*amaeru*) on them, only to end up feeling betrayed in the end. For example, thirty-year-old Kawano-san, after graduating from an elite university, mainly stayed home because of her depression. She described the nine doctors she had seen and how her "trust" was almost always "betrayed": "I think it's better not to tell them bad things that have happened. What you say comes back to haunt you . . . and you get hurt in a weird kind of way." Nagano-san, the librarian, spoke most eloquently about the intricate dynamics of power in psychiatric encounters. She said that she trusted Dr. Tanaka, her current doctor, because "he never tried to create an absolute relationship, where I would become dependent on him":

> You know how psychiatrists try to control patients; patients crave it as well because they want to get better easily. But if you get a piggyback ride, then the next thing you want is to be cradled in his arms. Dr. Tanaka avoided that; he never stepped into the core of my being.

While the men seemed to appreciate psychiatrists' benevolent paternalism and thrived under their protection, women repeatedly told stories where (even seemingly well-meaning) attempts by doctors to foster dependency appeared to reinforce their sense of powerlessness. Their desperate search for the right doctor thus became a way of recovering a sense of control (cf. Whyte 1997, Janzen 1978, Garro 1994). In some of the unfortunate cases I saw over the years, however, such women risked becoming—in the eyes of medical professionals—"problem patients," even "personality disorder patients," leading to a vicious circle of distrust on both sides.

Apparently, the difficulty that women had in building a trusting relationship with their doctors also had to do with the implicitly gendered nature of psychiatric encounters. The psychiatrists these women consulted with were mostly male, which seemed to create a problem in the realm of empathy in two aspects (see Luhrmann 2000, for a brilliant exploration of the use of empathy in American psychiatric training). On the one hand, there was a shortage of empathy on the part of psychiatrists because of gender difference. As some male psychiatrists admitted to me, they tended to be more empathetic and understanding regarding the struggles of their male patients. One thirty-seven-year-old doctor said that he just "knew"—without probing too much—the kinds of trouble that his middle-aged salarymen patients would complain of. Being a "middle-level manager" at the hospital himself, he felt that he shared with his male patients the same kinds of responsibilities and pressures that came with his job. In contrast, women's complaints—especially because most of the women in question did not appear to these doctors to have the same kinds of social responsibility that they could relate to—seemed less significant and the patients were therefore harder to empathize with. Interestingly, after I published a paper on the gendering of depression in a Japanese psychiatric journal, a number of psychiatrists made a point of coming up to me at conferences to tell me that it made them realize how "gender-biased" their empathy had been.

On the other hand, there is also a problem of excessive (or misdirected) empathy. As discussed above, some women pointed out how emotionally charged a psychiatric encounter could be, with its politics of intimacy and dependency.

Some of these women reminisced about a particular doctor they felt emotion-ally connected to for years, even if treatment had gone awry and ended in fail-ure. They often expressed ambivalent feelings toward these doctors, which, in some cases, made them especially cautious about entering another therapeutic relationship or expecting very much from a doctor. Yet because most Japanese doctors do not receive systematic psychotherapeutic training, they rarely ad-dress these psychological issues. Consequently, these women were left to deal with their ambivalence about their doctors by themselves, which also contrib-uted to unnecessary tension in therapeutic relationships and created a vicious circle of mistrust.

Lack of Meaning and the Question of Escape

Characteristically, these women's "depression" was long in healing, in part, no doubt, because the causes—and associated meanings—remained uncertain to the women themselves. Furthermore, their ideas about recovery were divided in two. On the one hand, the middle-aged women—despite their different ex-periences from men up to this point—sounded strikingly similar to their male counterparts when they talked about the need to relinquish control. Endo-san, the nursery director, said that through depression she was released from her "self-imposed pressure" (*kioi*) and was now able to "let things go, naturally." Nagano-san said she used to be "a bit of a perfectionist," difficult to deal with. Now she was much more easygoing, cheerful, closer to her family, and had more friends than ever: "Recovering from depression, I came to accept my own limitations. . . . I've gained the freedom by accepting my imperfections." On the other hand, the younger women I interviewed did not seem to find the same sense of "liberation" in such quiet resignation. Still early in their career, they could not comfortably claim the psychiatric master narrative about overwork as their own. Given their unstable job status, their battle with "depression" was often intertwined with their struggles to achieve professional identity. And while they desperately searched for a cure, they seemed to be constantly tor-mented by the fear that their "depression" might be of their own making—that it might be a disguised form of *escape*.

These tensions were evident in the narratives of Aoki-san, a thirty-four-year-old who was among the first generations of women to get a job after the imple-mentation of the Equal Employment Opportunity Law of 1985, which urged companies to end the quite common practice of setting restricted career tracks and implicit rules of early retirement (often for people in their twenties) for their female employees. As with many women of her generation, Aoki-san en-tered the workforce full of aspirations and expectations for her career. Her first job was at an extremely busy publishing company, where she enjoyed the inten-sity of the work and aspired to become like the experienced, senior female staff in the office. However, Aoki-san soon began to experience pain in the back of her eyes and excruciating headaches, for which she visited numerous doctors and received various treatments, none of which worked. Urged by her parents, she decided to quit work and seek out a cure. Repeatedly given the diagnosis of autonomic nervous system disorder with no prospect of recovery, she was eventually referred to a psychotherapist but remained doubtful of the effect of a "talking cure": "This doctor seemed to think that I would recover if he listened to the anguish of my heart (*kokoro no nayami*) and pointed to the psychological problem at the root. He wasn't concerned with the pain I was suffering at that moment." Aoki-san became so despairing that she "even went to see a man who was selling dubious "chlorella" (supplement) therapy. She was almost driven to believe him, she said with a laugh, when he told her that she needed to go through a "purification ceremony" for the ancestral curse that was causing her pain. Tormented by the feeling that she was being left behind by others, she kept thinking about what she would do when she turned thirty and "almost felt like killing [her]self."

When she was finally diagnosed with "masked depression" at a university hospital and prescribed antidepressants, her pain "miraculously went away." With a bona fide diagnosis, she said she initially felt "vindicated," especially before her father and brother, who had long insinuated that she was simply lazy. However, she soon began to feel the strain of the uncertain nature of her "depression." Now working at a small publishing company, she had recurrent symptoms and often wondered where to draw the line between a "real illness that required medical attention" and what was "only a headache." Similarly, thirty-one-year-old Noguchi-san, who had to abandon her dream profession as a nurse while battling with the illness, spoke of the "ambiguity of depression": "There is a core that is depression, but there are many gray areas around it, like feeling down, being socially withdrawn, not being able to get up in the morning, and being unable to go to work." The uncertainty of a psychiatric diagnosis seemed to torment many women I met: thirty-year-old Kawano-san, who had stayed home after graduating from university, talked about her frustration for not "having a career" and expressed doubt about her own "depression": "I don't know if I became sick because I wanted to become sick and so created the illusion that I was sick." Given the polymorphic symptoms and the lack of a ready diagnosis, these women seemed torn between their desire to have their "depression" legitimized and their doubts about the nature of their ailment.

These women's uncertainty may also have been intensified by the doubts that psychiatrists expressed over the authenticity of their depressions. During the years I did my fieldwork, I often encountered psychiatrists who were frustrated with the increasing number of people coming to see them for what they dismissively called "self-proclaimed depression" (*jishō utsubyō*). Psychiatrists working in the 1970s had discussed similar types of patients increasingly seen in clinics, whose illnesses were said to differ from traditional types of endogenous depression. They named such "neurotic" forms of depression: "escaping depression" (Hirose 1977) and "immature-type depression" (Miyamoto 1978). The patients they discussed at the time were often young salarymen, whose depressions seemed only to worsen when they had to work. These young workers, in the eyes of these psychiatrists, lacked the same sense of traditional Japanese work ethic and thus remained a deviation from Shimoda's model of the depressed (see chapter 5). With the introduction of SSRIs and a new wave of depression patients in the 1990s, psychiatrists were again confronted with the question of who had a "true depression." One frustrated psychiatrist even wrote an entire book on what he termed, "mimic depression" (*gitai utsubyō*) in order to make people aware of the distinction between a true (biological) depression and a mere (psychological) depressive state (Hayashi 2001). While psychiatrists often problematized the personality of the latter types of patients, such discourses were, it seems to me, dangerously moralizing. Particularly for stay-at-home, "unproductive" women, diagnoses lacked the moral certainty of the "true depression" of overworked salarymen. And lacking the culturally fitting terms to articulate their plight, women did not, and could not, discuss their pain as a public product of structural injustice as some men did, but attributed it largely to private matters.

The struggles of the young women discussed here may be a prefiguring of what is more broadly to come for all Japanese, however, who face the increasing uncertainty of their place in the work force. Lifetime employment and the seniority system, which had characterized the postwar employment system and set the basis of public life, have begun to crumble. Younger people are facing the risk of unemployment in the emerging society, even if this means they do not have to endure the suffocating sense, as the older generations did, of being bound to an organization that seeks to act as their benevolent family (Dore 1958, Rohlen 1974a). Younger women caught in this transition cannot seem to settle for a kind of quiet resignation and acceptance of their place in society. Their experience of depression remains intricately intertwined—and invested—with the question of their professional identity, and the family no longer serves as the major source of psychological fulfillment as it may once have (see Lock 1993). In this context, the local indigenous notion of recovery as relinquishing control may no longer provide these people with the same kind of liberation, as it seems increasingly at odds with the global "Prozac Narrative" of the current medicalization. As Jonathan M. Metzl (2003) points out, the Prozac Narrative is a "productivity narrative," which urges people to take pills and to bring out assertiveness and competitiveness, enhancing their ability even beyond their limits in order to take control of their lives. The younger women discussed here certainly seem to sense underlying tensions evoked by this psychiatric expansion. They thus draw upon psychiatric diagnoses to demand care and recognition for their pain, all the while being uncertain of what kind of "cure" this will ultimately bring.

The Politics of Causality in De-gendering Depression

Starting with the question of what may lie behind the peculiar gendering of depression in Japan, this chapter has suggested how the Japanese psychiatric master narrative about depression may have produced uneven hegemonic effects on men and women, possibly leading to under-recognition of female depression. On the one hand, it is striking how Japanese psychiatrists have created powerful and sympathetic descriptions of depressed men—how, for instance, a man's devotion to a company is no longer rewarded in the emergent neoliberal economic order. As if to reflect this psychiatric master narrative, depressed men mainly discussed their depression as caused by work stress, some explicitly linking their personal ailment with a recognizable form of collective pain. They seemed to recover by submitting themselves to the familiar, protective relationship with a psychiatrist and by accepting the psychiatric diagnosis of "depression" that provided, particularly for these overworked men, an institutionally legitimized form of temporary "escape." On the other hand, this psychiatric master narrative has created a curious void in the Japanese understanding of female suffering, bringing about real-life consequences on women's subjective experiences. Women rarely attributed their suffering to straightforwardly recognizable structural causes of depression. Instead, they placed their resistance more explicitly on medical paternalism, criticizing the kind of clinical encounters that they saw as reinforcing their own sense of powerlessness. These women's persistent quest for the right doctor thus became a way of gaining a sense of control, yet it also brought the risk of their being labeled as problem patients. Lacking public legitimacy for their "depression," some of these women were tormented by the fear that their illness might be a prolonged—even self-defeating—form of "escape." In such ways, the experience of depression—as well as the kind of reflexivity that it brings—takes on different forms according to gender, not because Japanese women suffer more than Japanese men or vice versa, but because the nature of their social suffering is structured differently.

This is rapidly changing with the global move to de-gender depression. The Prozac Narrative, as Metzl (2003) points out, is not only a productivity narrative but also an "equal-opportunity one," particularly in workplaces, where depression has emerged as an object of public anxiety linked to presumed loss of productivity.[7] Thus, while male depression is rapidly gaining a new sense of

---

[7] The centrality of work as the perceived cause of depression is in fact not limited to Japanese men. A recent broad-scale epidemiological study on depression in Europe (called DEPRES) has

urgency in North America, in Japan, where depression has long been linked to men at work, it is women who are now bombarded with information designed to make them aware of their "hidden" depression. As they are told by psychiatrists (who usually draw upon Western data) that it is women who are much more prone to this illness, women are becoming more accustomed to articulating their everyday distress in terms of "depression." And as general practitioners are also adjusting their own assumptions, "depressed" women—who might have gone undiagnosed before—are now seeking *and* receiving medical care (to be discussed in chapter 10). Some women are also actively resorting to the emerging system of social security, whereby depression is increasingly recognized as a "work hazard" and a legitimate reason for economic compensation. This is exemplified in a recent legal victory of a female worker, who successfully held Toshiba, Inc. (a megaelectronic company) liable for firing her after she took three years of sick leave from the depression that the court determined had been caused by excessive work stress (*Asahi*, May 19, 2009a). The fact that women are more visible in the *public* realm of work is helping instill the awareness that depression can afflict both men and women, bringing, somewhat ironically, gender equality to the realm of psychic suffering.

As the gender representations of depression begin to shift, How will this affect the *politics of causality*? Contrasting the discourses on menopause in North America and Japan, Lock (1993) has demonstrated that, despite the biomedical insistence on the body universal, the making of female maladies is in no way a uniform process. In particular, Lock has illuminated the moralized discourse about the female fragility in North America, which has served to pathologize women by emphasizing their "inherent" biological vulnerability, which also long underlined the gynecological discourse. While a similar discourse about female vulnerability seems historically much less pronounced in Japanese medicine (for reasons that remain to be investigated), I am also tempted to ask to what extent the peculiarly "socializing" discourse about the cause of depression in Japan owes to the fact that depression has long been treated as a male malady in Japanese psychiatry. In other words, can it be that the Japanese psychiatry's rather sympathetic discourse about the depressed—which has often emphasized social stress over individual vulnerability—is, after all, a product of a traditionally masculinized understanding of depression? And if so, as women are attracting more psychiatric attention, will they receive the same kind of "master narrative" from psychiatry that has done so much to legitimize male suffering?

---

also shown that while women were "characteristically more distressed by relationship problems and illness or death in the family," men "more frequently attributed the onset of depression to problems at work and unemployment " (Angst et al. 2002:205). Thus, the theme of work stress as the cause of depression may well in fact be universal; what may be distinctive in Japan is the extent to which work stress has been highlighted, both in popular and medical discourses, as the legitimate cause for depression.

Or, as some feminist critics in the West have expressed concern, will these women find that psychiatry will simply pathologize them by urging them to take pills without fully understanding their social predicaments? While the current medicalization will certainly make more women aware of their distress, whether this will bring social recognition of their pain, or end up silencing claims by the depressed by placing the blame on individual biological vulnerability, still remains uncertain. Perhaps, the question that needs to be carefully examined in the years to come is how psychiatry, in conjunction with the new legal system that recognizes depression as a work hazard, can provide an alternative framework for understanding complex causes of depression as it attempts to go beyond the monolithic dichotomizing of the social versus the biological.

PART THREE

Depression in Society

IN PART III, I turn to the effects of medicalization beyond the walls of clinics and examine how lay people and other professionals draw upon psychiatry as a framework for expressing—and interrogating—social ills. In particular, I examine the changes brought on by medicalization in the realms of legal debates concerning overwork depression and suicide, public debates about the nature of psychopharmacology, and the emergence of psychiatric science of work in industry.

Chapter 9 demonstrates how claims for the social origins of depression have gained force through a series of workers' legal victories against overwork depression and overwork suicide. Anthropologists have of late called attention to emergent forms of "biosociality" (Rabinow 1996) and "biological citizenship" (Petryna 2002), whereby a medical diagnosis or a patient identity becomes a means for the socially weak to collectively claim their victimhood and gain legitimacy for their suffering. Here, I examine the brief history of overwork depression and suicide in Japan in order to discuss how this new form of legitimation has been made possible. By illuminating the link between depression and work stress, psychiatrists have become engaged in a social movement against overwork that has brought doctors, lawyers, and depressed workers and their families together. Psychiatry is thus at the heart of important social changes, at times used to urge Japanese to question the status quo, particularly where model workers who have internalized a strong work ethic are driven to suicide. However, psychiatrists' attempts to address social causality are also creating epistemological tensions within the medical community, where doctors—faced with moral, rather than scientific, arguments about the nature of workers' psychiatric suffering—ultimately remain unsure of how to conceptualize the "social."

In chapter 10, I analyze the overall effects of the decade-long medicalization in three realms—legal/policy changes, public debates about antidepressants, and industrial management—based on follow-up fieldwork I conducted in 2008 and 2009. Discussing the contradictory effects of medicalization, I particularly focus on the rise of the "psychiatric science of work," whereby medical experts are increasingly called upon by government and industry to cultivate a system of scientific management for depressed workers. The political implications of this science remain highly ambiguous as the various actors—including doctors, lawmakers, and industrial managers—assert different ideas about the nature of individual vulnerability, what kind of causality exists between work stress and psychopathology, and how best to deal with depressed workers. By reflecting on historical attempts to conceptualize mental illness as social pathology, I consider future political implications of the emerging psychiatric science of work.

In closing reflections (chapter 11), I reconsider these local forces of medicalization in light of global political movements that are beginning to problematize the psychological burden of work through the discourse about depression. Questioning the allegedly sweeping effects of the ongoing medicalization, I ask in the end in what ways the Japanese articulation of social etiology of depression may be retained against the evidence of global, biological standardization.

CHAPTER NINE

Advancing a Social Cause through Psychiatry:
The Case of Overwork Suicide

Overwork Suicide

As DISCUSSED at the beginning of the book, overwork suicide and overwork depression have emerged as national concerns in 2000, when the Supreme Court ordered Dentsū, Inc., Japan's largest advertising agency, to pay the sum of 168,600,000 yen (approximately US$1,560,000 at the time) to the family of a deceased employee, Ōshima Ichirō.[1] This represents the highest amount ever paid for a worker's death in Japan. The Supreme Court determined that the cause of Ichirō's suicide was clinical depression, and that his depression had been produced by long and excessive overwork (*Asahi*, June 23, 2000). After the precedent-setting verdict, a number of similar lawsuits followed regarding the suicides of teachers, doctors, policemen, and employees of companies like Toyota, many of which brought victory (and economic compensation) to the families of the deceased workers (*Daily Yomiuri*, October 11, 1999, Amagasa et al. 2005). In the meantime, the government has implemented the Basic Law on Suicide Countermeasures in 2006, which pledges to reduce suicide rates by 2016 by 20 percent, while declaring that suicide should not be reduced to an individual problem but be seen as a "social problem" (*Asahi*, July 16, 2005).

Indeed, suicide has long been a battleground for arguments for and against social causality.[2] From the early 1900s, Japanese psychiatrists such as Kure Shūzō asserted that suicide be seen as a matter of individual pathology (see chapters 3 and 4). He criticized the Japanese popular idea that social predicaments drove people to suicide and claimed that the true cause lay in these people's diseased brains (Kure 1917). Though postwar psychiatrists had a reserved stance toward such genetic determinism, some even advocating social causes (Katō 1953, Ōhara 1975, Inamura 1977), psychiatrists' tendency to explain suicide in terms of mental illness rarely impacted the way Japanese had thought about suicide over a century. This has been fundamentally changing since the

---

[1] Hereafter referred to as "Ichirō." It is customary in such legal documents to use the first name so as to avoid confusion with other family members with the same last name.

[2] Note that it was in a dispute over the psychiatric argument of Esquirol (the originator of the modern notion of depression) that Durkheim advanced his social theory of suicide (Goldstein 1987).

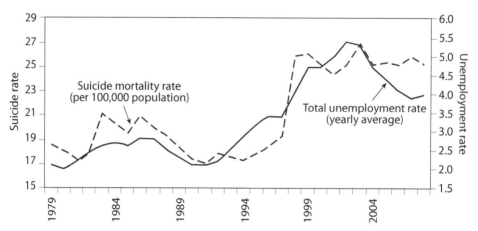

Figure 9.1. Changes in suicide mortality rate and total unemployment rate, 1979 to 2008. Source: Suicide statistics for 2008 by the National Policy Agency and labor force survey by the Ministry of Internal Affairs and Communication. Adapted from Kuwahara 2009, courtesy of Nikkei BP.

1990s, when the series of overwork suicide cases brought about a new awareness both in the government and the popular media. (Note that, although overwork suicide accounts for only a small segment of the total suicides in Japan, it has been disproportionally represented in the media and has played an important role, symbolically and politically, in changing the way Japanese deal with suicide.) Psychiatrists and lawyers involved in overwork suicide cases have argued that suicide is not a matter of individual will and intentionality—as the cultural view would assume—but rather needs to be understood as an unfortunate consequence of mental pathology. Yet, where their argument clearly departs from the traditional pattern of medicalizing suicide is the fact that they are using psychiatric ideas to argue for its social cause. Some of the psychiatrists actively involved in the overwork suicide cases are directly influenced by the antipsychiatry era of the 1970s, and together with socially oriented lawyers, they are changing the way Japanese think about suicide. By arguing for the pathological mechanism of suicide, they are directly asking how the corporations—and Japanese society itself—should take responsibility for these people's deaths (Kawahito 1996, Segawa 2001, *Asahi*, June 21, 2000).

In order to understand how psychiatry—which has been accused of biological reductionism—had come to be employed as a tool for advancing a social cause, I observed the proceedings of several overwork death/overwork suicide court cases at the Tokyo District Court, and attended conferences and a series of study groups held by the lawyers and psychiatrists involved in such cases. I also interviewed a number of psychiatrists at various medical institutions about their views on depression and suicide and conducted archival research on both psychiatric and legal papers on overwork suicide.[3] First, I will describe the history-making Dentsū Case, which established the social etiology by drawing upon psychiatric arguments. Second, I will illustrate how the government has responded to the social argument of suicide by introducing new ideas about "stress" and psychopathology. Third, I will examine the responses from psychiatrists and how they remain deeply conflicted over the conceptual transition from genetic determinism to social etiology. I ask, in the end, what may be the consequences—and problems—of advancing the social causality of suicide by way of psychiatry, and what implications this may have for the way Japanese think about those who are driven to take their own lives.

The Dentsū Case—How Lawyers Established the Social Cause of Suicide

The Dentsū Case verdict at the Supreme Court was undoubtedly a triumphant moment for social psychiatry as well as for workers' movements (T. Fujimoto 1996). As one of the plaintiff's attorneys, Kawahito Hiroshi said, for families to take such action against the employer for the suicide of their loved ones was almost inconceivable in the early 1990s. When people heard about the litigation, they would ask if it was the company, not the family, that was suing for the damage caused by the employee's suicide. Things have changed since then, and the verdict also sent a powerful message that suicide is a psychiatric problem. When the plaintiff's initial victory at the Tokyo District Court in 1996 was announced in the media, many Japanese heard, probably for the first time, that suicide could be caused by a mental illness called "depression" and that such an illness could affect anyone.

In the discussion that took place during the Dentsū case (see T. Fujimoto 1996, S. Fujimoto 2002), it emerged that Ōshima Ichirō, twenty-four years old at the time of his death, joined the company in 1990. He showed no abnormality in the medical examination taken two months prior to employment. He was healthy and athletic, and his personality was cheerful, honest, and responsible as well as tenacious and thorough. He was assigned to the Radio Department and eventually was put in charge of public relations for dozens of sponsors. On his usual working days, he would leave home by 8 A.M., commute for an hour, and spend the normal working hours dealing with clients and production companies. Because the daytime was taken up with such dealings, it was only after eating dinner at 7 P.M. that he could start tackling other tasks such as drafting proposals and researching new projects. Ichirō was given positive evaluations

---

[3] For archival research, I examined the *Japanese Journal of Psychiatry and Neurology* from its first issue in 1902 to the present, as well as a number of popular journals and a few of newspapers from the 1870s to the 2000s. I also used Japanese legal journals such as *Jurist* and *Hanrei Times* in order to investigate the legal discourses regarding overwork depression and overwork suicide.

by his bosses for his high incentive and enthusiasm. His tasks and responsibility gradually increased, and by August 1990 he began to come home past midnight or even spend the whole night in the office. In March 1991, his boss, having heard of Ichirō's all-nighters, urged him to go home at night. His workload was not reduced, however, with no new hires for his section that April. By the summer of 1991, his boss noticed that Ichirō seemed despondent, lacking energy and looking pale with an unstable gaze. Ichirō himself told the boss at the time that he was feeling a lack of confidence and was unable to sleep. Preparing for a big summer public relations event, Ichirō, weeks prior to his death, was working even longer hours, staying in the office all night every four days. Around this time, he was heard making pessimistic utterances, such as "I'm no use," "I'm no good as a human being." On August 23, Ichirō came home at 6 A.M., only to leave again at 10 A.M. to head for Nagano, where the public relations event was to take place. During the drive to Nagano, his boss noticed Ichirō's strange behavior: he was weaving while driving and talking about a "spirit" possessing him. After spending the next few days at the event and seeing it to its completion, Ichirō left Nagano on August 26, and reached home the following day around 6 A.M. He called in sick at about 9 A.M., and within an hour hanged himself in the bathroom.

In establishing that Ichirō's death had been a result of overwork, the plaintiff's attorneys had to clear three points of dispute: (1) the level of stress, (2) the presence and the nature of his depression, and (3) the nature of his suicide. First of all, the plaintiff's attorneys had to demonstrate the severity of the stress by showing how many hours of overwork Ichirō was engaged in. This seemingly straightforward task proved to be difficult when they looked into Ichirō's self-reported hours of work. According to this report, Ichirō's overtime fluctuated between 48 and 87 hours per month, and seldom went over the limits set up by the labor union at Dentsū. This clearly contradicted the testimonies indicating that Ichirō spent many nights in the office, even coming home at 6:30 A.M. only to leave for work again at 8:00 A.M. The reason for this gap was because it was customary for Dentsū workers to under-report the actual overtime they had worked (this practice in Japan is commonly referred to as "service overtime"). The plaintiff's attorneys therefore resorted to the building security reports by night guards, who kept the record of the times and the names of the employees who were still within the building at the time of their routine patrols. Based upon these reports, the attorneys calculated that the actual overtime Ichirō spent at night was 147 hours per month. This meant that Ichirō was in the office for double the amount of time of his normal working hours. The defense argued that (a) Ichirō's workload was not necessarily more than that of his colleagues; (b) Ichirō must have spent these hours doing other activities; and (c) Ichirō must have avoided going home for personal reasons. However, the judges added in the fact that Ichirō's daytime was already filled with scheduled meetings and communications with sponsors, which left him little choice but to stay up to finish his job. Considering that Ichirō was pressured by his boss to keep deadlines, the judges concluded Ichirō's consequent overwork was done under "general and comprehensive orders" from the company.

Second, having established Ichirō's stress from excessive overwork, the plaintiff's attorneys then had to prove that, as a result of overwork, he began to suffer *depression*. According to Fujimoto Tadashi, one of the plaintiff's attorneys, this seemingly "commonsensical idea"—that too much stress may cause mental illness—turned out to be extremely difficult to prove when they resorted to psychiatric theories for explaining such a mechanism (Fujimoto 1997:162). Ichirō never consulted a psychiatrist while he was alive, and the defendant asserted that Ichirō never suffered depression, that fatigue did not cause depression, and that he killed himself because of the failing relationship with his girlfriend. The plaintiff's attorneys, however, sought out psychiatrists' expert opinions and proved that Ichirō was, by August 1991, exhibiting typical depressive symptoms such as despondency, low energy, and pessimism. The attorneys particularly relied on the expert opinion of Kaneko Tsuguo (then-current director of Matsuzawa Hospital), who cited German psychiatrist P. Kielholz in arguing that Ichirō suffered "fatigue depression" caused by long-term chronic fatigue, sleep deprivation, and work stress. The plaintiff also pointed out other psychological stress caused by the inhumane work culture at Dentsū. They cited, for instance, how at one drinking party, Ichirō's superior poured beer in his own shoe and forced Ichirō to drink out of it, hitting him when Ichirō refused to obey his orders (Fujimoto 1997). Illustrating how Ichirō was gradually driven to the edge physically and psychologically, the plaintiff demonstrated successfully that the work stress produced his depression.

Lastly, the dispute remained over where the responsibility lay for Ichirō's *suicide*—whether or not Dentsū could have foreseen such a risk and how much the company, as opposed to the worker himself, should have been responsible in managing their employee's health (Segawa 2001). As a legal scholar Okamura points out, companies had rarely been held responsible for a worker's suicide because in Japan the legal definition of suicide itself had been based on the idea of "intentionality and free will" (Okamura 2002). Public administrators had also assumed suicide to be, in principle, an "intentional and deliberate" act of killing oneself, and thus outside such compensation coverage (*Hanrei Times*, 1998). The rare cases in which worker's compensation was granted were when suicides occurred as a result of clear accidents on the job. These included a case of a truck driver who caused a crash and impulsively committed suicide from the (false) belief that he had killed someone. In such cases, the deceased were judged to have been in such an extreme psychological state (called "non compos mentis") that they were driven to the act without fully comprehending its consequences.[4] In the Dentsū case, however, because Ichirō had not seemed to

---

[4] Such psychological states are called "non compos mentis" and include the condition of (a) stupor (clouding of consciousness), (b) delirium tremens (stupor accompanied by psychomotor agitation), and (c) psychotic/dissociative state accompanied by xenopathic experience (governed by hallucination and delusion or severe depressive state) (see Kuroki 2002).

be in such a psychotic state prior to his death, the question remained if his suicide was of a pathological nature or out of free will. The Supreme Court determined that Ichirō's suicide was a result of his reactionary depression by accepting the plaintiff's argument that it was caused by chronic overwork. In the verdict, the judges even ventured into Ichirō's psychological state before his death, and pointed to the significance of the fact that Ichirō killed himself on the morning right after the completion of the important project. The verdict stated that the project completion suddenly relieved him of the psychological burden (*kata no ni ga orita*), while at the same time created in him the dreadful anticipation (and despair) for the kind of life that awaited him from that day on. The judges concluded that Ichirō thus committed suicide impulsively and accidentally, under the influence of the depression that had affected his way of thinking. The Supreme Court pointed out Dentsū's negligence in having taken no concrete measures to adjust Ichirō's workload even after his superiors became aware of his deteriorating health. As legal scholars have emphasized, the Supreme Court verdict was intended as a public warning for employers to be responsible for not letting their employees' stress accumulate beyond a reasonable limit and for protecting their mental health at the workplace.

The Emerging System for Protecting Workers' Mental Health

Creating the New Guidelines

The rising number of such lawsuits led to the establishment of the new guidelines of mental health in workplaces (Kuroki 2003). After the Dentsū verdict, the Ministry of Labor became increasingly concerned with the fact that juridical decisions were directly challenging and overruling the decisions made by its Labor Standard Inspection Offices. For instance, the very first application for worker's compensation for overwork suicide had been submitted in 1989 by the wife of a (metal) press operator who died from hanging himself (Nishimori 2002). The man was routinely working till 2 or 3 A.M., only to return to work after a short nap at home. In fact, his overwork time—90 to 150 hours per month—had been so excessive that his company even arranged to have part of his salary paid to his wife's bank account so as to avoid officially violating labor regulations. Although he had talked about quitting the job, his strong sense of responsibility kept him at work, especially after he was promoted to unit leader. (Note that people who kill themselves from overwork are often regarded by their peers and superiors to be highly responsible and dutiful. Some even leave a suicide note with minute directions for unfinished work and with apologies to their company for not having done better [Kamata 1999]). Left with young children, his wife filed the application for workers' compensation for his suicide, but heard nothing from the inspection office for years. Finally she was notified in 1995 that her request had been turned down (as it was revealed later, despite the fact that consulting psychiatrists diagnosed his death as having been caused by overwork). The wife decided to take the inspection office's decision to court, finally winning the compensation in 1999 after a long battle (*Nihon Keizai Shimbun* [*Nikkei*], March 12, 1999). As similar legal decisions followed, it was apparent that there was an undeniable gap between the governmental policies and juridical decisions, and the government was under increasing criticism about the lack of transparency in the process of granting workers' compensation. And for other families who were making such legal actions, overwork litigations have become a way of finding out how their father or husband had been driven to such extreme mental state and reaching the "truth" about their death (Fujimoto 1997, Kawahito 1996, 1998).

Standardizing Stress

In response to mounting public criticism, the Ministry of Labor in 1998 solicited legal scholars' and psychiatrists' input and set up a special committee in order to create a new standard for approving workers' compensation for the mentally ill, which was issued and distributed to all the Labor Standard Inspection Offices nationwide in September 1999 (*Monday Nikkei*, December 27, 1999). The guidelines on mental illness caused by psychological stress at work give a flowchart and tables to aid the examiners to measure workers' stress and determine the causal relationship between overwork and mental illness. For compensation to be granted in a case, it has to be demonstrated that (1) the employee suffered mental illness; (2) there was strong (psychological) stress at work within half a year before they became ill; and (3) their mental illness was not caused by nonwork-related stress or personal reasons (and that they did not have a previous history of mental illness and alcoholism). Having met these conditions, the level of stress that workers were exposed to is measured according to the newly created Stress Evaluation Tables (see Okamura 2002). These tables list thirty-one items respectively both for work and nonwork-related stressful events. Work stress includes categories such as (1) accidents and disasters; (2) failures and excessive responsibilities on the job; (3) changes in the quantity and quality of work; (4) changes in employment status; (5) changes in job roles and ranks; (6) troubles in interpersonal relationships; and (7) changes in interpersonal relationships. Each item under these categories describes a specific event, which is given a predetermined number of points. For example, the events that are considered the severest stress and thus given 3 points (the highest score) include: having a major injury or a traffic accident, or making a big mistake on the job and being forced to quit work. The events given the lowest points (1) are: promotion, a change of boss, trouble with a client, and increases or decreases in the number of subordinates to oversee. There is also a similar table for nonwork-related psychological stress, which includes events such as a death in the family (3), divorce (3), pregnancy (1), personal illness (2), financial loss (3), child's school entrance examination (1), worsening environment at home (2), relocation (2), and betrayal by a friend (2). Adding up these points to calculate the total score for stress, the consulted expert is then expected to determine if such stress actually led to some changes in work or in interpersonal relationships at work, and if the work stress significantly outweighed that of personal stress. If it is then determined that there was a strong level of work stress and that the worker suffered a mental illness as a consequence, then such cases are approved for compensation. These Stress Evaluation Tables are supposed to standardize and speed up the process of examining each case, so that judgments can be made not only by the Ministry itself (which used to examine all such applications) but also by respective inspection offices (*Asahi*, July 31, 1999, Okamura 2002). These stress tables make it clear that the government is now ready to accept the causal link between stress and mental illness.

Challenging the Traditional Psychiatric Nosology

The second change implemented—and what most shocked the psychiatrists—was that the guidelines officially abolished Japanese psychiatry's conventional nosology. Previously, consulting psychiatrists would use the traditional notions of endogenous versus reactionary depressions in determining the cause of suicide. If psychiatrists gave the diagnosis of endogenous depression, then there was small chance for workers' compensation because the blame was implicitly placed on the worker's predisposition. This actually became a point of contestation in the Dentsū Case, particularly in the second set of proceedings at the Tokyo High Court, when the defense lawyer drew on the authority of Japanese psychiatry to argue that Ichirō's serious and overly meticulous personality (Typus Melancholicus) was a sign of endogenous depression. Taking into consideration the argument made by the defense that the company should not be held responsible for the worker's weak constitution, the Tokyo High Court introduced a measure of comparative negligence and reduced the original amount of compensation by 30 percent. The 1997 verdict clearly reflects this traditional psychiatric theory of depression:

> Not everyone becomes depressed from being overworked or being in a stressful situation. The individual constitution and personality are also factors involved in causing depression. Ichirō was serious, responsible, thorough, and a perfectionist; he had the tendency to voluntarily take up a task and responsibility for it beyond his capacity. It cannot be denied that his so-called melancholic premorbid personality resulted in increasing the amount of his own work, leading to delays and inappropriate methods of managing the work, and creating situations where he worried

about the outcome of tasks that were beyond his control. (Tokyo High Court 1997)[5]

Though this premorbid personality theory had been routinely applied in over-work depression/suicide cases, the Supreme Court rejected this argument and stated that personality factors should not be used as reasons for comparative negligence as long as the worker's personality remains within the expected range of variance among the group of workers engaged in the same type of work. The Supreme Court added that employers have the obligation to accom-modate workers' different types of personalities and assign them to appropriate tasks accordingly. This decision challenged the psychiatrists' traditional concept of "endogeneity" in Japanese psychiatry, which, because it is etiology-based, had served to predetermine the cause of illness before the legal decisions could be made (Kuroki 2000a).

In response to such verdicts, the government adopted the "stress-diathesis" model of mental illness so that each illness could be clearly conceptualized as a product of interactions between individual factors and social factors. In addi-tion, the government adopted the ICD-10 as the standard nosology for examin-ing cases of workers' compensation, and thereby significantly expanded the range of mental illness that could be considered for workers' compensation (*Daily Yomiuri*, April 11, 1999); the guideline now includes all of those mental illnesses categorized under the ICD-10's F0 to F4.[6] This is truly a radical move (particularly for traditional Japanese psychiatrists), as the international nosol-ogy has mostly abolished the notion of assumed etiology and thus opens up possibilities for almost all forms of mental illness to be legally examined for their social cause. This has the implication of seriously challenging the prevail-ing notion in traditional Japanese psychiatry that some illnesses—such as en-dogenous depression and schizophrenia—are genetically based (Kuroki 1999, 2002).

Redefining Suicide of Resolve

Another important change—which was extensively reported in the popular media—is the way suicide was now redefined in the guidelines (Watanabe 2002). As Okamura points out, legal scholars long held that suicide was a mat-

[5] The verdict adds, in parentheses, "Even though, in society in general, such a [melancholic pre-morbid] personality and behavioral tendencies are usually regarded as virtues, and thus this point should not be overemphasized," but nonetheless used this argument for comparative negligence.

[6] These include: F0: organic, including symptomatic, mental disorders; F1: mental and behav-ioral disorders due to psychoactive substance use; F2: schizophrenia, schizotypal and delusional disorders; F3: mood (affective) disorders; and F4: neurotic, stress-related and somatoform disorders.

ter of "intentionality and free will" and thus excluded it from workers' compensation (Okamura 2002). As discussed above, the only suicides that would be considered for compensation were acts committed in an acute psychotic state (non compos mentis) when the worker failed to comprehend the consequences of their act. If a worker left a suicide note, this was seen as a proof of mental competency and was automatically assumed to lie outside of compensation coverage, regardless of individual circumstances. The new guidelines' broader definition of mental illness also brought changes in this regard. Even if workers were not severely psychotic and even appeared to be acting normally—if they were suffering some form of mental illness that affected their cognition and behavior—then such suicides could be deemed pathologically driven. The media has emphasized this change, noting that "suicide of resolve" (kakugo no jisatsu) may be a result of depression and that the presence of a suicide note does not necessarily indicate that the person had acted normally and intentionally (*Asahi*, July 31, 1999; also see the discussion at the Labor Committee held in the Lower House in November 15, 2000). Apparently, the long-held legal—as well as cultural—assumptions about suicide were being transformed.

The effects of these changes were immediate. Over the twelve years from 1983 to 1995, the Ministry of Labor approved workers' compensation for only 7 cases of mental illness (3 of which were suicides) (*Nikkei*, May 23, 2002). Both in 1996 and 1997, the number remained a modest 2, and then went up to 4 in 1998. In 1999, however, the number notably increased to 14 cases (11 suicides). After the guidelines came out, the number of approved cases suddenly went up to 26 (19 suicides) in 2000, 100 (43 suicides) in 2002 (*Nikkei* June 18, 2005), and as many as 269 (66 suicides) in 2008 (*Asahi*, June 9, 2009).

Further Points of Contestation

Can Stress be Objectified?

Even with these policy changes, the juridical world was producing even more drastic decisions, further pushing the government—and the traditional psychiatrists—to accept a broader range of social causes for the mentally ill. In the meantime, the first contestation emerged with regard to the definition of "stress." Psychological stress, like pain, is notoriously difficult to measure. One worker can feel stressed out about his or her promotion while another might simply enjoy the challenge. Also, any one individual worker may take trouble with a client more seriously one day than s/he would on another day. As psychiatrists involved in overwork suicide cases have often emphasized, psychological stress is subjective and how the worker experiences the stress remains ultimately unknowable. Despite such psychiatrists' concerns, the Ministry of Labor seemed intent to define stress as objectifiable and not as a subjective experience. Probably in attempt to avoid the slippery slope such a relativist argument could take, the guidelines are explicit on this point of objectivity:

> In evaluating the stress level, examiners must base their judgment not on how the person subjectively responded to the event ... but on how the same ranks of workers (engaged in the same kinds of work, position with the same kind of experience), would generally respond to it. (Ministry of Labor 1999, cited in Okamura 2002:382)

This notion of "objective stress," however, was immediately questioned by the judges presiding in the overwork suicide case of a Toyota employee (*Nikkei*, March 12, 1999). This is a controversial case in many ways. Though the final verdict in 2001 was often reported in the newspaper as a "victory for the weak" (e.g., *Asahi*, June 18, 2001), the man in question was apparently an ideal "Toyota Man." According to the verdict, the assistant manager at Toyota killed himself in 1988 at age thirty-five. He was well liked by everyone and highly evaluated as a well-balanced, thorough, serious, cheerful, and easygoing person. He exhibited good leadership and was able to speak his mind while maintaining good relationships with people around him. He was also a bit of a perfectionist, meticulous, sensitive, and tended to carry the work burden by himself. He was healthy and highly athletic, having competed on the rowing team at the National Athletic Meet in high school; he played rugby in college and climbed mountains for a hobby. A good father and a dedicated worker, he had rarely complained about work and even seemed to thrive on challenges. Yet, around the time before his death, Toyota was trying to reduce the employees' overwork hours without necessarily reducing the workload, which soon began to affect this man's life. With the pressure under the "Just-in system," where a small delay in one section could profoundly affect the whole production system, the assistant manager was working with strict deadlines. While the number of subordinates he had to oversee doubled in a short time and there was a delay in his section, the man was distressed about having to draw up a plan that he knew would be hard to meet. Around this time, he also received an order for an overseas trip to be scheduled six months later (which coincided with a deadline) and another order to serve as a chairperson for the labor union, a task that would be highly time-consuming. Two months prior to his death, his wife noticed that he was beginning to complain that he could not finish his work; he would suddenly open up a design plan on the dinner table and wake up in the middle of the night to jot down ideas for work. On August 25th, he came home and told his wife that he could no longer "keep up with the Toyota way," and confessed that he had gone up to the company rooftop that day to jump off, only stopping himself when his children's faces came to his mind. That night, as his wife saw him bathing with their one-month-old daughter and weeping quietly in the tub, she made him promise to go see a doctor the following morning.

He left the apartment before dawn, however, and jumped to his death from a nearby building.

What immediately surfaced as the points of dispute were the level and the sources of his stress. Under the company policy to reduce overwork at the time, the man's timesheets did not show excessively long hours of overwork (though disputes remained as to the actual hours of "service overtime" and the time he spent working at home). Not surprisingly, the defense argued that the assistant manager's workload was no more than that of his peers and that it was his own weakness (his "melancholic premorbid personality") that was the true cause of his suicide. The plaintiff, however, argued that it is *not the quantity* but rather the *quality* of the work that should be considered, and the fact that his work had grown increasingly intense over a short period of time under the new company policy. The Nagoya District Court accepted this argument that what should matter is not how each stress is "objectively" scored—as in the Stress Evaluation Tables—but how the worker himself experiences the stress. The verdict went even further in arguing that the standards for work conditions should be set to accommodate not the "average" worker—as the Ministry's guidelines state—but rather those who are "most vulnerable to stress." The verdict is explicit that workplaces should not exclude those workers who might be more vulnerable to psychological stress than others, as long as their personalities remain within an acceptable range found among the workers doing the same kind of job and having a similar age and experience. The Nagoya District Court also added that the causal mechanism of depression is yet to be scientifically proven and that the government's guidelines fail to provide a clear and sufficient standard. In so doing, the Court was urging the government to reconsider its labor policies (*Daily Yomiuri*, March 30, 2004).

Whose Level of Stress Should be the Standard?

In challenging the government's definition of stress, then, the Toyota verdict also raised an important question about how much corporations—and perhaps society itself—have to change to accommodate the needs of the "weak." The dissenting government (or the Toyota Labor Standard Inspection Office) appealed to the Nagoya High Court, only to lose again on the same grounds (*Asahi*, July 9, 2003). After their defeat, the Minister of Health, Welfare, and Labor,[7] Sakaguchi Chikara, made a point of appearing in the media to say that they decided not to take the case to the Supreme Court because the High Court already accepted [their] argument that the Ministry's standards were appropriate (*Asahi*, July 18, 2003). However, the verdict is strangely ambiguous on this point; it only states that the District Court's decision that the people who are

[7] The Ministry of Labor and the Ministry of Health and Welfare merged to create the Ministry of Health, Welfare, and Labor in 2001.

"most vulnerable to stress" should be the standard for work environments, and is in essence the same thing as the High Court's idea that the standard should be for the "average" worker (the question of who is the "average" worker has since been raised). While this issue seems to have remained, in my eyes, largely unresolved, the psychiatrists I met through the study group on overwork suicide were clearly aware of the profound implication that the Toyota verdict could have, and some explicitly criticized it and said that it had "gone too far."[8] They knew that, if this decision was to be taken seriously, then work conditions in Japan must be fundamentally changed to accommodate a wider acceptance of the mentally ill, who had long been excluded from workplaces. This also had to do with accepting on a much broader scale collective and social responsibility for the mentally ill before asking about their individual responsibility (also see Fujikawa 2000, *Asahi*, February 23, 2001).

In fact, as they see their long-held assumption about the "endogeneity" of depression abolished by the policy change, some Japanese psychiatrists seemed uncomfortable about how far the argument for social causality should be extended. Regarding depression, the claim for social causality apparently has not troubled psychiatrists very much (though this is also changing), partly because the depressed—or at least the Japanese psychiatric representations of the depressed—provided a certain moral legitimacy for their suffering. As we have seen, Japanese psychiatrists have long asserted that it is the personality of the ideal Japanese worker (diligent, thorough, and responsible) that is most prone to depression. By arguing that the Japanese work culture itself reproduces and rewards such a personality, to the point that workers begin to take their responsibilities too much to heart (see chapter 5), psychiatrists see some justice in demanding corporate responsibility for these workers' suicides. However, psychiatrists have remained much more ambivalent about other illnesses, particularly schizophrenia, for which blame is implicitly placed on the individual in the diagnosis itself, in the form of assumed genetic vulnerability. Because the government's guideline adopted the ICD-10 criteria, extending the workers' compensation to most mental illnesses, psychiatrists are now faced with the inevitable question—is schizophrenia socially caused as well?

This question about personal vulnerability briefly surfaced as a potential problem over one of the first cases of overwork suicide (Nakazono 1998). In

---

[8] Some depression experts I interviewed complain of the simplistic model of depression that lawyers and judges use. On more than one occasion I witnessed, during an overwork suicide case being deliberated in the Tokyo District Court, how the presiding judges were asking doctors to pinpoint precisely on what date the worker's depression began (as if it were an infectious disease that has a clear moment of origin). And over the Toyota case, psychiatrists also wondered what exactly constituted the cause and effect, as some of the stressful events deemed to be the cause of his depression seemed to have occurred after the man was already manifesting depressive symptoms. Thus they have asked if these events were so stressful that the man became depressed, or if these events became particularly stressful because he was already depressed (Nomura et al. 2003).

another case, whose verdict was reached about a month after the initial Dentsū verdict in 1996, one psychiatrist argued that the worker had schizophrenia and clearly stated that it was a matter of predisposition and not of work stress. In this case, the worker was Kōno Jirō, who graduated from an elite university to join a steel manufacturer in Kobe in April 1983. In December of the same year, because of his good English skills, Jirō was sent on a business trip to India, near Bombay, scheduled for two months. He was to serve as an interpreter-cum-assistant for a Japanese engineer already in India and two other staff members to arrive on January 13th, who were to conduct business with an Indian company and a European company. Troubles awaited Jirō upon his arrival, however, as the Indian company's guesthouse rooms that the Japanese staff had been promised, suddenly became unavailable. Concerned about the unexpected expenses of having to stay at a hotel, Jirō tried to negotiate with the Indian company, to no avail, and his attempts to seek instruction from the Japanese office also failed because of poor conditions for telecommunication. At the time when the two Japanese staff arrived on January 13th, the engineer noticed that Jirō was becoming increasingly distressed and repeatedly and excessively apologizing for the accommodation inconvenience, blaming himself though it was not his fault. On January 15th, Jirō was seen staring blankly at the ceiling, acting strangely, and not remembering his (odd) behavior when asked about it later. On January 16th, the concerned engineer and another member of staff decided to drive Jirō to Bombay in order to establish communication with the Japanese office and to seek medical care for him. Jirō hardly spoke or responded to questions during the drive. After checking into the hotel, Jirō quarreled with the engineer, asking him why he was trying to send him back to Japan, telling the engineer to get out of their room. That night, Jirō jumped from his hotel room on the 16th floor and died instantly.

The three psychiatrists consulted in this case could not agree on the diagnosis. The first psychiatrist gave a diagnosis of reactive psychosis caused by work stress. The second psychiatrist stated that it was a brief reactive psychosis with depressed features and that his suicide was accidental. Notably, both of these doctors also added that the gravity of such stress was subjective and thus ultimately lay beyond a psychiatrist's knowledge. The third doctor, however, gave the diagnosis of schizophrenia, stating that it was a "personal illness"; Jirō's schizophrenia, he said, was not caused by work stress and that it merely triggered it (the true cause being his predisposition). The Court rejected the schizophrenic diagnosis, arguing that Jirō had shown no previous signs of delusions and hallucinations. They determined that Jirō had suffered a brief reactive psychosis or reactive depression caused by the stress of working in a difficult situation in a foreign country, and that his suicide had been committed in a state of non compos mentis. This verdict was later discussed by psychiatrists, in a roundtable discussion on overwork suicide, as one of the problematic cases where diagnoses had significantly differed among psychiatrists (Nomura et al.

2003). They brought up another case of a schizophrenic worker, which ended in an out-of-court settlement, where the company recognized his illness as having been caused by work stress. Then they raised the question of to what extent social stress could be seen as a cause of mental illness and how much individual predisposition and personality should be taken into account (Nomura et al. 2003, Nakazono 1998).

While at the moment arguments for the social etiology of mental illness have received much attention in the media, there have been cases—even after the Dentsū verdict—where the workers' own personal vulnerability has become an issue. Some judges have rejected claims for compensation or have adopted comparative negligence and significantly reduced the amount of compensation as a way of placing certain responsibilities on the part of the workers. For instance, in a case of a kindergarten teacher who became depressed and committed suicide after she had already quit the kindergarten, her personality and psychological factors were given much weight. In this case, the Osaka High Court introduced an argument for comparative negligence and reduced the original amount of compensation by 80 percent (Fujimoto 2002:145). The fact that "no history of mental illness" in the worker's life or in the family is stated as a prerequisite for compensation coverage in the guideline also suggests ambiguity as to what extent social causality can be argued for the mentally ill (Nishimura 2001). As Kuroki points out, the tension between genetic arguments and socially deterministic arguments is becoming more pronounced now as the distinction between "private illness"—which is dealt with as a personal and family problem—and "public illness"—for which social responsibility is demanded—begins to blur (Nomura et al. 2003, Kashimi 2001, Kuroki 2000a).

Who is Responsible for Workers' Suicides?

Though psychiatrists remain conflicted and divided over social causes, they are nonetheless increasingly implicated in the social management of mental illness and suicide. Up to the early 2000s, most of the overwork suicide cases for which they were asked expert opinions were cases where the "patients" died without having consulted a psychiatrist, for which psychiatrists could only provide a posthumous diagnosis. Now, psychiatrists are faced with an increasing number of depressed patients who seek them out hoping they can provide a cure for their illness, or by their families who expect them to avert the danger of suicide. Companies as well, concerned with the risk of employees' depression and suicides (and of potential litigations), are also urging sick leave and psychiatric consultation. The Ministry of Health, Welfare, and Labor has also revised labor safety laws, which make it mandatory for anybody working more than 100 overwork hours to be examined by a medical doctor (see chapter 10). With the Basic Law on Suicide Countermeasures of 2006, psychiatrists are increasingly expected to play the central role in preventing suicide (*Asahi* July 16, 2005).

This reflects the shift in Japanese attitude towards suicide, which has long been regarded with a certain sense of romanticism and aestheticization, but for which little practical intervention has occurred (e.g., Ōchi 2001). Given such rising expectations, how do psychiatrists themselves regard their role in the social management of suicide?

It may not be an exaggeration to say that, until recently, most Japanese psychiatrists have taken a "hands-off" approach to suicide. While the biologically oriented Japanese psychiatrists have, over a century, asserted that suicide is largely a product of mental illness, they have also been sensitive to the traditional, cultural sentiment that has regarded suicide as an act of individual free will. This ambivalence was once clearly manifested in the debate over the existential, humanistic perspectives of the 1960s and 1970s, when psychiatrists asked whether the existential angst that drove people to their own deaths could be understood and treated by a biological approach, and if it was acceptable that such people's subjective vulnerability should remain unknowable. This seemingly humanistic argument was also used, however, to emphasize the difficulty of preventing suicide (see chapter 7; also see *Hanrei Times* 1998). In a 1985 case, parents sued a mental hospital for having failed to prevent the suicide of their depressed son, who was hospitalized there. Echoing the humanistic discourse of the era, the judge ruled in favor of the doctors by emphasizing the "individuality" of the therapeutic relationships between respective doctors and patients:

> [Depression] is, after all, not a physical disease that merely affects partial organs but is something profoundly rooted in the depth of a person. As such, there is no mechanical, objective measure to evaluate mental symptoms and they can only be captured through personal interaction between the doctor and the patient. . . . In essence, psychiatric practice can only exist as an expression of such individuality and the personality of the therapist. (cited in Nishizono 1986:190)

Such reasoning would probably not work in the current context, when depression is being discussed as a "physical disease," and suicide as something treatable by antidepressants. Not surprisingly, though, most psychiatrists I interviewed at universities and mental hospitals seemed unenthusiastic about having to treat a much broader range of patients and becoming more responsible for the prevention of suicide. This is partly because of the difficulty of the tasks involved and of the uncertainty of their own "objective" knowledge of depression and suicide (Kuroki 2000b). As one suicide expert told me, writing a psychiatric expert opinion for an overwork suicide case is almost in the realm of "storytelling," where you already have a conclusion and piece together the information and build up a case to establish either the genetic story or social story. With much of their etiological theories of mental illness still open to dispute, they have little on which to go in terms of "hard science" in making either argument. They are also hesitant to get involved because they are strongly wary of the potential criticisms they face against the expanding web of psychiatric surveillance.

As I was finishing this book, the government announced that it would introduce mental health checkups as part of the standard health examination. This is a significant move, since the government had long been highly cautious about intruding into the realm of workers' mental health (not least because of the strong oppositions from leading psychiatrists, who argue that it could lead to stigmatization of the mentally ill) (*Asahi*, July 15, 2010).[9] Thus, there is an increasing dilemma as to what extent psychiatrists should be involved in managing mental health, as the success of overwork suicide cases shift the focus from asking about workers' "self-responsibility" to demanding "corporate responsibility" (*Nikkei*, November 8, 2004, Nakajima 2001, Amagasa 1999a, 1999b, 2005), and if such a demand for collective responsibility may in the end give rise to wider—possibly insidious—forms of social surveillance (to be discussed in the next chapter).

The Medicalization of Suicide as a Form of Social Movement

The medicalization of suicide is thus made possible in Japan by a social movement that does not negate the cultural argument but rather actively incorporates it. That is to say, psychiatrists involved in overwork suicide have created a kind of conceptual marriage between the psychiatric view that redefines it as biologically caused and the cultural view that asserts that suicide be seen as socially produced. The current medicalization has not (so far) translated into a kind of biological individualism, where the deceased are denied any existential ponderings and intentionality. On the contrary, psychiatrists have gained popular appeal by drawing upon the cultural idea that reads meaning into suicide —as the silent resistance of the oppressed.

Yet such a social movement in the form of medicalization poses certain contradictions. First of all, Japanese remain largely unaware of the serious implications involved in accepting the psychiatric argument for suicide. Though the questions about individual intentionality are, for the time being, left unexplored, there is clearly a contradiction in the way the deceased are said to be so ill that they are unable to tell what they are doing, and the way they are seen by their families as having performed a meaningful social action. A quick glance at the testimonies of the families who have sued the companies and held them responsible for the suicide of their loved ones attests to this implicit duality, as

---

[9] This was announced by a Democratic administration that came into power in 2009, which ended more than a half-century's predominance of the conservative Liberal Democratic Party.

they often seem accepting of the psychiatric argument that the deceased was clinically depressed while still expressing the idea that their loved ones were "making a protest" by taking their own lives, against the companies that had done them an injustice. These testimonies make clear that these families still find a certain level of intentionality and meaning in the act of suicide, even if they regard the immediate cause of death to be depression (Kawahito 1998, Kamata 1999, *Shimbun Akahata* 2003). This raises questions about the extent to which people "truly believe" the psychiatric explanation, as opposed to using it as a means of getting public recognition for suicidal individuals' suffering. Such contradictions are left unexamined because of the ways in which the medicalization of suicide in Japan has proceeded largely as a result of the social and juridical forces outside of psychiatry itself, as a means of getting public recognition for social injustice. But sooner or later, Japanese will have to face up to the real implications of accepting a psychiatric argument that could seriously compromise their cultural view of suicide as an intentional act.

The second problem has to do with the uncertain scientific nature of the psychiatric arguments used in overwork suicide litigations, where, as we have seen, the psychiatrists' interpretations are often in conflict. For the time being, most psychiatrists find the extremity of some of the conditions in Japanese workplaces (and the societal "common sense" that has allowed overwork suicides to happen in the first place) as reason enough to justify the use of psychiatric arguments about cause and effect, even if some of these explanations lack scientific rigor. As workers' compensation is distributed more widely than before to cover the mentally ill at work, psychiatrists are now increasingly confronting the century-old question of how to tell malingerers from the true patients (Nikkei, January 21, 2000, February 13, 2002).[10] When this problem surfaces on a much larger scale, the uncertain scientific status of the psychiatric theories about the social etiology of mental illness will have to be challenged (cf. Duncan 2003). For now, however, psychiatrists remain largely silent about these contradictions.

Importantly, while psychiatry is transforming the cultural notion of suicide in Japan, Japanese psychiatry itself is being transformed via the discourse on overwork suicide. That is, by asserting multiple layers of explanation for suicide, it may just be possible that these families, lawyers, and psychiatrists are relativizing both the romanticized cultural argument and psychiatry's naïve genetic determinism. The Supreme Court decision in the Dentsū Case, and many subsequent legal disputes about overwork suicide, have depicted suicide and depression not as manifestations of stark insanity but as states between normality and abnormality. The overwork suicide discourse has thus "normalized" de-

---

[10] Some psychiatrists I interviewed also suspected that the governmental policy change was due to the fact that the vast unused budget of the Ministry of Labor for workers' compensation needed to be spent somehow.

pression in a significant departure from the genetic determinism of the past and the popularly held assumptions about the biological deficiencies of the mentally ill. Coupled with the global rise of depression discourse, the psychiatric discourse about overwork suicide may thus be indicative of a more fundamental conceptual shift that Japanese psychiatry has been going through—as it tries to overcome its rigid dichotomy between biological and social approaches to diagnosis and treatment, and moves toward a more complex, nuanced understanding of how people are driven to take their own lives.

CHAPTER TEN

The Emergent Psychiatric Science of Work:
Rethinking the Biological and the Social

Psychiatry as an Agent of Liberation

It's almost as if an entire town is disappearing every year.
Last year, 32,249 people took their own lives. . . . These
were 32,249 regular lives; 32,249 people in unbearable
pain. Each of the 32,249 had family and friends. The suicide rate of the "lost generation"—those who entered the
job market during a time of limited prospects for employment—has increased. Suicides caused by unemployment
and financial difficulties can be eliminated by appropriate
measures. Not to take these measures is nearly equivalent
to willful negligence.
—("Soryūshi," *Asahi*, May 15, 2009; also see figure 9.1)

BACK IN THE 1990s, my North American colleagues would appear incredulous
upon hearing me talk about overwork depression and suicide in Japan. They
would ask how it is that Japanese could be so blind and so unreflective as to
work themselves into depression, even driving themselves to suicide? In France,
the idea of "overwork death" itself was apparently curious enough that *Le
Monde* ran a number of articles about this Japanese phenomenon (e.g., Brice
1999). A decade later, however, the news of a spate of suicides among employees
of France Telecom made headlines around the world—suicides that were attributed to work stress that these employees were under due to the company's
radical restructuring (*BBC News*, September 12, 2009). Rising rates of suicide
and psychopathology in the workplace have also raised public concern elsewhere in Europe—most notably Italy, Germany, and Finland—where these are
often discussed as products of the increasing pressure people face in the new
neoliberal economic order. Like their Japanese counterparts, European commentators tend to emphasize how typical victims are not "deviants" but people
who have led well-adjusted lives, and that their pathologies should not be explained away by their individual biological/psychological weakness but rather
be interpreted, à la Durkheim, as social problems, even forms of social protest
(Moerland 2009). As depression and suicide in workplaces are becoming a

global concern, Japanese psychiatrists are now invited to other Asian countries to introduce the psychiatric criteria they have helped create for diagnosing the psychopathology of overwork. An idea that seemed strange only a decade ago—that one could be driven to depression by work stress—is now becoming a global reality as people increasingly experience the effects of a massive economic meltdown with a resulting "sense of vulnerability in being part of a world system" (Lupton 1999:49). This has given new energy to the theoretical foundation of psychiatry with a social perspective, which attests to how suicide and depression must be understood as social pathologies, although, paradoxically, this shift is taking place at a time when psychiatry in Japan is increasingly making use of antidepressants.

This growing psychiatric attention paid to the social causes of depression contrasts with the situation in the United States back in the 1990s, during which time the advent of new antidepressants such as Prozac created optimism for biological treatments for depression. The hype around Prozac then led to the proclamation that it would not only cure depression but also bring "pain-free happiness," even enabling one to somehow discover one's "authentic self" (see Rose 2007). However, as Carl Elliott (2003⁴) demonstrates, it is important to realize that this hype was also accompanied from an early stage by deep-seated anxiety (or what Gerald Klerman called "pharmaceutical Calvinism") as well as heated controversies among intellectuals (Healy 1997, Kramer 1993). There was debate at the time over whether the increase in the prescribing of antidepressants—encouraging individuals to use pills to fix their personal "defects"—would instill in them a false sense of control and reduce attention paid to possible social, structural causes of their distress. These critics asked if such technology might foster a desire for even more potent forms of biological self-enhancement, all the while constraining people's capacity for critical reflection and personal transformation (Degrazia 2000). It is thus not surprising that, as the initial hype has subsided in the United States, there has also been growing public debate in the media about how such an expansive role for pharmaceutical self-enhancement is in fact becoming a reality (Carey 2008). For instance, a 2008 article in *Nature* reported that a surprising number of scientists are now taking antipsychotic drugs to boost their productivity, even though many remain uneasy about the side effects and the moral implications of their act (Maher 2008). As these scientists even seem pressured to *voluntarily* take drugs in order to actualize the desirable selfhood, more and more people are beginning to wonder if acts like this may soon take on an inevitable, iron-cage-like quality in a society that demands the endless pursuit of personal growth and advancement (cf. Franklin and Roberts 2006).

I have argued throughout this book that the socializing discourse about depression and suicide in Japan of the last two decades—which is also rapidly evolving in Europe and other parts of Asia—provides a strikingly different picture of medicalization from that of the United States. These differences partly

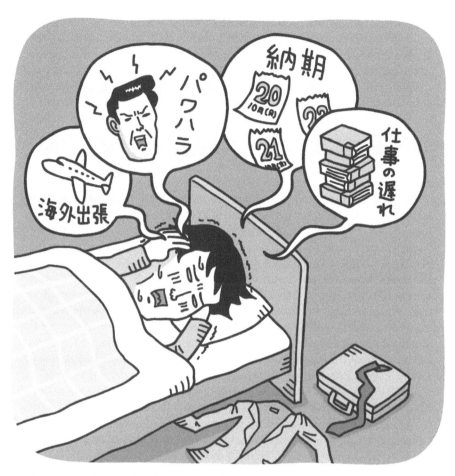

Figure 10.1. A depressed and insomniac salaryman, tormented by thoughts of work delays, looming deadlines, "power harassment" from his boss, and the prospect of an upcoming business trip overseas, featured in the column "Legal Advice for Workers" on compensation for work-induced mental illness (courtesy of Imai Yōji and The Asahi Newspaper; *Asahi*, October 27, 2008).

stem from the historical contexts, whereby the advent of Prozac occurred in the United States during an era of economic expansion, which set the stage for a characteristically optimistic discourse about the infinite possibilities that biological technology would bring for individual enhancement and national advancement. In contrast, the new antidepressants were introduced to Japan in the late 1990s, during what economists now call "Japan's lost decade." At that time, Japanese, who had relished the manic phase of the bubble economy, plunged into a deep recession and ensuing political stagnation. The following decades, replete with bankruptcy, unemployment, and suicide, created an at-mosphere of social stagnation and uncertainty—even hopelessness—that some commentators have compared to the eve of the fatal collapse of the feudal state in the nineteenth century (Hirai 1999). It is in this historical context that Japa-nese psychiatrists have been able to capture the Japanese imagination by ex-plaining the rise of depression as a product of the interplay between biology and the economy. By linking recession, depression, and suicide, they have cre-ated a culturally infused image of collectively depressed bodies under siege, while crystallizing people's prevailing sense of loss and anxiety in the name of depression. It is not surprising then that the kind of themes that characterize the dominant American discourse on depression—such as the psychological discovery of the "real self," the relentless appetite for individual self-enhance-ment, and the desire to transcend nature by means of pharmaceutical technol-ogy—are nearly absent in Japan. Instead, the rising discourse about depression in Japan does not seem to negate suffering (which is still accepted as part of normality [Borovoy 2008]) inasmuch as it encourages people to recognize and articulate their distress, and to do so via a new *psychiatric language of expe-rience*. This psychiatric discourse—in sharp contrast to the psychologizing and individualizing discourse in the United States—gives Japanese a language to express their suffering in a "socializing" manner.

What I want to ask, however, is what consequences this "socializing" form of medicalization could ultimately bring about? I am particularly concerned with unpacking the extent to which psychiatry—a branch of biomedicine that has long been accused of biological reductionism—can truly take on the task of creating social approaches to depression, and what vision of society this will promote.

On the one hand, it seems undeniable that psychiatric language has helped bring significant social change by altering the way Japanese talk about psycho-pathology. The current discourse about depression has reversed the meaning of mental illness by turning it from a mark of inherent individual defect to an evocative sign of existential crisis that calls for critical reflexivity and social ac-tion. At the individual level, the psychiatric discourse has prompted not just burned-out workers but fatigued housewives, the isolated elderly, and even exam-drained children to reflect on the nature of their "depression" and con-sider the possibility that excessive social pressure can lead them to mental breakdown, even suicide. This has even led some Japanese to contemplate on how their own unreflexive immersion in the pathogenic system has pushed them beyond a limit and numbed their ability to "feel their own emotions" (e.g., *Asahi*, June 27, 2007). In this regard, psychiatrists have highlighted depression as a failsafe mechanism for protecting one's body and mind from total col-lapse—possibly a means of adaptation in a time of social upheaval (see chapter 5). Through this discourse, they seem to be creating a kind of "structural pos-sibility" (Corin 1998a) that allows Japanese to distance themselves from the social norms and cultural commonsense that may have bounded those who are driven to psychiatric breakdown.

At the institutional level, psychiatrists have helped build a public platform upon which these individuals have come to protest social injustice—particularly in the workplace—by calling attention to social stress as a significant cause of depression. Working together with socially conscious lawyers, some psychiatrists have linked biological depression to economic depression concretely by demonstrating how depression can be a manifestation of accumulated work stress and excessive fatigue. Through litigations that have successfully held companies and the government liable for workers' distress, psychiatrists have transformed people's private narratives of depression into forms of a public language of pain. This suggests the potentially subversive political power that psychiatry could take in the post–antipsychiatry era, where it has reemerged as a means for the socially weak to articulate dissent, voice collective anger, and insert social critique. By linking with the grassroots movements that question Japan's status quo, psychiatrists have emerged as unlikely *agents of liberation*.

On the other hand, however, the rapid spread of antidepressants and the emerging biopolitics—with its evolving web of psychiatric surveillance by government and industry —also raise questions about the potential ill effects of medicalization. During my follow-up fieldwork in 2008 and 2009, it became apparent to me how aggressively the pharmaceuticalization of everyday distress has penetrated Japanese society (also see Healy 2004, Applbaum 2010). Sales of antidepressants rose from approximately 17 billion yen in the 1990s to exceed 90 billion yen by 2007, and the number of depressed patients is now over a million, an increase of 2.4 times in the last ten years (*Yomiuri*, January 6, 2010). This is notable especially for a society whose own psychiatrists had assumed until a decade ago that depression was a rare occurrence. Suicide rates, which the government pledged in 2006 to reduce by 20 percent by 2016, have so far shown little sign of declining. Despite the "advancement" of psychiatric care, Japanese seem to be at increasing risk for psychopathology.

This grim picture prompts us to ask if this medicalization has simply served to make people's sense of vulnerability all the more prevalent and imminent, while socializing language has functioned as little more than a commodity employed by the pharmaceutical industry for cultivating a wide market for antidepressants. In other words, there may be a dual structure, whereby a socializing language serves as a rhetorical device for breaking down local resistance to psychiatry and psychopharmacology, while actual intervention continues to work at the level of biological reductionism that induces individuals to simply take pills for what ails them so as to quiet their dissent. Given such concerns, we have to ask what kind of role the socializing language of depression now plays in the expanding web of psychiatric practice, what place it has in the ongoing restructuring of Japanese society, and if there is any possibility that this social movement, beyond being local knowledge, generates a new theoretical framework in psychiatry that can seriously address the *social* nature of depression?

Making Depression *Real*: Changing Debates in the Realms of Medicine, Law, and Policy

The rapid success of the medicalization of depression in Japan is due in large part to psychiatrists' successful attempts to change the terms of the debate regarding psychopathology. In disseminating a new medical model of depression, they have combined physiological, neurochemical accounts with social, existential narratives that place it in both a scientific and experiential illness category. Particularly through their successful destigmatization campaigns, psychiatrists have emphasized that depression is not a sign of genetic weakness or a mere psychological problem but a *physiological disease*—a "cold of the heart" that one becomes susceptible to when placed under excessive stress. Redefining depression as a problem of somatic and social origins, they have offered both antidepressants and ample rest as the cure—a persuasive prescription for people who feel thoroughly overworked and wish to have it recognized. Also notable is the way in which psychiatrists have existentialized—even historicized—depression by linking it to the prevailing sense of fatigue and stress that set in during the economic meltdown in the 1990s. Elaborating on the psychiatric discourse of the 1970s about social change—and the prevailing sense of alienation it creates—as an important cause of depression (see chapter 5), some Japanese psychiatrists have explained the sudden rise of depression in Japan by contrasting two kinds of fatigue (Kanba 2005). The first is a fruitful and gratifying sense of fatigue, which psychiatrists claim was common during the decades of Japan's economic expansion, when a worker could endure long hours of overwork, even unreasonable demands and pressure, because they knew that such fatigue would bring psychological and economic fulfillment in the end. The other is a futile, even alienating sense of fatigue (called *torō* or wasted effort), which, psychiatrists say is pervasive in Japanese society today. This occurs when people feel unappreciated for the work they do, when they face fragmentation in the workplace, unsure if their hard work will bear fruit in the end. Given the perpetual uncertainty that they feel about the future, this futile sense of fatigue becomes damaging, even *traumatic*, as it leaves individuals feeling excluded from social bonds and left with little meaning. Here, fatigue goes well beyond its physiological dimension and begins to take on social and existential connotations. This collective sense of fatigue among Japanese has also raised a political, economic concern, prompting the government to take initiatives by creating a nationwide intervention in the form of depression and suicide prevention programs.

Furthermore, this medical model began to have another social career when it was adopted by a group of lawyers to consolidate a *forensic model of depression*. It has rapidly evolved in Japan since the 1990s, when lawyers began to politicize depression by challenging the preexisting conceptual boundaries between individual vulnerability and social causality. Up to the 1990s, it was rare that workers would even imagine suing companies for their own psychiatric breakdown because psychopathology, including depression, was understood as resulting from individual vulnerability. All this changed after the worker's victory in the Dentsū case, when lawyers began to systematically challenge cases where, previously, workers' individual vulnerability would have been simply assumed. Over the last fifteen years, the workers' side has continued to accumulate legal victories by arguing for corporate responsibility over individual vulnerability. For instance, a worker with a history of recurrent depression, who before would have surely been thought of as innately weak biologically, was judged to have been driven to depression from overwork (Hirata 2007). The family of an anesthesiologist who had a history of epilepsy was likewise awarded compensation for her overwork depression and suicide (*Rōdō Keizai Hanrei Sokuhō* 2007). As the notion of individual biological vulnerability becomes reconceptualized in terms of social causality, the range of definitions of "pathogenic stress" has also expanded. In 2003, a worker who had become depressed not because of excessive work but lack of work (his company had deprived him of any meaningful work as a way of pressuring him to resign) successfully held his company liable by arguing that this was a form of *psychological bullying* (Okada 2003). Other similar cases involving sexual harassment (*Asahi*, May 18, 2007) and what Japanese call "power harassment" (a term that signifies a wide range of harassments that occur particularly in workplaces and often take the form of verbal abuse) have also brought victories to workers (Hozumi 2007, *Asahi*, October 16, 2007). In 2009, two postal workers were awarded compensation after arguing that they developed depression from doing consecutive night shifts. Notably, depression is here conceptualized primarily as a physical condition triggered by fatigue and the disturbance of "life rhythms"—with little consideration for psychological aspects (*Asahi*, May 19, 2009b). These highly publicized lawsuits, some of which have successfully mobilized grassroots support for the depressed through the Internet, have helped disseminate the idea to the public that depression can be a product of excessive work stress.

These medical and forensic debates have also set the tone for subsequent policy changes since the 1990s. The Ministry of Health, Welfare, and Labor, which once routinely turned down workers' compensation claims for mental illness, began to fundamentally change its stance after facing a series of humiliating losses in court. In reformulating its policies, the government has turned to psychiatric experts for advice, who subsequently helped establish the Stress Evaluations Tables in 1999, the revised Labor Safety and Health Acts in 2005, the national incentives for "Building Mental Health" in 2006, and the revised guideline for the Labor Standards Acts in 2009 (Kōsei Rōdōshō 2010). The government has further responded to the legal challenges by commissioning its own empirical survey on pathogenic stress, interviewing 6,000 employees about what kind of events are subjectively experienced as most stressful (see Kuroki 2007). Based upon these findings, the government revised the Stress Evaluation Tables in 2009, upgrading events such as "making a major mistake on the job" and "being urged to quit a job" to the category of "the most stressful events," which are supposed to rarely happen in one's life. The government also added to the Stress Evaluation Tables new criteria for sexual harassment and power harassment, thereby significantly expanding the notion of what counts as pathogenic stress (*Asahi*, March 20, 2009). By incorporating workers' own voices into its policies, the government appears to be countering the lingering criticism that it is using psychiatric measures to instill another apparatus of social control.

Through changes that encompass the realms of medicine, law, and policy, medicalization has brought a fundamental shift in the way Japanese conceptualize depression. Hacking (1990) has shown how the rise of statistics as a moral science has created conceptual and institutional possibilities in which people come to concretely imagine, and start interacting with, formerly unthought of (or merely abstract) groups beyond their immediate experience. In a parallel manner, psychiatric discourse has made depression *real*, first by cultivating a new popular language for it and second, by creating intermingled linkages and networks of different forces—conceptual, technological, institutional, political, and economic—which are assembled to embody a new form of power. Thus, it is not surprising that left-leaning psychiatrists I interviewed up to the mid-2000s told me how excited and proud they were of all the developments that were taking place: some of them, who were known to have been fierce fighters during the antipsychiatry era, proclaimed to me that after years of struggle their social vision was finally beginning to be realized. Also, I kept hearing optimistic statements in conferences on industrial mental health not just from these psychiatrists but also from industry managers, who all seemed to be harboring hope that psychiatric management will somehow contain, if not entirely eradicate, the rapid spread of depression. These changes were bringing the whole profession to a new era of scientific biological psychiatry with a social conscience—or so it seemed at the time.

(Bio)looping Effect

It did not take long, however, for this therapeutic optimism to wane in the latter half of the 2000s, when Japan, after brief economic elation, again slid into a deep recession triggered by the economic crisis in the United States. As became apparent during my fieldwork in 2008 and 2009, the once-popular medical model was beginning to expose its limits. Administrators, general practitioners, patients, and their families, began to realize that depression, after all, was not the straightforward illness with a linear recovery timeline like a "cold of the heart" that it was supposed to be. Psychiatrists as well, many of whom initially appeared pleasantly surprised by the success of their own depression campaigns, were starting to worry about the careless use of the "depression" diagnosis and the increasing use and abuse of antidepressants. As I have demonstrated in the ethnography of clinical practices (chapters 6 through 8), Japanese psychiatrists, even those who are psychotherapeutically inclined, have traditionally resorted to medication as *the* primary treatment for depression. (This approach is reinforced by the institutional makeup of Japanese medicine, where psychotherapy is poorly reimbursed and the time for consultation is limited). Especially given psychiatrists' prevailing "somatism," where they generally believe that the body is the central medium by means of which the mind can be cured, administering medication—even when they are fully aware of the underlying psychological issues and/or social origins of patients' distress—remains the primary choice for treating depression. With the increasing popularization of antidepressants to treat depression (now prescribed to patients by internists and other specialists), however, this treatment approach has slipped into "biologism," a form of biological reductionism that exclusively focuses on the body without much consideration for social and existential dimensions of depression (see chapters 6 and 7). This has become a pronounced problem, particularly now that the growing patient population includes ever more diversified types of "depressed" people with complex psychological and social problems—for which antidepressants often prove ineffective, at times even detrimental (Healy 2004, Horwitz and Wakefield 2007).

Thus, at various conferences from the mid-2000s, psychiatrists began to organize panels addressing the clinical confusion brought on by the flood of patients into clinics and the rapid increase in the number of "intractable" patients. With these concerns, some psychiatric leaders—who read my work on depression and suicide, gender politics in the clinic, and the history of neurasthenia—started asking me to speak at their conferences and publish in their journals about the ill effects of medicalization. As they heard me discuss the ominous parallels between the rise and fall of neurasthenia a century ago and what was happening with depression today, these psychiatrists heatedly debated whether they might be repeating the same mistake as their forebears by gradually turning depression from an "illness of overwork" into an "illness of personality" (see chapter 4). They pointed out that the changes via medicalization might be occurring far more widely and rapidly today than at the time of neurasthenia because of the alluring promise of antidepressants and the prevailing influence of the media. As I demonstrate below, it was clear to psychiatrists that the medical model was beginning to spin off its contradictions, rapidly reshaping the "social course of illness" (Kleinman 1986), while antidepressants were beginning to create their own biological realities.

Indeed, some of the "depressed" people I met in 2008 and 2009 had entered patienthood on the basis of a scientific definition of depression on which experts are now increasingly casting doubt and had done so without fully realizing the economic, social, and psychological costs of becoming a "depressed patient." While some patients told me that they had self-diagnosed their "depression" before going to a doctor, others said that they were initially surprised when they received the diagnosis, for they had thought depression as something more serious than the kind of symptoms they were experiencing. One such patient, a thirty-eight-year-old contract nurse, Kawai-san, remembered feeling uneasy about the diagnosis. Deeply fatigued at the time, she was nonetheless relieved to know that this would give her a legitimate reason to take time off from the extremely busy diathesis unit she was in charge of, and glad to be told that depression "is like a cold of the heart" and would go away with "ample rest and antidepressants." Being a firm believer in the power of biomedical technology, she did not hesitate to take all the pills prescribed to her. Yet, she became gradually anxious as both the amount and the variety of medications prescribed to her increased, and nothing she was taking seemed to work: "Once things started to go wrong, it all went straight downhill." She did not expect that, instead of returning to work in a few months as she had planned, she would end up being a "depressed" patient for more than three years.

After a year of treatment with the internist, Kawai-san found herself uncured, unemployed, and on welfare. By then, the doctor, who was growing impatient with the lack of her recovery while on antidepressants, began to treat her dismissively, telling her that she must be not depressed but simply neurotic, thereby reproducing the familiar gender politics in Japanese medical encounters I described in chapter 8. What the internist certainly did not tell her (if he was indeed aware of this himself) was the fact that antidepressants do not always cure and often show modest—even insignificant— success rates, particularly for milder forms of depression (Carey 2010). The second doctor she saw was a neurologist, who impressed Kawai-san as a "genuine and caring" doctor. He was nonetheless inept at curing her, as he responded to her every complaint by strictly following the pharmaceutical algorithm (perhaps all too diligently) with the result of pushing the amount of her medication beyond excess. By then completely devoid of energy, socially withdrawn in her tiny apartment, and feeling more and more "removed from [her]self," Kawai-san finally decided to seek a psychiatrist, who, alarmed by the amount and the assortments of pills she was on, took her off medication entirely (though gradually) in order to ascertain the "real shape of the underlying depression." To their surprise, they discovered that she was, at least by then, hardly depressed at all (her doctor told me he could not tell if she had ever been truly "depressed"). As she began to regain energy, she made her first-ever trip abroad—a trekking trip to Nepal—where she felt reinvigorated by the beautiful scenery, a healthy regimen of daily walking, and the warmth of the local people; it was a transformative experience that seems to have lifted her out of depression altogether. I met her just when she was starting to work again: "Off medication, I've felt myself coming back to me." It was apparent to her that antidepressants had literally and fundamentally altered both her body and her sense of identity.

Social scientists have long discussed the ill effects on people of their being labeled, as well as the ways in which a socially stigmatized identity becomes internalized, even eroding a person's core sense of self (Becker 1960, Goffman 1963). What the current medicalization has brought seems even more complex: what Ian Hacking calls a "looping effect," in this case where the nature of "depression" is altered by the way people start to live as (and conform to the idea of) "depressed patients." As they do so, these people's lives also evolve in ways that alter the classifications, descriptions, and the experiences of "depression" itself (Hacking 1999). This process is further convoluted by what Hacking (1999) calls a "biolooping effect," whereby the act of taking antidepressants literally alters the chemical condition of patients' brains. Kawai-san, like some of the other people I met in 2008 and 2009, was diagnosed as "depressed" and given antidepressants by an internist who probably would have been more careful with such a diagnosis ten years prior to that. Kawai-san as well, despite her initial uncertainty about the diagnosis, accepted it and continued to take antidepressants, despite her sense that these pills were not helping but simply aggravating her condition. As she became homebound and eventually lost her job, she became one of the growing numbers of "intractable patients," for whom the straightforward psychiatric treatment of antidepressants and ample rest did not seem to work. As psychiatrists are confronted with these "new types" of patients, they are having to critically reexamine their own assumptions about depression and the limits of their traditional approach.

This increasing clinical uncertainty was graphically revealed in a much-discussed TV program that aired in March 2009 and was later published in book form (NHK 2009), signaling a shift in the popular perception of depression and psychopharmacology in Japan. The program was produced by NHK, which up to that point had done much to popularize the medical model of depression. This time, however, NHK called attention to the growing confusion surrounding the diagnosis and treatment of depression. The program illuminated how an increasing number of patients are becoming dysfunctional, socially withdrawn, and housebound from overmedication. Some of these patients were taken to a psychopharmaceutical expert, who examined their prescriptions and found them to be cases of excessive polypharmacy. When the expert drastically reduced both the number and dosage of patients' medication, the effect was dramatic: they either returned to the same level of mild symptoms they had initially complained of or, in some cases, completely recovered. In another segment of the program, in a manner reminiscent of the 1973 Rosenhan experiment with pseudo-patients' successful entry into mental hospitals (Rosenhan 1973), a woman with depressive symptoms went to five different doctors only to be prescribed five different sets of medication, some of which suggested (to the psychopharmaceutical expert) competing diagnoses among these doctors. The message was clear: antidepressants were not necessarily curing people but may well be producing chronically depressed, "intractable" patients, and medical professionals cannot even agree on what depression is. As these patients' struggles with depression are increasingly publicized, the biomedical cure that involves mild-altering drugs has become morally suspect, leaving psychiatry's therapeutic power and its promise of rational control increasingly in doubt.[1]

In the meantime, psychiatrists, despite their smooth and upbeat medicalization campaigns in public, are deeply troubled and internally divided about the nature of the current confusion. Some psychiatrists blame the diffusion of the depression diagnosis, for which they hold the media and pharmaceutical companies responsible. They are critical of how "depression" is being used by workers as a convenient means of getting out of work, as well as by some of their medical colleagues (who lavishly dispense the diagnosis) to expand their lucrative clinics. In frustration, some have even published popular books, with titles like *People who like to say 'I'm depressed'* (Kayama 2008), thereby implicitly placing the blame on the "new types" of the depressed and their (supposedly illegitimate) claim for patienthood. As if to repeat the history of neurasthenia, some of them are trying to impose an intellectual boundary control, preaching to the public to strictly distinguish the *real* (biological) depression from other, mere (psychological) depressed states. Given that such boundaries had long dissolved when psychiatrists adopted the DSMs, however, such attempts seem belated, even futile. Other psychiatrists are explicitly critical of the way in which they themselves have become complicit in fueling therapeutic optimism and giving rise to a massive number of what Ivan Illich (1975) called "iatrogenesis"— a *false* illness of doctors' own making. The psychiatrists involved in suicide prevention are aghast at the growing gap between the grand vision of prevention proposed by the government and their meager daily practice that has borne little result. Feeling defeated, they lament that, all too frequently, what they need to stop people from committing suicide is not a medical consultation or even antidepressants but a couple of hundred-thousand yen (a few thousand dollars) to help them pay off their debts. Psychiatrists have become keenly aware of the limit of biomedical intervention into what they regard as social and political

---

[1] One change that I noticed in the field was that doctors now spend far more time explaining the possible side effects of antidepressants, with the heightened concern of the increasing incidents of litigation over the lack of such explanations.

problems (see chapter 7). Yet they seem increasingly helpless as they watch the machinery of medicalization at work, trapped in the contradiction they themselves have been complicit in creating.

Managing Depression as Collective Risk: The Emergence of the Psychiatric Science of Work

> In all countries . . . the science of work was based on the premise that greater productivity would lead to social happiness.
> —Anson Rabinbach (1990:203)

> Whenever [the science of labor] goes beyond the economic-technical dimension . . . [labor] is seen essentially as a psychological problem. Psychology, however, cannot adequately deal with the problem of labor since . . . labor is an ontological concept.
> —Herbert Marcuse (1973:11[1933])

Partly in response to the increasingly exposed limits of the medical model, there is now developing a field of science—or what I would like to call, following Anson Rabinbach (1990), the *psychiatric science of work*. While occupational medicine as a whole has been mainly concerned with "physical" illnesses, the psychiatric science of work is a loosely jointed field that involves scientists from various fields—including psychiatrists, internists, epidemiologists, and policymakers—who are trying to assess the nature of psychopathology in the workplace. As the field remains a bundle of different theoretical and methodological orientations, it is perhaps premature to determine what directions this science will be taking. While it could easily evolve into a system of biological management and surveillance used to select out the fit and the unfit for the labor system, it is also open to the possibility of building a more humane, socially oriented caring space for the mentally ill in the workplace. For now, this field is beginning to address what has been left unresolved in medical and legal debates—that is, the question of individual *agency*. If medical and forensic experts have done much to shift responsibility from the depressed, instilling a "blame-free self of the therapeutic model" (Douglas 1992:230), the people involved in the prevention and treatment of depression seem to be re-addressing it by re-conceptualizing depression as a form of risk that every worker is subjected to. Depression defined in this way becomes something preventable by rational management both at collective and individual levels—an idea that is increasingly adopted by the government and corporations as they search for effective means of dealing with the rapid increase in the number of depressed workers.

Regarding depression as an imminent risk in the workplace, the government in 2006 took a step toward the prevention of depression by endorsing the idea of "Four Levels of Care" (Kōsei Rōdōshō 2010). This principle states that the responsibility for preventing and treating workers' psychopathology lies with the four parties involved: medical practitioners at large, medical practitioners within the organization, workers' units (called "line-care"), and workers themselves (called "self-care"). As one concrete measure for actualizing such "care," the government has also proposed stricter time management. Operating from the premise that fatigued workers are likely to become depressed, particularly after excessive hours of overwork, the government has restricted overwork hours while requiring companies to provide employees who do more than 100 hours of overwork in a given month (or an average of 80 hours within the preceding two to six months) with medical consultation upon their requesting it. This policy is based on a government-commissioned epidemiological survey, which found that workers who do more than 80 hours of overwork per month—who consequently secure less than 60 hours of sleep at home—are at increased risk for depression. Workers are also encouraged to keep a healthy balance between their time at work (calculated by the hours of overwork) and at home (often measured in terms of hours of sleep). Conceptualizing depression in this way has enabled medical experts, personnel staff, and workers themselves to approach the complex problem of psychopathology by breaking it down into a series of risk factors and chain causalities that are easier to objectify and control.

However, some psychiatrists involved in this field have expressed the concern that these policy changes may prove to be a double-edged sword for workers. While these policies have given corporations concrete guidelines for preventing depression, they are also generating a more restrictive, bureaucratic system of evaluation and of complaint processing (cf. Petryna 2002, 2004), thereby bringing to the care of the depressed new expectations and demands. This is suggested in the way depressed workers' recovery is now assessed in terms of *industrial time*, rather than in *clinical time*. Before mental health became strictly mandated in workplaces, Japanese corporations (particularly those beyond a certain scale) once offered highly generous and flexible systems of sick leave. Workers were allowed to spend a long stretch of time in hospital as a way to rest, a kind of down time for recovering from both physiological and psychological fatigue that was deemed almost inevitable during a lifetime of employment. This system operated with the Parsonian idea of a *sick role*—where fatigued workers were expected to recover under the jurisdiction of medical experts who determined what the "natural" recovery process should be and when these workers were well enough to return to their job with their personhood fully restored. Today, as mental health comes to be seen as not only a matter of medical jurisdiction but also an object of corporate risk management, some companies are introducing much more rigorous and standardized systems for evaluating workers' mental health. They constantly monitor those afflicted and scrutinize their recovery with the aim of promptly restoring their health as well as productivity. Given the prolonged recession, where both personnel staff and workers are coming under increasing pressure to return the afflicted to a healthy state, they have to negotiate between the ideals of *clinical time* that prioritizes a "natural" recovery and the demands of *industrial time* that constantly seeks, even for a therapeutic process, the principle of *efficiency*.

The ideal of efficient recovery may also be relegating those who remain out of line with industrial time into new categories of Otherness. This is suggested by the fact that industry is now taking steps of dealing with depressed workers using means that introduce various degrees of estrangement. First of all, instead of trying to take care of the depressed within the company under the guidance of contracted company doctors or letting workers take care of themselves, more and more companies are now choosing to outsource the care of the depressed to specialized clinics that have sprung up since the 1990s. These clinics provide not only medical care but also occupational training specifically designed to restore and improve the work skills of the depressed. While such specialized care may have beneficial effects on ailing workers, depression experts also express concern that this has become a way for the industry to deal with depression as a problem of "individuals" without having to confront pathogenic work conditions. Secondly, these companies (as well as other smaller companies that cannot afford to give such service to their employees) are also exploring ways to let go of workers who do not easily recover and who refuse to "voluntarily" resign. While I repeatedly heard such stories of disemployment during my fieldwork in the late 2000s, this move can also be risky and costly for companies when they are legally challenged. Tension of this kind surfaced in 2009, when a female worker took Toshiba (one of the biggest electronic corporations in Japan) to court and successfully challenged its decision to fire her after she had been on sick leave for three years (*Asahi*, May 19, 2009a). As the impact of the court decision swept over the nation, companies have begun to explore other "safer" measures.

A third tactic that has recently emerged is to rehire depressed workers through the category of *disability employment*. This is now much talked about because of recent legislative changes that the government has made in order to pressure the companies (above a certain scale) to fulfill the 1.8 percent disability employment quota, while imposing penalties on those who fail to meet this criterion. Whereas disability employment usually implied physical and intellectual disabilities, the government introduced various measures in 2006 in order to expand this category to incorporate a wider range of *mental* disabilities. According to Teruyama Junko, a University of Michigan-trained anthropologist working on disability in Japan, some company personnel are hoping to fulfill the required quota with depressed workers, preferably those who are already employed through a "normal" route and who have since become ill and obtained a disability certificate from the government. While they think it would be easy to fill up the quota this way (as there are already so many depressed workers), they cannot urge employees to obtain a disability status (or to "come out" and declare that they actually applied for the certificate) as this would be inappropriate and might even be taken as a violation of their human rights. Some psychiatrists have also told me that some depressed patients are now voluntarily asking doctors to process the paperwork for a disability certificate (given the economic support it would bring), while many others remain hesitant to do so not only because of its stigmatizing implications but also because they do not wish their depression to become a chronic state. Indeed, given the scientific uncertainty of its definition, depression as a form of disability is still in the making, leaving the afflicted vulnerable to competing interpretations about their social, economic, and political status beyond their control (cf. Petryna 2002; on the politics of disability in Japan, see Nakamura 2006, 2008).

Part of the ensuing confusion that I found in the industry in the late 2000s stems from the overly homogenized and simplified "rational" assumptions about depression that psychiatrists have done much to popularize. In attempts to normalize depression and dispel its residual image as a genetic disease marked by irrationality, psychiatrists have gone to the other extreme of portraying depression as a straightforward, all-too-rational illness that can be easily induced by excessive fatigue. Lawyers have also contributed to constructing this image by arguing that the depressed are not to blame but instead are legitimate victims of inhumane work conditions. This picture has become widely accepted by general practitioners and lay Japanese, as it does not challenge the preexisting boundaries between the normal and the pathological or commonsensical ideas about human nature. Contrary to this popularized image, however, depression, like other forms of psychopathology, is far more complicated in its etiology and often leaves a mark on the afflicted, at times fundamentally altering their body and their sense of identity. This is especially the case with chronic patients, for whom "depression" remains irregular, irrational, unpredictable—and ultimately in the realm of the *incomprehensible*, where a certain period of social disengagement and detachment may be crucial for recovery. Yet, because of the generally simplified and optimistic understanding of depression, workers who long remain depressed appear to staff as puzzling and unpredictable. Staff say it is difficult to differentiate malingerers from those who are trying hard to recover. Some staff also complain that depressed workers are even more difficult to manage than traditional types of mentally ill workers (by which they mean schizophrenics), with whom they already have some familiarity and established measures to take (see Okazaki et al. 2006). Thus, the overly normalized understanding of depression generates new forms of stigmatization against those who fail to live up to the idealized view of the depressed. By remaining disengaged for too long, they risk being reclassified as a *moral threat* to the labor-obsessed society.

Conclusion: Rethinking the Biological and the Social in the Age of Global Medicalization

These developments lead us to consider the tensions evoked by today's biomedical expansion, where people are encouraged to use medical technologies to enhance their autonomy and realize their desires, while tinkering with troubling suspicions about the unseen consequences of compliance and potential risks for subjugation (Lock 1993, 1998, 1999, Haraway 1997, Mol and Berg 1998). The variety of information that is generated urging people to "recognize" and take care of their depression—to become more informed, responsible, and autonomous beings—clearly reflects an era of disillusionment, where workers are now having to look out for themselves as well as demand public, legal protection when corporations may no longer provide them with the security of lifetime employment. Yet, as Adriana Petryna has shown in her ethnography of medicalization of the nuclear disaster victims in Ukraine (Petryna 2002), this use of biomedical categories depends on a delicate moral balance, as those who claim legitimacy for their social suffering through a biomedical category are also subject to experts' competing interpretations about the nature of their distress and shifting politics that can at any time redefine what *really* lies behind their pathology. Thus, the increasing calls for psychiatric care for the depressed in Japan should not be naively celebrated as an advancement in health care and/ or social policy, but has to be carefully examined in light of the legal, social apparatuses that have legitimized—indeed necessitated—the move to make the depressed the agents of their own management and more "productive" citizens (cf. Rose 1990).[2]

Such concerns are also heightened by the fact that, although similarly "socializing" discourses have recurred in the history of psychiatry, they have often brought ironic consequences. Historians have shown that left-leaning doctors' attempts to address social ills through the biomedical language of "nerve diseases" gained political force in the late nineteenth century, particularly as these doctors began to link up with workers' movements. While they made significant contributions by helping establish workers' compensation and welfare laws, they also ended up placing the workers under the control of medical experts and insurance associations (Rabinbach 1990). The ideological tension

---

[2] Also note that there seems to be a growing biopolarization in psychiatric treatment, that is, between care for the depressed and care for people diagnosed with schizophrenia, many of who still remain subject to long-term hospitalization. There have been important developments in the latter realm as well, however, as seen in patients' movements towards de-stigmatization and normalization (see Nakamura 2008, Ukigaya 2009).

built up as more and more workers began to claim welfare status on the basis of nerve diseases, which had the effect of gradually turning workers' *"right to health"* into *"duty to health"* (Schmiedebach 1999:53). The rise of work-related neurosis also led to what people then regarded as an increase in self-claiming neurotics, and to a new label of "compensation neurosis," with the idea that it was not the burden of work but the Welfare State itself that was creating mass addiction to neurosis among "weak" individuals (Schmiedebach 1999).

Also, as anthropologists have pointed out, the rise of medical holism in the 1950s allowed medical professionals to regard patients not as "isolated, individual bodies" but as "psychosocial entities located in an 'ecological' system" (Martin 1991:499). Yet, this supposedly more socially oriented, humane approach soon turned into another hegemonic means of control as it began to approach patient's psychology as a new entry point to more thorough medical, psychological management (Martin 1991, Arney and Bergen 1984:68, also see Taussig 1980). Equally disturbing is the way that "social" discourse can be used—as elucidated by Kleinman (1986), in his ethnography of medicalization in post–Cultural Revolution China—by the state as a means for collectively managing people's dissent. The use of "neurasthenia" both as a medical and political category allowed people to express their *anger* against political injustice while serving to funnel their potentially disruptive emotional force into an officially sanctioned discourse that would keep the political machinery intact. This sort of employment of the "socializing" discourse serves to assemble an inchoate mass of realities as an "illness" and place dissenting individuals under the supervision of medical experts, who then provide (and at times overdetermine) the meaning of patients' suffering while keeping them from fundamentally challenging the status quo.

These historical recurrences should prompt us to reexamine the consequences of the ongoing medicalization in Japan. On the one hand, it has certainly been demonstrated that the biologization of depression does not necessarily have to be individualizing or depoliticizing, but can be socializing and even liberating. On the other hand, however, it is unclear to what extent this socializing form of medicalization has the power to fundamentally alter the way psychiatry operates. As Lock (2002) has shown through her work on the medicalization of death in Japan, biomedicine, when faced with local discourses that raise epistemological questions, often resolves such ambiguities by establishing stricter criteria and standardization of diagnoses. Scientists' flat acceptance that they indeed lack the epistemological grounds (in Lock's work, for defining what death means socially) often does little to stop the process of this standardization. Biomedicine then begins to produce knowledge invested with a scientific aura of neutrality that subsequently gains popular currency. This serves to conceal social contradictions as it takes on the status of universal knowledge seemingly devoid of the particularities of its local production (Lock 2002, also see Young 1995). If this culture of science prevails in the medicalization of depression as well, then it may begin to reshape "depression" within the discursive limits of biopsychiatry, with its tendency to depoliticize illnesses and promote ideologies of individual responsibility and the rational manipulation of health (Comaroff 1982, Gordon 1988). If so, particularly in a time of economic uncertainty, Japanese may become more concerned about their own somatic and psychological vulnerabilities rather than structural injustices, and end up strengthening their commitment to individual management and commodified mental health. This is a likely scenario, particularly considering that such an individualizing approach would be beneficial for the fast-growing mental health industry, which is also finding fuel in the global pharmaceuticalization of everyday distress (for a parallel discussion of "Healthism" in the United States, see Crawford 1984). Especially given the fact that psychiatric interventions—even by seemingly socially conscious experts— have too often ended up reproducing the dominant social structure without challenging the system itself, we have to seriously ask in what ways the disillusionment of people in Japan can become a motor for fundamental social change.

CHAPTER ELEVEN

The Future of Depression:
Beyond Psychopharmaceuticals

Ironies of Medicalization

I BEGAN THIS BOOK with the question of how Japanese have come to embrace the psychiatric view of depression so suddenly, despite their long resistance to psychiatric intrusion into everyday life. As the book has demonstrated, this is partly due to the way psychiatry in Japan has been able to create a language of depression that speaks to people's sense of social distress (cf. Kleinman 1986, Lock 1987, Young 1980, 1995). By linking with grassroots movements, psychiatry has come to provide a means by which people can seek social legitimation of their distress and challenge the increasingly oppressive culture of the workplace in the neoliberal economic order. Funneling people's dissent and private emotions into a public narrative of injustice, psychiatrists have effectively politicized depression.

Despite the seemingly redemptive role it has played in Japan, however, psychiatry continues to be characterized by a dual structure: while providing a socializing language that has helped popularize depression, psychiatry retains its biological principles at the core of its practice. Without fundamentally altering the way it operates—or generating a new theoretical and clinical framework to address the social nature of people's "depression"—psychiatry has relegated the depressed to the pharmaceutical management of everyday distress. Such a split in the therapeutic process—whereby the "biological" is divorced from the "psychological" and "social" aspects of the ailment—remains a deep-seated problem of psychiatry more generally in industrialized countries. The irony of this duality is perhaps all the more pronounced in Japan, where, behind the social rhetoric, the diffusion of the depression diagnosis and the aggressive pharmaceuticalization of everyday distress are rapidly producing contradictions,[1] which can have

[1] Neurobiological metaphors prevalent in the United States—such as explaining depression as a matter of "chemical imbalance" in the brain—do not seem to have the same explanatory power or salvatory implication in Japan. Instead, through their distinctive set of "holistic" bodily metaphors (such as "cold of the heart"), Japanese psychiatrists have effectively turned depression into an object of aggressive pharmaceuticalization. As I hope to have shown, this calls for an ethnographic investigation into what "makes sense" as an illness account in different societies (Evans-Pritchard 1937), and what ideological forces go into making it a socially and politically legitimate explanation.

serious ill effects on those who suffer (see chapter 10).[2] Also, as the discourse about depression has evolved over the last decade, the depressed are made even more vulnerable to shifting politics of causality (cf. Petryna 2002), where medical, legal, and policy experts continue to debate exactly where the responsibility lies for the psychiatric breakdown of the depressed. Given the prolonged recession that produces various political and economic pressures, the experience of depression itself is subject to fundamental changes, leaving the future of depression in Japan in a highly uncertain state.

Three Changes via the Ground-up Medicalization

Granted that these uncertainties exist, there are three positive signs I find in the ongoing medicalization of depression that indicate potential for bringing about important social transformation. First, this medicalization has brought to Japanese alternative understandings of the *biological* nature of mental illness by illuminating its fundamentally *social* nature. Second, it has also cultivated—via the localized psychiatric science of work—a new public awareness about the burden of *psychological labor*. Third, this local science is further gathering force by creating linkages with other local grassroots movements that are beginning to address the psychopathology of work on a global scale.

Redefining the "Biology" of Depression

First of all, what the emerging psychiatric language of depression has done is to radically liberate the psychiatric meaning of the "biological" for Japanese from its century-old adherence to genetic determinism. Throughout the twentieth century, psychiatrists, despite their initial hope that approaching mental illness as a biological disease would soon liberate the afflicted from their suffering, ended up inflicting more pain on them by instilling a profound disconnection between the normal and the pathological. This is because the "biological" nature of mental illness came to signify an essential difference, a condition of Otherness that was assumed to remain beyond the realm of rationality, empathetic understanding, and social connectedness. This biological perspective, by reducing depression to an isolated disease entity triggered by internal brain defects, discouraged Japanese from seeing it as something intrinsically connected to themselves and to the context of their social life. It also introduced a radical and unfortunate disjuncture from the traditional medical perspective that once em-

---

[2] In this regard, Japanese psychiatry's traditionally "somatic" approach, with its strong reservations about intruding into the realm of the psychological (see chapters 6 and 7), seems to have only intensified the move toward broad-scale pharmaceuticalization.

phasized the interrelatedness of the mind and the body as well as individuals and their (natural and social) environment (see chapters 2 through 5).

However, through the conceptual debates about depression both within and outside medical domains, Japanese psychiatrists are now officially reassessing their genetic determinism, an important shift indicated in recent discussions about "vulnerability." In 1999, when psychiatric leaders were asked by the government to establish objective criteria for measuring social stress at work, they decided not to produce a similarly "objective" scale for assessing individual vulnerability. These leaders agreed that it would be nonsensical to call those who were prone to depression "vulnerable" (with its negative connotation of weakness), as the depressed often embody what is normal, even ideal in Japanese society.[3] Psychiatrists have also reasoned that vulnerability to depression can be rooted in socialization as much as it is in genetics, and might only manifest itself as pathology when the vulnerable are placed in an unaccommodating environment or at a time of social change. In other words, vulnerability here has come to be conceptualized not as something inherent, static, and frozen in time but rather something *collective, relational*, and even *historical*. Vulnerability as such resides as much in society as it does in individual biology, thereby potentially shifting the target of medical intervention (see chapter 5). This reconceptualization signals a fundamental change in Japanese psychiatry from the era of absolute geneticism to the age of "susceptibility," or the realization that we all carry "genomic vulnerabilities to different conditions" (Rose 2007:204). This parallels the emergent understanding of (epi)genetics, where a gene is increasingly conceptualized not as a rigid entity but rather as something dynamic and flexible that manifests itself in different ways as a result of interaction with the environment (Lock 2005). By insisting on how the biological is simultaneously social, this medicalization process may enable Japanese to finally overcome psychiatry's negative legacy of crude genetic determinism and instead to understand "depression" once more as something bodily, tangible, and familiar.

Problematizing the Psychological Labor

Second, beyond mere private reflections, such critical awareness is becoming institutionalized as a public language through the psychiatric science of work that calls attention to the hazards of *psychological labor*. This indicates the emergence of a new historical sensibility for Japanese: through the discourse about overwork depression and suicide, they are beginning to talk about not only the burden of physical labor—which has long been recognized and paid

[3] On a similar note, one management expert wrote in *Asahi Shimbun* recently that hiring people who are "resilient" to depression—by choosing those who score high on the stress-resilience test, for instance—would be a waste of resources, as these people would be so insensitive in interpersonal relations that they would perform poorly in the Japanese workplace (Ozawa 2010).

for—but of psychological and emotional labor, a subject that has, despite the serious cost it incurs on workers' health, long been neglected. Arlie Hochschild (1983), who first proposed the notion of emotional labor, contrasted today's labor with that of the early phase of industrialization described by Karl Marx, where factory workers were in the process becoming alienated from their own bodies and themselves. Hochschild argued that despite the fact that the nature of work has shifted from manual labor to service labor in contemporary societies, the kind of psychological and emotional labor increasingly demanded of workers (such as being forced to sell one's "smile" for free at McDonald's or to use one's imagination so one can "empathize" with a customer who is unjustifiably rude) has remained largely unrecognized and undertheorized. Analyzing various ways in which workers are implicitly urged to commodify their own emotions, Hochschild also explores the alienating effects on their psyches even as they remain at times unaware of the serious toll it has taken on their sense of themselves. This form of exploitation remains particularly salient in societies like Japan, where such psychological labor has long been justified and naturalized as a virtue, even aestheticized as part of "Japanese culture" (in the name of *kizukai* or *omoiyari*, for instance, which indicate consideration for others). By telling people how depression tends to afflict those who work too hard, who go out of their way to be considerate to others, the psychiatric language of depression may be beginning to work as an antidote against this hegemonic cultural discourse.

With this new reflexivity, some depressed people are also opening up a public space in Japan to collectively ask, beyond the technicality of how to treat depression, what makes them vulnerable and what it *means* to be depressed. This change can be seen in the number of publications, websites, and support groups related to depression that have mushroomed in the past decade. Through such media, they are beginning to talk about how depression is not simply a biological defect or a distortion in cognition but a kind of bodily insight that is calling for a change in the way they live (cf., Obeyesekere 1985). Echoing the narratives I heard through my interviews (see chapter 8), many of these people find positive meaning in depression as a retreat from social engagements and obligations that were cornering them. Such a discourse parallels what Amy Borovoy (2005) has described regarding an American psychotherapy movement transplanted to Tokyo, whose notion of "codependency" had a subversive effect on the wives of alcoholics. Borovoy illustrates intriguing ways in which these women use this psychotherapeutic language to question the Japanese virtue of "interdependence" cultivated in the postwar era, which prompts them to also contemplate the nature of their own self-subjugation (Borovoy 2005, also see Ong 1987). Used in similar ways, the psychiatric language of depression—with its power of relativization and destabilization—may help people to address the fundamental question of modernity—that is, if their relentless quest for personal advancement through the current system is really the way to pursue happiness.

Globalizing the Psychiatric Science of Work

Third, what is also notable is that the emergence of this critical awareness about depression in Japan is not an isolated local occurrence but part of the global movement happening concurrently in many nations to protest alienation in the workplace. For instance, as discussed by Daena Funahashi (2010), the increase of psychological problems in the workplace in Finland has been tied to the deterioration of labor relations and the decline of the Finnish welfare state. As shown by Noelle Mole (2008), for Italians, debate over workplace bullying (what Italians call "mobbing") and rising psychopathology among workers has become a means by which they question the rapid change brought on by neoliberalism that they see as destroying their traditional culture of work. Similar discourses have emerged in other parts of Europe, including France and Germany, as well as in Asia, where the growing incidence of psychopathology in the workplace is discussed as the ill effect of global neoliberalism and changing labor relations (e.g., Jolly and Saltmarsh 2009). Such local resistance may well be, as Mole (2010) points out, a product of the transitional period when the system of lifetime employment is in the process of being replaced by short-term labor contracts that will soon impose more pressure on individual workers to be responsible for their own mental health. For now, however, these counterdiscourses both in Japan and Europe reflect the ways in which people are reexamining the directions that their societies are taking under the banner of globalization. By linking depression to the "social ills" brought on by neoliberalization—including the perils of privatization, the collapse of lifetime employment, and the crisis in national health care—people seem to be addressing their sense of alienation as real and concrete, as something that requires resolution through political intervention. This suggests a form of *ground-up* medicalization in the age of globalization, when both local psychiatrists and their patients increasingly use psychiatric language to mediate the immense tensions involved in global-formation and strive to find avenues for asserting their local agency.

The Future of Depression

Despite the concern that the Prozac Narrative is sweeping the globe, instilling the single vision of the "neurochemical self" fit for the new economic order, global medicalization has instead emerged as a fertile ground for local critiques against the imposition of a homogenizing view of personhood (Rose

2007). These local developments also fly in the face of technological determinism, as they demonstrate how the effects of drugs are never simply given but produced by both their neurochemical components and by cultural desires (Rose 2007:100). If the American discourse prompts people to take antidepressants to recover (and discover) their *real* self (Kramer 1993), the Japanese discourse has sold them as a relief from the debilitating sense of fatigue that comes from living in a society with an uncertain future. In India, where sales of antidepressants have expanded over the years, some psychiatrists in Calcutta have successfully promoted antidepressant use as *moner khabar* ("mind's food"), an idea that taps into widely held ideas about food, nutrition, digestion, and rebalancing of the body (Ecks forthcoming). In Nepal, antidepressants are being used as a pill for all sorts of "nerve disease"—a term that in itself is highly ambiguous and malleable in meaning (Kohrt and Harper 2008). In other words, when we examine respective local discourses about "depression," what is discussed is so diverse and so specific to each locale that one even begins to wonder if they are talking about the same thing at all. As Alain Ehrenberg points out, depression's popular appeal lies in its having both "maximum universality" and "extremely heterogeneity" (Ehrenberg 2010:74). While its seeming universality renders it into a common term of biological, scientific investigation, the concept's plasticity leaves it wide open to creative local interpretations.

These diverging local responses to ongoing medicalization may also be shaped by the way local psychiatries have evolved in the post–antipsychiatry era, where they have adopted contrasting approaches to the *political* dimensions of people's distress, at times drawing strikingly different boundaries between what constitutes "biomedical" and "social" realms (Davis in press, Lakoff 2005, Lloyd 2008, Raikhel 2010). At one end of the spectrum is the self-consciously "apolitical" stance that American biopsychiatry has adopted. As illuminated by the works of Tanya Luhrmann (2000) and Jonathan Metzl (2009), the increasing biologization of American psychiatry can be understood in part as a response to the turbulent period of the 1960s and 1970s, when psychiatrists ventured into the social realms that they now regard as having had little expertise over. The subsequent confusion led many psychiatrists to instead turn their scientific commitment to the more strictly "biological" realm, with the whole profession becoming "apolitical about national matters almost to a fault" (Metzl 2009:206). At the other end are various forms of community psychiatry that have sprung up in places like Italy, Greece (Davis in press), Argentina (Lakoff 2005), and Brazil (Béhague 2008, 2009), where concerns about political injustice continue to shape knowledge and practice. For instance, Dominique Béhague's exquisite account of community-based psychiatry in southern Brazil shows the ways in which local psychiatrists transform their therapeutic encounters into a site of empowerment for youth with behavioral problems, urging them to reflect upon the impact of social inequalities on their lives. By also analyzing the contradictions these psychiatrists face in trying to mediate political injustice via biomedical means, Béhague shows medicalization to be a conflicted process whereby local actors try to articulate local forms of oppression while exploring locally grounded forms of agency (Béhague 2008, 2009, see also Abu-Lughod 1990, Gal 1991, and Tsing 1993 on these themes). As I hope to have shown in this book, the Japanese approach to politicizing depression falls somewhere in between these two poles in the sense that psychiatrists are keenly aware of the limits of their practice and the danger of intruding into social realms. While they remain critical of reducing mental illness to a homogenized (and unjustly politicized) symbol for social suffering or a mere instrument for social transformation, they also seek ways to engage with people's sense of social distress by questioning their own rigid dichotomy between the biological and the social. By juxtaposing globalizing medicalization and local formation of subjectivity as occurring in a dialogic process, anthropologists of medicine are beginning to go beyond the straightforward domination/resistance model and instead to explore the transformative possibilities that both biomedicine and local subjectivity face (see Brotherton 2008, 2012).

Of course, this may be too optimistic and premature an assessment of ongoing medicalization, particularly when we think about the fact that its power of imposing a universal view of personhood stems not only from pharmaceuticalization but from biological science. Given the strong incentives within psychiatry to get to the bottom of mental illness by way of genetic and neurobiological research, methodological individual reductionism will likely continue to be an important part of its scientific endeavor. The evolving paradigm of biological psychiatry, as Young (1995) has observed, is establishing an even firmer division of mental labor and hierarchy by moving the data further away from the realm of local clinical practice (see chapter 5). Also important is the possibility that younger generations of psychiatrists, who are trained to draw on DSM-IV or ICD-10 diagnostic categories, are becoming dismissive of localized clinical theories and are keen to reestablish the depression concept as a universally applicable notion devoid of its social, cultural meanings.

At the same time, however, psychiatry continues to be a field of medicine where all the contradictions of society come to the fore (Kleinman 1988a, 1995, Good 1994, Young 1995, Rhodes 1995, Luhrmann 2000). This fact keeps psychiatric practitioners and patients from safely settling with a reductionist view of causality or a single view of personhood (Kleinman 1988b). Now that biomedicine as a whole has begun to move away from the old, simplistic version of genetic determinism toward multifaceted ideas of causality (Lock 2005), psychiatry seems best fit for experimenting with approaches that encompass complex views of personhood (Kirmayer and Gold 2011). Furthermore, given the politics of medicalization today, depression is no more "owned by psychiatry" (to paraphrase Allan Young [see Duclos 2009:111]) than it is by a bundle of institutions and actors—including legal, industrial, pharmaceutical, administrative, as well as various forms of grassroots movements—each of whom promotes their own ideas about what "depression" represents. Such realities constantly destabilize the assertion that there is only one true, universal vision of human nature and urge us instead to explore a language to express a more nuanced view of mental illness—one that remains simultaneously biological, psychological, and thoroughly *social*.

References

Abu-Lughod, Lila. 1990. The Romance of Resistance: Tracing Transformations of Power through Bedouin Women. *American Ethnologist* 17, no.1: 41–55.

Akimoto, Haruo. 1976. *Seishinigaku to Hanseishinigaku* (*Psychiatry and Antipsychiatry*). Tokyo: Kongō Shuppan.

———. 1985. *Meisai no Michishirube: Hyōden Nihon no Seishiniryō* (*Signposts in the Winding History of Japanese Psychiatry*). Tokyo: Nova Shuppan.

Althusser, Louis. 1971. *Essays on Ideology*. London and New York: Verso.

Amagasa, Tadashi. 1999a. Karō Jisatsu no Mekanizumu to Sono Konzetsu ni Mukete (The Mechanism of Overwork Suicide and How to Eradicate It). *Chōsa Jihō* (*Research Report*) 444 (December): 41–49.

———. 1999b. Rōdōsha no Jisatsu to Sono Haikei (Workers' Suicides and the Background). *Kikan Hatarakumono no Inochi to Kenkō* (*The Life and Health of Workers*) June: 32–39.

———. 2005. Seishinshōgai Hasshō no Seishinigaku ni Miru Gendankai to Rōsai Ninteikijun (The Current Psychiatric Knowledge of and the Standards for Workers' Compensation for Mental Illness). *Hataraku Mono no Inochi to Kenkō* (*The Life and Health of Workers*) 22: 19–31.

Amagasa, Takashi, Takeo Nakayama, and Yoshitomo Takahashi. 2005. Karojisatsu in Japan: Characteristics of 22 Cases of Work-Related Suicide. *Journal of Occupational Health* 47, no.2: 157–64.

Ambaras, David R. 1998. Social Knowledge, Cultural Capital, and the New Middle Class in Japan, 1895–1912. *Journal of Japanese Studies* 24: 1–33.

Angst, J., A. Gamma, M. Gastpar, J. P. Lepine, J. Mendlewicz, and A. Tylee. 2002. Gender Differences in Depression: Epidemiological Findings from the European DEPRES I and II Studies. *European Archives of Psychiatry & Clinical Neuroscience* 252, no.5: 201–9.

Applbaum, Kalman. 2006. Educating For Global Mental Health: American Pharmaceutical Companies and the Adoption of SSRI in Japan. In *Pharmaceuticals and Globalization: Ethics, Markets, Practices*, eds. Adriana Petryna, Andrew Lakoff, and Arthur Kleinman. Durham, NC: Duke University Press.

———. 2010. Shadow Science: Zyprexa, Eli Lilly and the Globalization of Pharmaceutical Damage Control. *BioSocieties* 5, no.2: 236–55.

Arima, Akito. 1990. *Ki no Sekai* (*The World of Ki*). Tokyo: Tokyo Diagaku Shuppankai.

Armstrong, David. 1983. *Political Anatomy of the Body: Medical Knowledge in Britain in the Twentieth Century*. Cambridge: Cambridge University Press.

Arney, William R. and Bernard J. Bergen. 1984. *Medicine and the Management of Living: Taming the Last Great Beast*. Chicago: University of Chicago Press.

Arnold, David. 1993. *Colonizing the Body: State Medicine and Epidemic Disease in Nineteenth-Century India*. Berkeley: University of California Press.

Asada, Shigeya. 1985. *Shiritsu Seishin Byōin no Yakuwari: Furansu no Seishiniryō Seido ni Terashite* (*The Role of Private Mental Hospitals: a Comparison With the French Psychiatric System*). Tokyo: Makino Shuppan.

Asahi Shimbun. 1956. "Torikoshi Gurō" no Shinyaku (New Drug For "Worrying Too Much"). September 15.

———. 1965. Seishinanteizai no Jōyō ni Akashingō (Red Light to Casual Use of Minor Tranquilizers). November 21.

———. 1974. Pari no Panda Lilly Kun Shinkeisuijakude? Shinu (Lilly the Panda in Paris Zoo Dies of Neursthenia?). April 24.

——— 1999. Jisatsushita Etō Jun shi no Isho Kōhyō (The Suicide Note of Etō Jun), July 23.

———. 1999. Jisatsu no Rōsai Nintei Kanwa: Taishō "Kokoro no Shippei" mo (Relaxed Regulations for Work-Related Suicide Compensation: Broader Inclusion of Mental Illness). July 31.

———. 2000. Karō Jisatsu Rōsai no Monko wa Hirogattaka (Overwork Suicide: Has the Gate For Workers' Compensation Really Widened?). June 21.

———. 2000. Karō Jisatsu Soshō de Wakai, Dentsu Shain Izokugawa "Zenmenshōri no Naiyō" (Resolution for Overwork Suicide Lawsuit: Dentsu Employee's Family "All-Out Victory"). June 23.

———. 2001. "Sutoresu" Mitomeru Nagare, Kyōyo no Jisatsu "Rōsai" Nintei ("Stress" Increasingly Given Consideration: Suicide of a Teacher to Be Granted Worker's Compensation). February 23.

———. 2001. Shokuba no "Jakusha" ni Hikari, Karō Jisatsu ni Rōsai Nintei Hanketsu (Light on the "Weak" in Workplaces: Workers' Compensation Granted in Overwork Suicide Lawsuit). June 18.

———. 2003. Rōkishogawa ga Jōkoku Dannen e, Toyota Kakarichō Karō Jisatsu Soshō (Labor Standard Office Decides Not to Appeal to Higher Court: The Overwork Suicide of Toyota's Assistant Manager). July 18.

———. 2003. Rōsai Nintei no Handan Shishin "Gutaiteki ni", Toyota Karō Jisatsu Soshō (The Standard for Determining Workers' Compensation "Should Be More Concrete": Toyota Overwork Lawsuit). July 9.

———. 2005. Jisatsu Yobō e Sōgō Taisaku (Comprehensive Measures for Preventing Suicide). July 16.

———. 2005. Sazae-San o Sagashite (Looking for Sazae-San). May 14.

———. 2007. "Pawahara Jisatsu" Rōsai Nintei: Jōshi kara Bōgen "Kyūryō Dorobō" "Mezawari, Kiete kure" ("Power Harassment Suicide" to Receive Workers' Compensation: Insulted by Boss "Goldbricker" "Eyesore"). October 16.

———. 2007. Mado: Shitsukanjōshō (Window: Alexithymia). June 27.

———. 2007. Rōsai Nintei Josei Denīzu ni Baishōseikyū "Ijime, Sekuhara de Utsubyō" (Workers' Compensation Granted to a Female Worker, "Bullying and Sexual Harassment Led to Depression"). May 18.

———. 2008. Hataraku hito no Hōritsu Sōdan: Kokoro no Yamai Saiban dewa Rōsai Nintei ga Zōka (Legal Advice for Workers: Mental Illness, Increasingly Recognized and Compensated through Lawsuits). October 27.

———. 2009. Mottomo omoi Yōin ni Pawahara Tsuika e (Power Harassment Added to the Severest Factor). March 20.

———. 2009. Soryūshi (Particles). May 15, Evening.

———. 2009a. Tōshiba Shain Utsubyō Kajūgyōmu ga Genin (Toshiba Employees Depressed: Overwork is the Cause). May 19.

———2009b. Yūbinkyokuin Futari Shinyakin de Utsu (Two Post Office Workers Depressed after Late Night Shifts). May 19.

———2009. Kokoro no Yamai Rōsai Saita (The Highest Number of Worker's Compensation Ever Granted for Mental Illnesses). June 9.

———. 2010. Seishin Shikkan Chōsa Gimuka Miokuri (Mandatory Mental Health Examination Deferred). July 15.

Asai, Kunihiko. 1999. History and Present State of Psychiatric Care. In *Images in Psychiatry: Japan,* eds. Yoshibumi Nakane and Mark Radford. World Psychiatric Association.

Asano, Hirotake. 2000. *Seishin Iryō Ronsōshi (The History of Disputes in Psychiatry).* Tokyo: Hihyōsha.

Ashikawa Keishū, 1982. *Ashikawa Keishū,* eds. Keisetsu Ōtsuka and Dōmei Yakazu. Tokyo: Meicho Shuppan.

Atkinson, Paul. 1995. *Medical Talk and Medical Work.* London: Sage.

Azai, Teian, 1981. *Azai Teian,* eds. Keisetsu Ōtsuka, and Dōmei Yakazu. Tokyo: Meicho Shuppan.

Bakhtin, Mikhail M., and Michael Holquist. 1981. *The Dialogic Imagination: Four Essays.* Austin: University of Texas Press.

Barrett Robert J. 1988. Interpretations of Schizophrenia. *Culture, Medicine and Psychiatry* 12, no.3: 357–88.

———. 1996. *The Psychiatric Team and the Social Definition of Schizophrenia: An Anthropological Study of Person and Illness.* Cambridge, England/New York: Cambridge University Press.

Barthes, Roland. 1982. *Empires of Signs.* Translated by Richard Howard. New York: Hill and Wang.

Battaglia, Debbora. 1995. Problematizing the Self: A Thematic Introduction. In *Rhetorics of Self-Making,* ed. Debbora Battaglia. Berkeley: University of California Press.

BBC News. 2009. French Unease at Telecome Suicides. September 12.

Becker, Howard. 1960. *Outsiders: Studies in the Sociology of Deviance.* New York: Free Press.

Béhague, Dominique Pareja. 2008. Psychiatry and Military Conscription in Brazil: The Search for Opportunity and Institutionalized Therapy. *Culture, Medicine and Psychiatry* 32, no.2: 140–51.

———. 2009. Psychiatry and Politics in Pelotas, Brazil: the Equivocal Quality of Conduct Disorder and Related Diagnoses. *Medical Anthropology Quarterly* 23, no.4: 455–82.

Benedict, Ruth. 1946. *Chrysanthemum and the Sword: Patterns of Japanese Culture.* Boston: Houghton-Mifflin.

Boddy, Janice. 1989. *Wombs and Alien Spirits: Women, Men, and the Zar in Northern Sudan.* Madison: University of Wisconsin Press.

Bordo, Susan. 1993. *Unbearable Weight.* Berkeley: University of California Press.

Borovoy, Amy. 1995. *Good Wives and Mothers: The Production of Japanese Domesticity in a Global Economy.* Ph.D. Dissertation, Stanford University.

———. 2005. *The Too-Good Wife: Alcohol, Codependency, and the Politics of Nurturance in Postwar Japan.* Berkeley: University of California Press.

———. 2008. Japan's Hidden Youths: Mainstreaming the Emotionally Distressed in Japan. *Culture, Medicine and Psychiatry* 32, no.4: 552–76.

Bourdachs, Michael K. 1997. Shimazaki Toson's Hakai and Its Bodies. In *New Directions in the Study of Meiji Japan,* eds. Helen Hardacre and Adam L. Kern. Leiden/New York/ Koln: Brill.

Bourdieu, Pierre. 1977. *Outline of a Theory of Practice*. Cambridge: Cambridge University Press.

Breslau, Joshua A. 1999. *Learning to Locate the Heart: An Apprenticeship in Japanese Psychiatry*. Ph. D. Dissertation. Harvard University.

Brice, Pedroletti. 1999. Au Japonpersonne ne Respecte Les Limites Légales. *Le Monde*. May 22.

Brotherton, Sean P. 2008. "We Have To Think Like Capitalists But Continue Being Socialists": Medicalized Subjectivities, Emergent Capital, and Socialist Entrepreneurs in Post-Soviet Cuba. *American Ethnologist* 35, no. 2: 259-274.

Brotherton, Sean P. 2012. *Bodies in States of Crisis: The Biopolitics of Health in Post-Soviet Cuba*. Durham: Duke University Press.

Brown, Norman O. 1959. *Life Against Death: The Psychoanalytical Meaning of History*. New York: Vintage Books.

Burns, Susan L. 1997. Contemplating Places: the Hospital As Modern Experience in Meiji Japan. In *New Directions in the Study of Meiji Japan*, eds. Helen Hardacre and Adam L. Kern. Leiden: Brill.

Bynum, W.F. 1985. The Nervous Patient in Eighteenth- and Nineteenth-Century Britain: the Psychiatric Origins of British Neurology. In *The Anatomy of Madness: Essays in the History of Psychiatry*, eds. W. F. Bynum, Roy Porter, and Michael Sepherd. London and New York: Tavistock Publications.

Carey, Benedict. 2008. Brain Enhancement is Wrong, Right? *New York Times*, March 9.

———. 2010. Popular Drugs May Benefit Only Severe Depression, New Study Says. *New York Times*, January 6.

Castel, Robert, Francoise Castel, and Anne Lovell. 1982[1979]. *The Psychiatric Society*. Translated by A. Goldhammer. New York: Columbia University Press.

Clarke, Adele, and Theresa Montini. 1993. The Many Faces of RU486: Tales of Situated Knowledges and Technological Contestations. *Science, Technology & Human Values* 18, no.1: 42–78.

Clarke, Edwin, and L. S. Jacyna. 1987. *Nineteenth-Century Origins of Neuroscientific Concepts*. Berkeley: University of California Press.

Cohen, Lawrence. 1995. The Epistemological Carnival: Meditations on Disciplinary Intentionality and Ayurveda. In *Knowledge and the Scholarly Medical Traditions*, ed. Don Bates. Cambridge: Cambridge University Press.

———. 1998. *No Aging in India: Alzheimer's, the Bad Family, and Other Modern Things*. Berkeley: University of California Press.

Comaroff, Jean. 1982. Medicine: Symbol and Ideology. In *The Problem of Medical Knowledge*, eds. Paul Wright and Andrew Treacher. Edinburgh: Edinburgh University Press.

———. 1985. *Body of Power, Spirit of Resistance: The Culture and History of a South African People*. Chicago: University of Chicago Press.

Conrad, Peter and Joseph W. Schneider. 1980. *Deviance and Medicalization: From Badness to Sickness*. St. Louis: C.V. Mosby.

Cooper, David. 1967. *Psychiatry and Anti-Psychiatry*. London/New York: Tavistock Publications.

Corin, Ellen. 1990. Facts and Meaning in Psychiatry: An Anthropological Approach to the Lifeworld of Schizophrenics. *Culture, Medicine and Psychiatry* 14, no.2: 153–88.

———. 1998a. The Thickness of Being: Intentional Worlds, Strategies of Identity and Experience Among Schizophrenics. *Psychiatry* 61, no. 2: 133–46.

———. 1998b. Refiguring the Person: the Dynamics of Affects and Symbols in an African Spirit Possession Cult. In *Bodies and Persons: Comparative Perspectives from Africa and Melanesia*, eds. Michael Lambek and Andrew Strathern. Cambridge: Cambridge University Press.

Corin, Ellen and Gilles Lauzon. 1992. Positive Withdrawal and the Quest For Meaning: The Reconstruction of Experience Among Schizophrenia. *Psychiatry* 55, no.3: 266–78.

Crawford, Robert. 1984. A Cultural Account of Health: Self Control, Release and the Social Body. In *Issues in the Political Economy of Health Care*, ed. J. Mckinlay. *New York: Travistock Publications.*

Daily Yomiuri. 1999. Courts Becoming More Open to Work-Related Suicide Suits. October 11.

———. 1999. Government to Establish Criteria For Work-Related Suicides. April 11.

———. 2004. Worker's Comp Claim Filed Over Osaka Judge's Suicide. March 30.

Davis, Elizabeth. 2008. *Bad Souls: An Ethnography of Madness and Responsibility in Greek Thrace.* Durham: Duke University Press.

Degrazia, David. 2000. Prozac, Enhancement, and Self-Creation. *Hastings Center Report*, March-April.

Doi, Takeo. 1954. Seishinbunseki Hihan no Hanhihan (Critique of the Critique of Psychoanalysis). *Seishin Shinkeigaku Zasshi (Journal of Psychiatry and Neurology)* 55, no. 7: 748–51.

———. 1966. Utsubyō no Seishin Rikigaku (Psychodynamics of Depression). *Seishinigaku (Clinical Psychiatry)* 8, no. 12: 978-81.

———. 1973. The *Anatomy of Dependence.* Tokyo/New York: Kodansha International.

———. 1990. The Cultural Assumptions of Psychoanalysis. In *Cultural Psychology: Essays on Comparative Human Development*, eds. James W. Stigler, Richard A. Shweder, Gilbert H. Herdt, and University of Chicago Committee on Human Development. Cambridge/New York: Cambridge University Press.

———. 2000. Noirōze, Ki no Yamai, Kichigai (Neurosis, Illness of Ki, Insanity). In *Doi Takeo Senshū 6 (Collected Works of Doi Takeo Vol. 6)*. Tokyo: Iwanami Shoten.

Dore, Ronald P. 1958. *City Life in Japan: A Study of a Tokyo Ward.* Richmond, Surrey: Japan Press.

Douglas, Mary. 1992. *Risk and Blame: Essays in Cultural Theory.* London: Routledge.

Duclos, Vincent. 2009. When Anthropology Meets Science: An Interview with Allan Young. *Altérités* 6, no. 1: 110–18.

Duden, Barbara. 1991. The *Woman Beneath the Skin: A Doctor's Patients in Eighteenth-Century Germany.* Cambridge, MA: Harvard University Press.

Duncan, Grant. 2003. Workers' Compensation and the Governance of Pain. *Economy and Society* 32, no. 3: 449–77.

Ecks, Stefan. 2003. Is India on Prozac?: Sociotropic Effects of Pharmaceuticals in a Global Perspective. *Curare* 26, no.1–2: 95–08.

———. 2005. Pharmaceutical Citizenship: Antidepressant Marketing and the Promise of Demarginalization in India. *Anthropology and Medicine* 12, no. 3: 239–54.

———. Forthcoming. *India on Prozac.* London: Routledge.

Eguchi, Shigeyuki. 1987. Shigaken Koto Ichisanson ni Okeru Kitsunetsuki no Seisei to Henyō (The Production and Alteration of Fox Possession in a Mountain Village in Shiga Prefecture). *Kokuritsu Minzokugaku Hakubutsukan Kenkyū Hōkoku (National Ethnological Museum Research Report)* 12, no. 4: 1113–79.

Ehrenberg, Alain. 2010. *The Weariness of the Self: Diagnosing the History of Depression in the Contemporary Age*. Montreal and Kingston: McGill-Queen's University Press.

Ejima, Kiseki and Tsuyoshi Hasegawa. 1989. *Keisei Irojamisen; Keisei Denju-Gamiko; Seken Musume Katagi (The Vocal Shamisen of the Courtesan)*. Tokyo: Iwanami Shoten.

Elliott, Carl. 2003. *Better than Well: American Medicine Meets the American Dream*. New York: W. W. Norton.

Elliott, Carl and Tod Chambers. 2004. *Prozac as a Way of Life*. Chapel Hill: University of North Carolina Press.

Estroff, Sue E. 1981. *Making It Crazy: An Ethnography of Psychiatric Clients in an American Community*. Berkeley: University of California Press.

———. 1993. Identity, Disability, and Schizophrenia: The Problem of Chronicity. In *Knowledge, Power & Practice*, eds. Shirley Lindenbaum and Margaret Lock. Berkeley: University of California Press.

Evans-Pritchard, Edward Evan. 1937. *Witchcraft, Oracles and Magic Among the Azande*. Oxford: Clarendon Press.

Foucault, Michel. 1973. *Madness and Civilization: A History of Insanity in the Age of Reason*. New York: Vintage Books.

———. 1975. *The Birth of the Clinic: An Archeology of Medical Perception*. New York: Vintage Books.

———. 1977. *Discipline and Punish: The Birth of the Prison*. New York: Vintage Books.

Fox, Renée C. 1979. *Essays in Medical Sociology: Journeys into the Field*. New Brunswick/ Oxford: Transaction Books.

Franklin, Sarah and Celia Roberts. 2006. *Born and Made: An Ethnography of Preimplantation Genetic Diagnosis*. Princeton: Princeton University Press.

Freidson, Eliot. 1970. *Profession of Medicine: A Study of the Sociology of Applied Knowledge*. New York: Dodd, Mead & Company.

French, Howard W. 2000. A Postmodern Plague Ravages Japan's Workers. *New York Times*, February 21.

Fujikawa, Hiroaki. 2000. Iwayuru Karō Jisatsu to Anzen Hairyo Gimu Hōri (So-Called Overwork Suicide and the Obligation of Safety Doctorine). *Bessatsu Jurist: Shakai Hoshō Hanrei Hyakusen (Jurist Supplement: Social Security 100 Precedents)* 153: 150–51.

Fujimoto, Shigeru. 2002. Karō Jisatsu to Shiyōsha no Songai Baishō Sekinin (Overwork Suicide and the Liability of Employers). *Bessatsu Jurist (Jurist Supplement)* 165 (November): 142–43.

Fujimoto, Tadashi. 1996. *"Jisatsu Karōshi" Saiban 24 Sai Natsu Adoman no Ketsubetsu ("Overwork Suicide" Lawsuit: 24-Year-Old Advertisement Man's Departure)*. Tokyo: Daiamond Sha.

———. 1997. Nihongata Kigyō no Byōri to Seinen no Shi: Dentsū Jisatsu Karōshi Jiken (Pathology of Japanese-Style Corporate Society and the Death of a Young Man: Dentsu Overwork Suicide Case). *Kikan Rōdōsha no Kenri (Workers' Rights)* 220: 158–63.

Fujisaki, Kazuhiko. 1995. Ishi (Doctors). In *Gendai Iryō no Shakaigaku: Nihon no Genjō to Kadai (Sociology of Modern Medicine: the Present Condition and Issues in Japan)*, ed. Kōichiro Kuroda. 33–58. Kyoto: Sekai Shisōsha.

Fukuoka Chihō Saibansho (Fukuoka District Court). 1982. *Songai Baishō Seikyū Jiken (Appeal for Compensation for Damage)*, No.27405686.

Funahashi, Daena Aki. 2010. "Wrapped in Plastic": Metamorphosis and Burnout in Finland. Unpublished manuscript.

Furusawa, Satoshi. 1998. Nihon ni okeru Shinrigaku(sha) to Shakai (Psychology[ists] and Society in the Prewar and Interwar Japan). In *Nihon Shinrigakushi no Kenkyū* (*Studies of the History of Japanese Psychology*), eds. Shinrigaku Kenkyūkai and Rekishi Kenkyūbukai. Kyoto: Hōsei Shuppan.

Gaines, Atwood D., ed. 1992a. *Ethnopsychiatry: The Cultural Construction of Professional and Folk Psychiatries*. Albany: State University of New York Press.

———. 1992b. From DSM I to III-R; Voices of Self, Mastery and the Other: A Cultural Constructivist Reading of U.S. Psychiatric Classification. *Social Science and Medicine* 35, no.1: 3–24.

Gal, Susan. 1991. Between Speech and Silence: The Problematics of Research on Language and Gender. In *Gender at the Crossroads of Knowledge: Feminist Anthropology in the Postmodern Era*, ed. Micaela di Leonardo. Berkeley: University of California Press.

Garon, Sheldon M. 1997. *Molding Japanese Minds: The State in Everyday Life*. Princeton, NJ: Princeton University Press.

Garro, Linda C. 1994. Chronic Illness and the Construction of Narratives. In *Pain as Human Experience: An Anthropological Perspective*, eds. Mary-Jo Delvecchio Good, Paul E. Brodwin, Byron J. Good, and Arthur Kleinman. Berkeley: University of California Press.

Gates, Barbara T. 1988. *Victorian Suicide: Mad Crimes and Sad Histories*. Princeton, NJ: Princeton University Press.

Giddens, Anthony. 1991. *Modernity and Self-Identity: Self and Society in the Late Modern Age*. Cambridge, England: Polity Press.

Gijswijt-Hofstra, Marijke and Roy Porter. 2001. *Cultures of Neurasthenia from Beard to the First World War*. Amsterdam/New York: Rodopi.

Gilbert, G. Nigel and Michael Mulkay. 1984. *Opening Pandora's Box: A Sociological Analysis of Scientists' Discourse*. Cambridge: Cambridge University Press.

Gluck, Carol. 1985. *Japan's Modern Myths: Ideology in the Late Meiji Period*. Princeton, NJ: Princeton University Press.

Goffman, Erving. 1961. *Asylums: Essays on the Social Situation of Mental Patients and Other Inmates*. Garden City, NY: Anchor Books.

———. 1963. *Stigma: Notes on the Management of Spoiled Identity*. Englewood Cliffs, NJ: Prentice-Hall.

Goldsmith, S. K. et al., eds. 2002. *Reducing Suicide: A National Imperative*. Washington, D.C.: National Academic Press.

Goldstein, Jan. 1987. *Console and Classify: the French Psychiatric Profession in the Nineteenth Century*. Cambridge: Cambridge University Press.

Good, Byron J. 1994. *Medicine, Rationality, and Experience: An Anthropological Perspective*. Cambridge: Cambridge University Press.

Good, Mary-Jo Delvecchio, Paul E. Brodwin, Byron Good, and Arthur Kleinman, eds. 1992. *Pain as Human Experience: An Anthropological Perspective*. Berkeley: University of California Press.

Gordon, Andrew. 1998. *The Wages of Affluence: Labor and Management in Postwar Japan*. Cambridge, MA: Harvard University Press.

———. 2009. *A Modern History of Japan: From Tokugawa Times to the Present*. Oxford/New York: Oxford University Press.

Gordon, Deborah R. 1988. Tenacious Assumptions in Western Medicine. In *Biomedicine Examined*, eds. Margaret Lock and Deborah Gordon. Dordrecht: Kluwer Academic Publishers.

Gosling, Francis G. 1987. *Before Freud: Neurasthenia and the American Medical Community, 1870–1910*. Urbana: University of Illinois Press.

Gotō, Konzan. 1971. *Shisetsu Hikki (Transcription of [Gotō's] Ideas). Kinsei Kagaku Shisō (Premodern Scientific Thought)*. Tokyo: Iwanami Shoten.

Habermas, Jürgen. 1987. *The Theory of Communicative Action. Vol. 2: Lifeworld and System: a Critique of Fundamental Reason*. Boston: Beacon Press.

Hacking, Ian. 1982. Language, Truth and Reason. In *Rationality and Relativism*, eds. Martin Hollis and Steven Lukes. Oxford: Blackwell.

———. 1986. Making Up People. In *Reconstructing Individualism: Autonomy, Individuality, and the Self in Western Thought*, eds. Thomas C. Heller, Morton Sosna, and David E. Wellbery. Stanford, CA: Stanford University Press.

———. 1990. *The Taming of Chance*. Cambridge: Cambridge University Press.

———. 1995. *Rewriting the Soul: Multiple Personality and the Sciences of Memory*. Princeton, NJ: Princeton University Press.

———. 1999. *The Social Construction of What?* Cambridge, MA: Harvard University Press.

———. 2002. *Historical Ontology*. Cambridge, MA: Harvard University Press.

Hanrei Times. Rōdō Saiban Rei (Labor Court Cases). 1998. no.962: 145–52.

Haraway, Donna J. 1997. *Modest_Witness@Second_Millennium.FemaleMan_Meets_OncoMouse: Feminism and Technoscience*. New York and London: Routledge.

Hattori, Toshirō. 1978. *Edojidai Igakushi no Kenkyū (A Study on the History of Medicine in the Edo Period)*. Tokyo: Yoshikawa Kōbunkan.

Hayashi, Kimikazu. 2001. *Gitai Utsubyō (Mimic Depression)*. Tokyo: Takarajimasha.

Healy, David. 1997. *The Antidepressant Era*. Cambridge, MA: Harvard University Press.

———. 2000. Some Continuities and Discontinuities in the Pharmacotherapy of Nervous Conditions Before and After Chloropromazine and Imipramine. *History of Psychiatry* Xi: 393–412.

———. 2002. *The Creation of Psychopharmacology*. Cambridge, MA: Harvard University Press.

———. 2004. *Let Them Eat Prozac: The Unehealthy Relationship Between the Pharmaceutical Industry and Depression*. New York: New York University Press.

Hendin, H., A. Lipschitz, J. T. Maltsberger, A. P. Haas, and S. Wynecoop. 2000. Therapists' Reactions to Patients' Suicides. *The American Journal of Psychiatry* 157, no.12: 2022–27.

Henriques, Julian, Wendy Hollway, Cathy Urwin, Couze Venn, and Valerie Walkerdine. 1984. *Changing the Subject: Psychology, Social Relation and Subjectivity*. London and New York: Methuen.

Herman, Ellen. 1995. *The Romance of American Psychology: Political Culture in the Age of Experts*. Berkeley: University of California Press.

Hirai, Yoshinori. 1999. *Nihon no Shakaihoshō (Social Security in Japan)*. Tokyo: Iwanami Shoten.

Hirasawa, Hajime. 1966. *Keishō Utsubyō no Rinshō to Yogo (Clinical Practice and Prognosis of Mild Depression)*. Tokyo: Igaku Shoin.

Hirata, Tsuneko. 2007. Hanpukusei Utsubyōsei Shōgai de atta Rōdōsha ni yoru Jisatsu to

Gyōmukiinsei (A Suicide by a Worker Who was Suffering Recurrent Depressive Disorder and Its Causal Attribution to Work). *Chingin to Shakaihoshō* (*Wage and Social Security*) 1435: 33–42.

Hiroi, Yoshinori. 1996. *Idenshi no Gijutsu, Idenshi no Shisō* (*Technology of Genetics, Epistemology of Genetics*). Tokyo: Chūkō Shinsho.

Hirose, Kyoko. 1972. Seishin Eisei Sōdan no Tachiba Kara (From a Viewpoint of a Mental Hygiene Consultant). *Kokoro to Shakai* (*Mind and Society*) 3, no.3–4: 135–41.

Hirose, Tetsuya. 1977. "Tōhigata Yokuutsu" ni Tsuite (On "Escaping Depression"). In *Sōutsubyō no Seishin Byōri II* (*Psychopathology of Manic Depression II*), ed. Tadao Miyamoto. Tokyo: Kōbundō.

———. 1979. Utsubyō no Seishin Ryōhō (Psychotherapy for Depression). *Rinshō Seishinigaku* (*Clinical Psychiatry*) 8, no.11.

Hirota, Isoo. 1981. *Seishin Byōin* (*Mental Hospital*). Tokyo: Iwasaki Gakujutsu Shuppansha.

Hiruta, Genshirō. 1999a. Edojidai Kanpōi no Seishinbyōkan (The Concept of Mental Illness among Physicians in the Edo Era Japan). *Seishinigakushi Kenkyū* (*Journal of History of Psychiatry*) 2.

———. 1999b. Nihon no Seishin Iryōshi (History of Psychiatric Practice in Japan). In *Seishin Iryō no Rekishi* (*The History of Psychiatry*), eds. Masaaki Matsushita and Genshirō Hiruta. Tokyo: Nakayama Shoten.

Hochschild, Arlie R. 1983. *The Managed Heart: Commercialization of Human Feeling.* Berkeley: University of California Press.

Hoff, Paul. 1996. *Kraepelin to Rinshō Seishinigaku* (*Kraepelin and Clinical Psychiatry*). Tokyo: Seiwa Shoten.

Holmes, Mary. 2004. The Importance of Being Angry: Anger in Political Life. *European Journal of Social Theory* 7, no.2: 123–32.

Honda, Yutaka. 1983. DSM-III in Japan. In *International Perspectives on DSM-III*, eds. Robert L. Spitzer, Janet B. W. Williams, and Andrew E. Skodol. Washington, D.C.: American Psychiatric Press.

Horwitz, Allan V. and Jerome C. Wakefield. 2007. *The Loss of Sadness: How Psychiatry Transformed Normal Sorrow into Depressive Disorder.* Oxford: Oxford University Press.

Hozumi, Masashi. 2007. Rībokku Japan Rōsai Nintei Jiken: Otona no Ijime Taishoku Kyōyō de Utsubyō wa Rōsai (The Reebok Japan Workers' Compensation Case: Workers' Compensation for Depression Caused by Bullying and Coerced Resignation). *Rōdōhōritsujunpō* (*Labor Law Report*) 1650: 51–53.

Hubert, Susan J. 2002. *Questions of Power: The Politics of Women's Madness Narratives.* Newark: University of Delaware Press.

Igarashi, Yoshio and Kazuhiko Ishii. 2000. Seishinka Byōin deno Jisatsu no Jittai (Suicide in Psychiatric Hospitals). *Igaku no Ayumi* (*Journal of Clinical and Experimental Medicine*) 194, no.6: 529–33.

Iida, Shin. 1973. Sōutsubyō no Jōkyōron to Kongo no Kadai (Situational Cause of Depression and New Issues). *Seishin Shinkeigaku Zasshi* (*Journal of Psychiatry and Neurology*) 75: 274–79.

———. 1974. Sōutsubyō (Manic depression). *Gendai no Esupuri* (*L'esprit d'aujourd'hui*) 88: 5–15.

Iida, Shin. 1978. Sōutsubyō no Jōkyōiron (Theories of Situational Cause for Manic Depression). In *Seishinigaku Ronbunshū* (*Papers on Psychiatry*). Tokyo: Kongō Shuppan.

Ikeda, Mitsuho and Junichi Sato. 1995. Kenkō Būmu (Health Boom). In *Gendai Iryō no Shakaigaku: Nihon no Genjō to Kadai* (*Sociology of Modern Medicine: the Present Condition and Issues in Japan*), ed. Kōichirō Kuroda. 263–78. Kyoto: Sekai Shisōsha.

Illich, Ivan. 1975. *Medical Memesis: The Expropriation of Health*. London: Calder & Boyars.

Inamura, Hiroshi. 1977. *Jisatsugaku: Sono Chiryō to Yobō no Tameni* (*Suicidology: Treatment and Prevention*). Tokyo: Tokyo Daigaku Shuppan.

Ingleby, David. 1980. *Critical Psychiatry: The Politics of Mental Health*. New York: Pantheon.

Ishida, Hidemi. 1989. Body and Mind: The Chinese Perspective. In *Taoist Meditation and Longevity Techniques*, eds. Livia Kohn and Yoshinobu Sakade. Center for Chinese Studies, The University of Michigan.

Ishida, Noboru. 1906. *Shinsen Seishinbyōgaku* (*New Psychopathology*). Tokyo: Nankōdō.

Ishikawa, Kiyoshi. 1962. Seishin Byōrigaku no Shotaikei to Ryōkai Seishin Byōrigaku Teki Hōhō (The Systems of Psychopathologies and "Versthehens"-Psychopathological Approach). *Seishin Shinkeigaku Zasshi* (*Journal of Psychiatry and Neurology*) 64: 953.

Ishikawa, Sadakichi. 1925. Kurecchimeru Shi no Taikei Oyobi Kishitsuron (Kretschmer's Theories on Constitution and Temperament). *Shikeigaku Zasshi* (*Journal of Neurology*) 26: 259–70.

Itsumi, Takeru, Masaji Iwamoto, Kazuo Okagami, Kōtarō Nakayama, Kazuo Yamamoto, and Masao Anjiki. 1970. Seishin Eisei towa Nanika (What Is Mental Hygiene?). *Kokoro to Shakai* (*Mind and Society*) 3–4: 154–78.

Ivry, Tsipy. 2010. *Embodying Culture: Pregnancy in Japan and Israel*. New Brunswick, NJ: Rutgers University Press.

Jack, Dana Crowley. 1991. *Silencing the Self: Women and Depression*. Cambridge, MA: Harvard University Press.

Jackson, Stanely W. 1986. *Melancholia and Depression: From Hippocratic Times to Modern Times*. New Haven: Yale University Press.

Jannetta, Ann Bowman. 1997. From Physician to Bureaucrat: The Case of Nagayo Sensai. In *New Directions in the Study of Meiji Japan*, eds. Helen Hardacre and Adam L. Kern. Leiden: Brill.

Janzen, John M. 1978. *The Quest for Therapy in Lower Zaire*. Berkeley: University of California Press.

Jolly, David and Matthew Saltmarsh. 2009. Suicides in France Put Focus on Workplace. *New York Times*, September 29.

Kagawa, Shūan. 1982. *Kagawa Shūan*, eds. Keisetsu Ōtsuka and Dōmei Yakazu. Tokyo: Meicho Shuppan.

Kaibara, Ekiken. 1928. *Yōjōkun* (*Theory of Health*). Tokyo: Yūhōdō Shoten.

Kakimoto, Akihito. 1991. *Kenkō to Yamai no Episteme* (*Episteme of Health and Illness*). Kyoto: Mneruva Shobō.

Kamata, Satoshi. 1999. *Kazoku ga Jisatsu ni Oikomarerutoki* (*When a Family Member Is Driven to Suicide*). Tokyo: Kōdansha.

Kanba, Shigenobu. 2005. Gendai Shakai to Utsubyō (Contemporary Society and Depression). *Kumamoto Seishinka Byōin Kyōkaishi (Journal of Kumamoto Mental Hospital Association)* 125: 1–20.

Kanbe, Bunsai. 1973[1876]. *Seishinbyō Yakusetsu (On Psychopathology)* [Translation of a text by Henry Maudsley]. Chōfu: Seishinigaku Shinkeigaku Koten Kankōkai.

Kaneko, Junji. 1965. *Nihon Seishinbyō Gakushoshi (History of Psychiatric Texts in Japan).* Tokyo: Nihon Seishin Byōin Kyōkai (Japanese Association of Mental Hospitals).

Karatani, Kōjin. 1993. *Origins of Modern Japanese Literature.* Translated by Brett de Bary. Durham, NC: Duke University Press.

Kasahara, Yomishi. 1992. Byōzen Seikaku ni tsuite (On Premorbid Personality). In *Utsubyō: Kibun Shōgai (Depression: Mood Disorders),* eds. Kasahara Yomishi, Itaru Yamashita, and Tetsuya Hirose. Osaka: Shinryō Shinsha.

———. 1976. Utsubyō no Byōzen Seikaku ni Tsuite (On Premorbid Personality of Depression). In *Sōutsubyō no Seishin Byōri I (Psychopathology of Depression I),* ed. Yomishi Kasahara. Tokyo: Kōbundō.

———. 1978. Utsubyō no Shōseishinryōhō (Brief Psychotherapy for Depression). *Kikan Seishinryōhō (Japanese Journal of Psychotherapy)* 4, no.2: 6–11.

———. 1989. Utsubyō no Seishinryōhō. In *Seishinryōhō no Jissai (Practice of Psychotherapy),* ed. Yoshihiro Narita. Tokyo: Shinkōigaku Shuppansha.

———. 1991. *Gairai Seishinigaku Kara (From Outpatient Psychiatry).* Tokyo: Seikōsha.

———. 2003. Keishō Utsubyō ni Tsuite (On Mild Depression). *Rinshō Seishin Yakuri (Clinical Psychopharmacology)* 6: 147–53.

Kasahara, Yomishi and Bin Kimura. 1975. Utsujōtai no Rinshōteki Bunrui ni Kansuru Kenkyū (Clinical Classification of Depressive States). *Seishin Shinkeigaku Zasshi (Journal of Psychiatry and Neurology)* 77, no.10: 715–35.

Kasahara, Yomishi, Itaru Yamashita, and Tetsuya Hirose. 1992. *Utsubyō: Kibun Shōgai (Depression: Mood Disorders).* Osaka: Shinryō Shinsha.

Kashimi, Yumiko. 2001. Minpō 7: Chōjikan Zangyō ni Yoru Karō Jisatsu to Shiyōsha Sekinin (Civil Law 7: Overwork Suicide From Long Hours of Overtime and Employer's Responsibility). *Jurist* 1202: 71–73.

Katayama, Kuniyoshi. 1906. Jisatsu to Shakai (Suicide and Society). *Tokyo Asahi Shimbun,* October 22.

———. 1912. Jisatsu no Hōigaku Teki Yobōhō (Prevention of Suicide form a Forensic Psychiatric Perspective). *Shinkeigaku Zasshi (Journal of Neurology)* 10: 492.

Katō, Masaaki. 1953. Kattō Hannō to Shite no Jisatsu no Kisei ni Tsuite (The Mechanism of Suicide As a Response to a Conflict). *Seishin Shinkeigaku Zasshi (Journal of Psychiatry and Neurology)* 55, no. 4: 569.

———. 1976. *Shakai to Seishin Byōri (Society and Psychopathology).* Tokyo: Kōbundō.

Katsuki, Gyūzan. 1981. *Katuki Gyūzan,* eds. Keisetsu Ōtsuka and Dōmei Yakazu. Tokyo: Meicho Shuppan.

Kawahito, Hiroshi. 1996. *Karōshi to Kigyō no Sekinin (Overwork Death and Corporate Responsibilities).* Tokyo: Shakai Shisōsha.

———. 1998. *Karō Jisatsu (Overwork Suicide).* Tokyo: Iwanami Shoten.

Kawakami, Norito. 2000. Sangyō Mentaru Herusu Kenkyū no Genjō to Kadai (Research in Occupational Mental Health: Current Status and Future Direction). *Seishin Hoken Kenkyū (Mental Health Research)* 46: 37–41.

Kawakami, Norito, Takeshi Takeshima, Yutaka Ono, Hidenori Uda, Yukihiro Hata, Yoshibumi Nakane, Hideyuki Nakane, Noboru Iwata, Toshiaki A. Furukawa, and Take-hiko Kikkawa. 2005. Twelve-Month Prevalence, Severity, and Treatment of Common Mental Disorders in Communities in Japan: Preliminary Finding from the World Mental Health Japan Survey 2002–3. *Psychiatry and Clinical Neurosciences* 59, no.4: 441–52.

Kawakami, Norito, Yutaka Ōno, Hidenori Uda, Yoshibumi Nakane, and Tadashi Takeshima. 2002. *Chiiki Jūmin ni Okeru Kokoro no kenkō Mondai to Taisaku Kiban no Jittai ni Kansuru Kenkyū: 3 Chiku no Sōgō Kaiseki Kekka (Mental Health of Local Residents and the Policy Basis: Analysis of 3 Areas)*. Tokyo: Kōseirōdōshō (Ministry of Health, Welfare, and Labor).

Kawakami, Takeshi. 1961. *Nihon no Isha: Gendai Iryō Kōzō no Bunseki (Japanese Doctors: an Analysis of Modern Medical System)*. Tokyo: Keisō Shobō.

Kawamura, Kunimitsu. 1990. *Genshi Suru Kindai Kūkan: Meishin, Byōki, Zashikirō, Aruiwa Rekishi no Kioku (Ilusions of Modern Space: Superstitions, Illnesses, Private Confinement, or Memories of History)*. Tokyo: Seikyūsha.

Kawamura, Nozomu. 1990. Sociology and Socialism in the Interwar Period. In *Culture and Identity: Japanese Intellectuals during the Interwar Years*, ed. Thomas Rimer. Princeton, NJ: Princeton University Press.

Kayama, Rika. 1999. Atogaki (Afterward). In *Jisatsu (Suicide)*. Yu Miri. Tokyo: Bungeishunjū.

———. 2008. *"Watashi wa Utsu" to Iitagaru Hitotachi (People who like to say 'I'm depressed')*. Tokyo: PHP Kenkyūjo.

Kelly, William W. 1993. Finding a Place in Metropolitan Japan: Ideologies, Institutions, and Everyday Life. In *Postwar Japan As History*, ed. Andrew Gordon. Berkeley: University of California Press.

Kimura, Bin. 1975. Utsubyō no Rinshō Seishinigakuteki Kenkyū no Dōkō (Clinical Psychiatric Research on Depression: 1959–75). *Seishinigaku (Psychiatry)* 17.

———. 1979. Hikakubunkaronteki Seishinbyōri (Psychopathology from a Comparative, Cultural Perspective). In *Gendai Seishinigaku Taikei Vol. 9-B: Sōutsubyō II (Modern Psychiatry Vol. 9-B: Manic Depression II)*, ed. Ryō Takahashi. Tokyo.

Kinzley, W. Dean. 1991. *Industrial Harmony in Modern Japan: The Invention of a Tradition*. London/New York: Routledge.

Kirmayer, Laurence. 1992. The Body's Insistence on Meaning: Metaphor as Presentation and Representation in Illness Experience. *Medical Anthropology Quarterly* 6, no.4: 323–46.

———. 1993. Healing and the Invention of Metaphor: the Effectiveness of Symbols Revisited. *Culture, Medicine and Psychiatry* 17, no. 2: 161–95.

———. 1994. Improvisation and Authority in Illness Meaning. *Culture, Medicine and Psychiatry* 18, no. 2: 83–214.

———. 1999. Rhetorics of the Body: Medically Unexplained Symptoms in Sociocultural Perspective. In *Somatoform Disorders: a World Wide Perspective*, ed. Yutaka Ono. Tokyo: Springer.

———. 2000. Broken Narratives: Clinical Encounters and the Poetics of Illness Experience. In *Narrative and the Cultural Construction of Illness and Healing*, eds. Cheryl Mattingly and Linda C. Garro. Berkeley: University of California Press.

Kirmayer, Laurence and Ian Gold. 2011. Re-Socializing Psychiatry: Critical Neuroscience and the Limits of Reductionism. In *Critical Neuroscience: A Handbook of the*

Social and Cultural Contexts of Neuroscience, eds. S. Choudhury and J. Slaby. Oxford: Blackwell.

Kirmayer, Laurence, Trang Dao, Thi Hong, and Andre Smith. 1998. Somatization and Psychologization: Understanding Cultural Idioms of Distress. In *Clinical Methods in Transcultural Psychiatry,* ed. S. O. Okpaku. Washington, D.C.: American Psychiatric Press.

Kitanaka, Junko. 2003. Jungians and the Rise of Psychotherapy in Japan: a Brief Historical Note. *Transcultural Psychiatry.* 40, no. 2: 239–47.

———. 2008. Questioning the Suicide of Resolve: Disputes Regarding 'Overwork Suicide' in 20th Century Japan. In *A History of Suicide in the Modern World: International Perspectives,* eds. John Weaver and David Wright. Toronto: University of Toronto Press.

Kitazawa, Kazutoshi. 2000. *"Kenkō" no Nihonshi (Japanese History of "Health").* Tokyo: Heibonsha.

Kleinman, Arthur. 1986. *Social Origins of Distress and Disease: Depression, Neurasthenia, and Pain in Modern China.* New Haven: Yale University Press.

———. 1988a. *The Illness Narratives: Suffering, Healing, and the Human Condition.* New York: Basic Books.

———. 1988b. *Rethinking Psychiatry: From Cultural Category to Personal Experience.* New York: Free Press.

———. 1995. *Writing at the Margin: Discourse between Anthropology and Medicine.* Berkeley: University of California Press.

Kleinman, Arthur and Byron Good, eds. 1985. *Culture and Depression: Studies in the Anthropology and Cross-Cultural Psychiatry of Affect and Disorder.* Berkeley: University of California Press.

Kleinman, Arthur, Veena Das, and Margaret Lock, eds. 1997. *Social Suffering.* Berkeley: University of California Press.

Klerman, Gerald L. 1990. The Contemporary American Scene: Diagnosis and Classification of Mental Disorders, Alcoholism and Drug Abuse. In *Sources and Traditions of Classification in Psychiatry,* eds. Norman Sartorius, Assen Jablensky, Darrel A. Regier, Jr., Burke Jack D., and Robert M. A. Hirschfeld. Toronto: Hogrefe & Huber Publishers.

Kobayashi, Tsukasa. 1972. Nihon no Seishin Eisei Undō towa Nandeattanoka (What Was Mental Hygiene Movement in Japan?). *Kokoro to Shakai (Mind and Society)* 3, no. 3–4: 93–134.

Kohrt, Brandon and Ian Harper. 2008. Navigating Diagnosis: Understanding Mind-Body Relations, Mental Health, and Stigma in Nepal. *Culture, Medicine and Psychiatry* 32, no. 4: 462–91.

Koike, Jun and Takaharu Matsuda. 1997. Nihon Seishin Shinkeika Shinryōjo no Ayumi (The History of the Japanese Association of Neuropsychiatric Clinics). *Rinshō Seishinigaku (Clinical Psychiatry)* 26, no. 8: 947–54.

Koizumi, Kiyota and Paul Harris. 1992. Mental Health Care in Japan. *Hospital and Community Psychiatry* 43, no. 11: 1100–3.

Komine, Kazushige. 1996. Seishin Hoken Fukushihō eno Kaisei. *Kokoro no Kagaku (Science of the Mind)* 67.

Komine, Shigeyuki. 1938. Oyako Shinjū no Seiin ni Tsuite no Kōsatsu (On the Causes of Parent-Children Suicides). *Seishin Shinkeigaku Zasshi (Journal of Psychiatry and Neurology)* 42: 210–26.

Kondo, Dorinne K. 1990. *Crafting Selves: Power, Gender, and Discourses of Identity in a Japanese Workplace*. Chicago/London: University of Chicago Press.

Kondō, Kyōichi, ed. 1999. *Utsu o Taiken Shita Nakamatachi: Utsubyō no Serufu-herupu Gurūpu Jissenki* (*People Who Have Experienced Depression: Record of Depression Self-Help Group*). Tokyo: Seiwa Shoten.

Kōra, Takehisa. 1938. Shinkeishitsu no Mondai (On Shinkeishitsu). *Seishin Shinkeigaku Zasshi* (*Journal of Psychiatry and Neurology*) 42, no. 10: 755–96.

Kosaka, Fumiko. 1984. *Byōnin Aishi: Byonin to Jinken* (*Sad History of the Ill: the Ill and Human Rights*). Tokyo: Keisō Shobō.

Kōsei Rōdōshō (The Ministry of Health, Welfare, and Labor), ed. 2001. *Kōsei Rōdō Hakusho* (*The White Paper of the Ministry of Health, Welfare, and Labor*). Tokyo: Gyōsei.

———. 2010. Policies Regarding Mental Health. Kokoro no Mimi (Ears for the Soul). http://kokoro.mhlw.go.jp/hatarakukata/shisaku/mental.html#keika. December 13, 2010.

Kramer, Peter D. 1993. *Listening to Prozac*. New York: Viking.

———. 2005. *Against Depression*. New York: Viking.

Kure, Shūzō. 1900. Seishin Byōsha no Jisatsu oyobi Jisatu no Kishin (Suicide and Attempted Suicide Among the Mentally Ill). *Chūgai Iji Shinpō* (*Chugai Medical News*) 20.

———. 1913. Bunmei to Shinkei Suijaku (Civilization and Neurasthenia). *Yomiuri Shimbun*, May 20.

———. 1914. Sōutsubyō ni Tsukite (Manic Depression). *Shikeigaku Zasshi* (*Journal of Neurology*) 13: 54–55.

———. 1915. Rinshō Kōgi Sōutsubyō (Clinical Lecture on Manic Depression). *Shinkeigaku Zasshi* (*Journal of Neurology*) 14: 90–97.

———. 1917. Jōshi Kenkyū: Shōgi ni Shinjū no Ooi Riyū (Study on Love Pact: the Reason Why So Many Prostitutes Commit Dual Suicide). *Yomiuri Shimbun*. July 19.

———. 2002[1894–95]. *Seishinbyōgaku Shūyō* (*Psychopathology*). Tokyo: Sōzō Shuppan.

Kuriyama, Shigehisa. 1992. Between Eye and Mind: Japanese Anatomy in the Eighteenth Century. In *Paths to Asian Medical Knowledge*, eds. Charles M. Leslie and Allan Young. Berkeley: University of California Press.

———. 1997. Katakori Kō (Reflection on Katakori). In *Rekishi no Naka no Yamai to Igaku* (*Illness and Medicine in History*), eds. Keiji Yamada and Shigehisa Kuriyama. Kyoto: Shibunkaku Shuppan.

———. 1999. *The Expressiveness of the Body and the Divergence of Greek and Chinese Medicine*. New York: Zone Books.

Kuroki, Nobuo. 1999. Hoshō ni Okeru Jisatsu (Suicide and Compensation). *Sangyō Seishin Hoken* (*Occupational Mental Health*) 7, no. 3: 222–24.

———. 2000a. Kigyō ni Okeru Jisatsu to Rōsai Hoshō (Suicide in Workplace and Worker's Compensation). *Nihon Shokugyō Saigai Igaku Kaishi* (*Japanese Journal of Traumatology and Occupational Medicine*) 48, no. 3: 227–33.

———. 2000b. Rōsai Nintei ni Okeru Hannōsei Seishin Shōgai no Kangaekata (Perspectives on Reactive Mental Disorder in Terms of Workers' Compensation). *Seishinka Chiryōgaku* (*Journal of Psychiatric Treatment*) 15, no. 8: 843–49.

———. 2002. Jisatsu to Seishin Shikkan ni Kansuru Rōsai Hoshō no Dōkō (Recent Trends in Work-Related Compensation Involving Job-Related Suicide and Mental

Disease). *Seishin Shinkeigaku Zasshi (Journal of Psychiatry and Neurology)* 104, no. 12: 1215–27.

——. 2003. Karō Jisatsu no Rōsai Nintei (Workers' Compensation For Overwork Suicide). *Sangyō Seishin Hoken (Occupational Mental Health)* 11, no. 3: 236–42.

——. 2007. Shokuba no Mentaru Herusu to Shūrō Shien (Mental Health in Workplaces and Job Assistance). *Kenkōkanri (Health Management)* 6: 6–33.

Kuwahara, Susumu. 2009. Fukyō ga Jisatsu o Zōka saseru nowa Nazeka: Haikei ni aru 2 Dankai de Rōdōsha o Hōshutsu suru Mekanizumu (Why Recession Leads to an Increase of Suicide: The 2-Step Mechanism of Dumping Workers). *Nikkei Business Online*. June 12. Available from http://business.nikkeibp.co.jp/., September 1, 2010.

Labor Committee Held in the Lower House on November, 15, 2000 (The Proceeding of the Committee on Labor at the 150th Diet Session). 2000. Available from http://www.shugiin.go.jp/itdb_kaigiroku.nsf/html/kaigiroku/001315020001115002.htm, December 13, 2010.

Laing, R. D. 1969. *The Divided Self: An Existential Study in Sanity and Madness*. London: Tavistockk Publications.

Lakoff, Andrew. 2005. *Pharmaceutical Reason: Knowledge and Value in Global Psychiatry*. Cambridge: Cambridge University Press.

Landers, Peter. 2002. Drug Companies Push Japan to Change View of Depression. *Wall Street Journal*, October 9.

Lee, Dominic T. S., Joan Kleinman, and Arthur Kleinman. 2007. Rethinking Depression: An Ethnographic Study of the Experiences of Depression among Chinese. *Harvard Review of Psychiatry 15, no. 1: 1–8*

Lee, Sing. 1999. *Diagnosis Postponed: Shenjing Shuairuo and the Transformation of* Psychiatry in Post-Mao China. *Culture, Medicine and Psychiatry* 23: 349–80.

Lepine, J-P, M. Gastpar, and J Mendlewicz. 1997. Depression in the Community: the First Pan-European Study DEPRES (Depression Research in European Society). *International Clinical Psychopharmacology* 12: 19–29.

Lévi-Strauss, Claude. 1963a. *Structural Anthropology*. New York: Basic Books.

——. 1963b. The Effectiveness of Symbols. In *Structural Anthropology*. New York: Basic Books.

Lewis, Michael. 1990. *Rioters and Citizens: Mass Protest in Imperial Japan*. Berkeley: University of California Press.

Liang, Rong. 1997. Gotō Konzan no Igaku ni Tsuite (The Medicine of Gotō Konzan). In *Rekishi no Naka no Yamai to Igaku (Illness and Medicine in History)*, eds. Keiji Yamada and Shigehisa Kuriyama. Kyoto: Shibunkaku Shuppan.

Lifton, Robert J. 1979. *The Broken Connection: on Death and the Continuity of Life*. New York: Simon and Schuster.

Light, Donald. 1980. *Becoming Psychiatrists: The Professional Transformation of Self*. New York: Norton.

Littlewood, Roland and Simon Dein. 2000. *Cultural Psychiatry and Medical Anthropology: An Introduction and Reader*. London/New Brunswick, NJ: Athlone Press.

Lloyd, Stephanie. 2008. Morals, Medicine and Change: Morality Brokers, Social Phobias, and French Psychiatry. *Culture, Medicine and Psychiatry* 32, no. 2: 279–97.

Lock, Margaret. 1980. *East Asian Medicine in Urban Japan*. Berkeley: University of California Press.

Lock, Margaret. 1981. Japanese Psychotherapeutic Systems: on Acceptance and Responsibility. *Culture, Medicine, and Psychiatry* 5: 303–12.

———. 1982. Popular Conceptions of Mental Health in Japan. In *Cultural Conceptions of Mental Health and Therapy*, eds. A. J. Marsella and G. M. White. Dordrecht: D. Reidel.

Lock, Margaret. 1986. Plea For Acceptance: School Refusal Syndrome in Japan. *Social Science and Medicine* 23, no. 2: 99–112.

———. 1987. Protests of a Good Wife and Wise Mother: The Medicalization of Distress in Japan. In *Health, Illness, and Medical Care in Japan*, eds. Edward Norbeck and Margaret Lock. Honolulu: University of Hawaii Press.

———. 1988. A Nation at Risk: Interpretations of School Refusal in Japan. In *Biomedicine Examined*, eds. Margaret Lock and Deborah R. Gordon. Dordrecht/ Boston/London: Kluwer Academic Publishers.

———. 1991. Flawed Jewels and National Dis/order: Narratives on Adolescent Dissent in Japan. *The Journal of Psychohistory* 18, no. 4: 509–31.

———. 1993. *Encounters with Aging: Mythologies of Menopause in Japan and North America*. Berkeley: University of California Press.

———. 1997. Displacing Suffering: the Reconstruction of Death in North America and Japan. In *Social Suffering*, eds. Arthur Kleinman, Veena Das, and Margaret Lock. Berkeley: University of California Press.

———. 1998. Perfecting Society: Reproductive Technologies, Genetic Testing, and the Planned Family in Japan. In *Pragmatic Women and Body Politics*, eds. Margaret Lock and Patricia Kaufert. Cambridge: Cambridge University Press.

———. 1999. Genetic Diversity and the Politics of Difference. *Chicago-Kent Law Review* 75, no. 1: 83–111.

———. 2002. *Twice Dead: Organ Transplants and the Reinvention of Death*. Berkeley: University of California Press.

———. 2005. Eclipse of the Gene and the Return of Divination. *Current Anthropology* 46, no. 5: 47–70.

Lock, Margaret and Deborah Gordon, eds. 1988. *Biomedicine Examined*. Dordrecht/ Boston: Kluwer Academic Publishers.

Lock, Margaret and Vinh-Kim Nguyen. 2010. *An Anthropology of Biomedicine*. New York/London: Wiley/Blackwell.

Luhrmann, Tanya M. 2000. *Of Two Minds: The Growing Disorder in American Psychiatry*. New York: Knopf.

Lunbeck, Elizabeth. 1994. *The Psychiatric Persuasion: Knowledge, Gender, and Power in Modern America*. Princeton, NJ: Princeton University Press.

Lupton, Deborah. 1997. Consumerism, Reflexivity and the Medical Encounter. *Social Science and Medicine* 45, no. 3: 378–81.

———. 1999. *Risk*. London and New York: Routledge

Lutz, Catherine. 1997. The Psychological Ethic and the Spirit of Containment. *Public Culture* 9: 135–59.

Lutz, Catherine A. and Lila Abu-Lughod, eds. 1990. *Language and the Politics of Emotion*. Cambridge: Cambridge University Press.

Lutz, Tom. 1991. *American Nervousness, 1903: An Anecdotal History*. Ithaca, NY: Cornell University Press.

———. 1995. Neurasthenia and Fatigue Syndromes (Social Section). In *A History of Cli-*

nical Psychiatry: the Origin and History of Psychiatric Disorders, eds. G. E. Berrios and Roy Porter. New York: New York University Press.

MacDonald, Michael and Terence R. Murphy. 1990. *Sleepless Souls: Suicide in Early Modern England*. Oxford/New York: Oxford University Press.

Machizawa, Shizuo. 1997. PTSD no Seishin Ryōhō ni tsuite (On Psychotherapy for PTSD). *Seishin Ryōhō (Journal of Psychotherapy)* 24, no. 4: 28–29.

Maebayashi, Kiyokazu, Kōetsu Satō, and Hiroshi Kobayashi. 2000. *"Ki" no Hikaku Bunkashi: Chūgoku, Kankoku, Nihon (Cultural Comparisons of "Ki": China, Korea, Japan)*. Kyoto: Shōwadō.

Maher, Brendan. 2008. Poll Results: Look Who's Doping. *Nature* 452: 674–75.

Makino, Toshio. 1997. Mansei Utsubyō (Chronic Depression). In *Kanjō Shōgai: Kiso to Rinshō (Affective Disorders: Foundations and Clinical Practice)*, eds. Yomishi Kasahara, Masaaki Matsushita, and Hideji Kishimoto. Tokyo: Asakura Shoten.

Mamiya, Masayuki. 1998. Nihon no Rinshō Shinrigaku no Hatten (The Development of Clinical Psychology in Japan). In *Nihon Shinrigakushi no Kenkyū (Studies of the History of Japanese Psychology)*, eds. Shinrigaku Kenkyūkai Rekishi Kenkyūbukai. Kyoto: Hōsei Shuppan.

Manase, Dōsan. 1979. *Manase Dōsan*, eds. Keisetsu Ōtsuka and Dōmei Yakazu. Tokyo: Meicho Shuppan.

Manase, Gensaku. 1979. *Manase Gensaku*, eds. Keisetsu Ōtsuka and Dōmei Yakazu. Tokyo: Meicho Shuppan.

Marcus, George E., ed. 1995. *Technoscientific Imaginaries: Conversations, Profiles, and Memoirs*. Chicago: University of Chicago Press.

Marcuse, Herbert. 1970. *Five Lectures: Psychoanalysis, Politics, and Utopia*. Boston: Beacon Press.

———. 1973 [1933]. On the Philosophical Foundation of the Concept of Labor in Economics. *Telos* 16: 9–37.

Marsella, Anthony. 1980. Depressive Experience and Disorder across Cultures. In *Handbook of Cross-Cultural Psychology, Volume 6: Psychopathology*, eds. J. Draguns and H. Triandis. New York: Allyn & Bacon.

Martin, Emily. 1987. *The Woman in the Body: A Cultural Analysis of Reproduction*. Boston: Beacon.

———. 1991. The Egg and the Sperm: How Science Has Constructed a Romance Based on Stereotypical Male-Female Roles. *Signs* 16, no. 3: 485–501.

———. 2007. *Bipolar Expeditions: Mania and Depression in American Culture*. Princeton, NJ: Princeton University Press.

Maruyama, Naoko. 1998. Kōdo Keizai Seichōki ni okeru Shinrigaku no Ryūsei (Popularity of Psychology in the Period of Rapid Economic Growth). In *Nihon Shinrigakushi no Kenkyū (Studies of the History of Japanese Psychology)*, eds. Shinrigaku Kenkyūkai Rekishi Kenkyūbukai. Kyoto: Hōsei Shuppan.

Matsubara, Saburō. 1914. Shinkeisuijaku no Genin (Causes of Neurasthenia). *Shinkeigaku Zasshi (Journal of Neurology)* 13, no. 1: 1–9.

Matsubara, Yōko. 1998a. The Enactment of Japan's Sterilization Laws in the 1940s: A Prelude to Postwar Eugenic Policy. *Historia Scientiarum* 8, no. 2: 187–201.

———. 1998b. Senjika no Danshuhō Ronsō (The Wartime Debates Over Sterilization Law). *Gendai Shisō* 26, no. 2: 286–303.

Matsumura, Hidehisa. 1937. Sōutsubyō no Ippanteki Tōkei (General Statistics of Manic

Depression). *Seishin Shinkeigaku Zasshi (Journal of Psychiatry and Neurology)* 41, no. 10: 195.

Matsushita, Masaaki, ed. 1997. *Zadankai 21seiki no Seishinka Iryō o Mitsumeru (Round-table Discussion on Psychiatry for the 21st Century)*. Tokyo: Shinryō Shinsha.

Matsushita, Masao. 1997. Shinkeika (Seishinka) & Naika Kurinikku (Neurological [Psychiatric] & Internal Clinics). *Rinshō Seishinigaku (Clinical Psychiatry)* 26, no. 8: 1027–32.

Maudsley, Henry. 2002[1876]. *Seishinbyō Yakusetsu (Theories of Mental Illness)*. Tokyo: Sōzō Shuppan.

Metzl, Jonathan. 2003. *Prozac on the Couch: Prescribing Gender in the Era of Wonder Drugs*. Durham: Duke University Press.

———. 2009. *The Protest Psychosis: How Schizophrenia Became a Black Disease*. Boston: Beacon Press

Micale, Mark S. 1995. *Approaching Hysteria: Disease and Its Interpretations*. Princeton, NJ: Princeton University Press.

———. 2008. *Hysterical Men: The Hidden History of Male Nervous Illness*. Cambridge, MA: Harvard University Press.

Mitchell, Timothy. 1988. *Colonizing Egypt*. Berkeley: University of California Press.

Miwaki, Yasuo. 2000. Seishin Iryō no Saiseijika no Tameni (For Repoliticization of Psychiatry). In *Seishin no Kanri Shakai o dō Norikoeruka? (How Do We Overcome the Psychiatric Management of Society?)*, eds. Masaaki Sugimura, Yasuo Miwaki, and Mahoro Murasawa. Kyoto: Shoraisha.

Miyake, Kōichi. 1912. Shinkeisuijakushō ni Tsuite (On Neurasthenia). *Shikeigaku Zasshi (Journal of Neurology)* 11, no. 12: 517–18.

———. 1924. Seishin to Byōki tono Kankei (The Relationship between Mind and Illness). *Taiyō* 30, no. 8: 336–39.

———. 1927. Rinshō Kōgi: Shinkeisuijaku to Shinkeishitsu no Kata (Clinical Lecture: Neurasthenia and Types of Neurotics). *Shikeigaku Zasshi (Journal of Neurology)* 28, no. 1: 75–86.

Miyake, Shū. 1900. Seishinbyōsha ni Taisuru Kokka no Senmu (The Nation's Tasks with Regard to the Mentally Ill). *Taiyō* 9: 6–9.

Miyamoto, Tadao. 1978. Gendai Shakai to Utsubyō (Contemporary Society and Depression). *Rinshōi (Medical Clinics of Japan)* 4: 1771.

———. 1979. Sōutsubyōsha no Mōsōteki Disukūru (Delusional Discourse of the Manic-Depressive). In *Sōutsubyō no Seishin Byōri (The Psychopathology of Manic Depression) II*, ed. Tadao Miyamoto. Tokyo: Kōbundō.

Miyaoka, Hitoshi, ed. 1999. *Kokoro no Kagaku: Shinryō Naika (Human Mind: Psychosomatic Medicine)* 84. Tokyo: Nihon Hyōronsha.

Moerland, René. 2009. In France, Suicide Can be a Form of Protest. *NRC Handelsblad*. October 9, 2009.

Mol, Annemarie and Marc Berg. 1998. *Differences in Medicine: Unraveling Practices, Techniques, and Bodies*. Durham and London: Duke University Press.

Mole, Noelle. 2008. Living It on the Skin: Italian States, Working Illness. *American Ethnologist* 35, no. 2: 189–210.

———. 2010. *Labor Disorders in Neoliberal Italy: Mobbing, Well-being, and the Workplace*. Bloomington, IN: Indiana University Press.

Monday Nikkei. 1999. Karô de Jisatsu Rôsai Nintei Kijun wa: Sutoresu Dō 31kômoku De

Sokutei (What Are the Standards For Determining Overwork Suicide?: the Level of Stress Measured By 31 Items). December 27.

Morita, Masatake. 1930. Shinkeishitsu, Shinkeisuijaku (Shinkeishitsu, Neurasthenia). In *Gendai Igaku Daijiten Dai 23 Kan Seishinbyōkahen (Dictionary of Contemporary Medicine Vol. 23 Psychiatry)*. Shunjūsha: Tokyo.

Moriyama, Kimio. 1975. *Gendai Seishinigaku Kaitai no Ronri (The Theory for Dismantling Modern Psychiatry)*. Tokyo: Iwasaki Gakujutsu Shuppansha.

———. 1988. *Kyōki no Kiseki: Kōzōronteki Rekishishugi no Shiza (Trajectories of Madness: From the Perspective of Structural Historicism)*. Tokyo: Iwasaki Gakujutsu Shuppansha.

Morohashi, Tetsuji. 1984. *Daikanwa Jiten (Kanji Dictionary) Vol. 12*. Tokyo: Taishūkan Shoten.

Morris, Ivan. 1975. *The Nobility of Failure: Tragic Heroes in the History of Japan*. New York: Holt, Rinehart and Winston.

Munakata, Tsunetsugu. 1984. *Seishin Iryō no Shakaigaku (Sociology of Psychiatry)*. Tokyo: Kōbunsha.

———. 1986. Japanese Attitudes towards Mental Health and Mental Health Care. In *Japanese Culture and Behavior*, eds. T. S. Lebra and W. Lebra. Honolulu: University of Hawaii Press.

Muramatsu, Tsuneo. 1953. Shinkeishō ni kansuru Shomondai (Problems of Neurosis). *Seishin Shinkeigaku Zasshi (Journal of Psychiatry and Neurology)* 55, no. 4: 504–9.

Murase, Takao. 1995. Nihon no Rinshō Shinrigaku (Clinical Psychology in Japan). In *Rinshō Shinrigaku no Genten (Origins of Clinical Psychology)*, Tokyo: Seishin Shobō.

Naka, Shūzō. 1932. Shorōki Utsuyūshō (Presenile Depression). *Shinkeigaku Zasshi (Journal of Neurology)* 34, no. 6: 53–77.

Nakagawa, Shirō. 1947. Shinkeishitsu Shōjō no Yogo ni Kansuru Tōkeiteki Kenkyū (Statistical Study on the Prognosis of Shinkeishitsu Symptoms). *Seishin Shinkeigaku Zasshi (Journal of Psychiatry and Neurology)* 49: 76–79.

———. 1954. Shinkeishitsushō Narabi ni Sono Kinen Jōtai no Yogo ni Tsuite no Kenkyū (Statistical and Clinical Studies on the Prognosis of Neurasthenia-Like States). *Seishin Shinkeigaku Zasshi (Journal of Psychiatry and Neurology)* 56, no. 3: 135–86.

Nakai, Hisao. 1976. Saiken no Rinri to Shite no Kinben to Kufū (Deligence and Innovation as An Ethic of Reconstruction). In *Sōutsubyō no Seishinbyōri I (Psychopathology of Manic Depression)*, ed. Yomishi Kasahara. Tokyo: Kōbundō.

Nakai, Hisao et al. 1983. *Chiryō to Bunka (Therapy and Culture)*. Vol. 8. Iwanami Kōza: Seishin no Kagaku (Science of the Mind). Tokyo: Iwanami Shoten.

Nakai, Masakazu. 1995. Ke, Ki no Nihongo to Shite no Hensen (Changes of Ke and Ki in Japanese). In *Nakai Masakazu Hyōronshū*, ed. Hiroshi Nagata. Tokyo: Iwanami Shoten.

Nakajima, Shigeya. 2001. Gyōmujō no Kajū Fuka to Minji Baishō Sekinin (Excessive Stress of Work and Civil Liability for Reparation). *Jurist* 1197: 15–21.

Nakamura, Karen. 2006. *Deaf in Japan: Signing and the Politics of Identity*. Ithaca, NY: Cornell University Press.

———. 2008. Crazy in Japan: Schizophrenia, Traumas of Memory and Community Storytelling in Rural Japan. Paper Presented at the GCOE Symposium at Keio University, Tokyo, Japan. January 23.

Nakamura, Kokyō. 1930. *Shinkeisuijaku wa Dōsureba Zenchi Suruka* (*How to Completely Cure Neurasthenia*). Tokyo: Shufu no Tomosha.

Nakamura, Sin'ichirō. 1971. *Raisanyō to Sono Jidai* (*Raisanyō and His Era*). Tokyo: Chūō Kōronsha.

Nakane, Yoshibumi, Yoshifumi Koshino, Kazuhiko Kinoshita, M.H.B. Radford, and Lin K-M. 2004. Utsubyō oyobi Fuan Shōgai ni okeru Bunka no Eikyō (Cultural Influences on Depression and Anxiety Disorders). *Nihon Iji Shinpō* (*Japan Medical News*), 4179: 27–32.

Nakane, Yoshibumi, Misako Tsukahara, and Shunichirō Michitsuji. 1994. Utsubyō no Nihonteki Tokusei (The Characteristics of Derpression in Japan). *Rinshō Seishinigaku* (*Clinical Psychiatry*) 23, no. 1: 5–12.

Nakazawa, Masao. 1985. Seishin Iryō no Ayumi (History of Psychiatric Care). In *Seishin Eisei to Hoken Katsudō* (*Mental Hygiene and Social Work*), eds. Masao Nakazawa and Yuki Utsuno. Tokyo: Igaku Shoin.

Nakazono, Kōichirō. 1998. Chōki Kaigai Shucchōchū no Rōdōsha no Jisatsu ni Tsuite Gyōmu Kiinsei ga Kōtei Sareta Jirei (Case of Suicide of a Worker Sent Abroad on a Long-Term Basis Recognized As Having Caused By Work). *Hanrei Times* (*The Law Times Report*) 978: 296–97.

Narita, Ryūichi. 1990. Eisei Kankyō no Henka no Nakano Josei to Joseikan (Women and Views of Women in the Changing Hygienic Environment). In *Nihon Josei Seikatsushi* (*History of the Lives of Japanese Women*), ed. Josei Shi Sōgō Kenkyūkai. Tokyo: Tokyo University Press.

———. 1993. Kindai Toshi to Minshū (Modern Cities and People). In *Kindai Nihon no Kiseki: Toshi to Minshū* (*Trajectory of Modern Japan: Cities and People*), ed. Ryūichi Narita. Tokyo: Yoshikawa Kōbundō.

———. 1995. Shintai to Kōshūeisei: Nihon no Bunmeika to Kokuminka (Body and Public Health: Modernization and Nationalization of Japan). In *Kōza Sekaishi 4: Shihonshugi wa Hito o Dou Kaetekitaka* (*World History: How Capitalism Has Changed People*), ed. Rekishigaku Kenkyūkai. Tokyo: Tokyo University Press.

Natsume, Sōseki. 1986. *Sōseki Bunmeiron Shū* (*Sōseki's Ideas on Civilization*). Tokyo: Iwanami Shoten.

Negishi, Yasumori. 1972. *Mimibukuro Vol. 4.* Tokyo: Heibonsha.

New Current. 1999. SSRI Toujōgo no Kōutsuzai no Shijō to Shinyaku Kaihatsu (The Antidepressant Market and New Pharmaceutical Development after the Advent of SSRI) 10, no. 20: 2–7.

NHK. 2009. *NHK Supesharu: Utsubyō Chiryō Jōshiki ga Kawaru* (*NHK Special: Changing the Beliefs about Depression Treatment*). Tokyo: Takarajimasha.

Nichter, Mark. 1998. The Mission within the Madness. In *Pragmatic Women and Body Politics,* eds. Margaret Lock and Patricia A. Kaufert. Cambridge: Cambridge University Press.

Nihon Keizai Shimbun. 1999. Nagano Chisai Hanketsu Karô Jisatsu Rôsai to Nintei (Nagano District Court Rules Overowrk Suicide Be Subject to Workers' Compensation). March 12.

———2000. Rôsai Shinsei Seishinshōgai ga Kyūzō (Drastic Increase in the Number of Applications for Workers' Compensation for Mental Illness). January 21.

——— 2001. Kōsei Rōdōhakusho: Kokoro no Mondai ni Kikikan, Utsubyō Taisaku ga

Kyūmu (The White Paper of the Ministry of Health, Welfare, and Labor Says That Mental Health Is a Serious Concern, Depression An Urgent Issue). September 7.

——. 2002. Watashi wa Utsu ni Chigainai, "Byōmei Hoshii" Shōkōgun Hirogaru (I Must Be Depressed: "I Want to Have a Diagnosis" Syndrome Spreads). February 13.

——2002. Karōshi Nintei Saita no 143 ken (143 Cases of Overwork Death Granted, the Highest Ever). May 23.

——. 2004. 1 Kagetsu 100 Jikan o Kosu Zangyō Ishi no Mensetsu Shidō Gimuzuke (Overwork Exceeding 100 Hours Per Month: Doctors' Interview and Guidance Required) August 19.

——. 2004. Kokoro no Kenkō mo Kigyō ga Kanri: Shain no Utsu, Sekinin Towareru (Companies to Also Manage Workers' Mental Health: Owing Responsibility For Workers' Depression). November 8.

——. 2005. Seishin Shōgai no Rōsai Nintei Saita, Kōrōshō Matome, Sakunendo 130nin (130 Cases Approved For Workers' Compensation; the Biggest Number Last Year, Says the Ministry of Health, Welfare, and Labor). June 18.

Nishimori, Miyuki. 2002. Puresukō ga Hannōsei Utsubyō ni Kakari, Jisatsu Shita Koto ni Tsuite Gyōmu Kiinsei ga Mitomerareta Jirei (Case of a Press Worker Afflicted With Depression and Committed Suicide, For Whom Work Was Recognized As the Cause). *Hanrei Times* 1096: 282–83.

Nishimura, Kenichiro. 2001. Hōteki Mondai to Shite no Karōshi ni Tsuite (Death From Overwork As a Legal Issue). *Jurist* 1197: 2–7.

Nishizono, Masahisa. 1986. Seishin Ryōhō (Psychotherapy). *Seishinka Mook (Psychiatry Mook)* 13: 189–98.

——. 1988. Nihonjin no Seishin Iryō to Seishin Ryōhō (Psychiatry and Psychotherapy for Japanese). In *Nihon, Ajia, Kita America no Seishin Ryōhō (Psychotherapies in Japan, Asia, and North America)*, eds. Masahisa Nishizono and Joe Yamamoto. Tokyo: Kōbundō.

Nolan, Jr., James L. 1998. *The Therapeutic State: Justifying Government at Century's End.* New York/London: New York University Press.

Nomura, Yoshihiro, Naoki Kinomoto, Takaharu Hiranuma, Masahiko Sugita, Nobuo Kuroki, Masaharu Katō, Fumio Itō, Yasuji Kodama, and Yōkichi Ōno. 2003. Karōshi to Kigyō no Songai Biashō Sekinin: Dentsū Karōshi Jisatsu Jiken (Overwork Death and Corporate Liability: Dentsū Overwork Suicide Case). *Baishō Kagaku (Journal of Compensation Science)* 30: 115–36.

Nomura, Naoki, and Masami Miyamoto. 1996. Kanja-Kangosha no Komyunikêshon ni Okeru Akujunkan no Kozô (The Structure of the Vicious Circle in the Communication Between Patients and Nurses). *Kango Kenkyû (Japanese Journal of Nursing Research)* 28, no. 2: 5–22.

Nye, Robert A. 1984. *Crime, Madness, and Politics in Modern France: The Medical Concept of National Decline.* Princeton, NJ: Princeton University Press.

Obeyesekere, Gananath. 1985. Depression, Buddhism, and the Work of Culture in Sri Lanka. In *Culture and Depression: Studies in the Anthropology and Cross-Culutral Psychiatry of Affect and Disorder,* eds. Arthur Kleinman and Byron Good. Berkeley: University of California Press.

Ōchi, Naomi. 2001. "Karōshi" no Yobô Taisaku (Prevention Measures for Overwork Suicide). *Jurist* 1197: 23–27.

Ochiai, Taizō. 1883. *Kanyō Byōmei Taishōroku (Comparison Table for Japanese-Western Illness Terms)*. Tokyo: Eirandō.

Oda, Susumu. 1998. *Nihon no Kyōkishi (Records of Madness in Japan)*. Tokyo: Kōdansha.

———. 2001. *"Hentai Shinri" to Nakamura Kokyō: Taishō Bunka e no Shinshikaku ("Abnormal Psychology" and Nakamura Kokyō: A New Perspective on Taishō Culture)*. Tokyo: Fuji Shuppan.

Ōhara, Kenshirō. 1973. Sōutsubyō no Shakai Seishinigakuteki Apurōchi (Social Psychiatric Approach to Manic Depression). *Seishin Shinkeigaku Zasshi (Journal of Psychiatry and Neurology)* 74: 263.

———. 1981. *Utsubyō no Jidai (Depression Era)*. Tokyo: Kōndansha.

Ōhara, Kenshirō, ed. 1975. *Jisatsu to Bunka (Suicide and Culture)*. Tokyo: Shihōdō.

Ōhigashi, Yoshitaka. 1999. Fūkō to Hanseishinigaku (Foucault and Antipsychiatry). *Kokoro no Kagaku (Human Mind)* 86: 98–102.

Ōhira, Ken, and Shizuo Machizawa, eds. 1988. *Seishinigaku to Bunka Jinruigaku (Psychiatry and Cultural Anthropology)*. Tokyo: Kongō Shuppan.

Ohnuki-Tierney, Emiko. 1984. *Health and Illness in Contemporary Japan*. Cambridge: Cambridge University Press.

Okada, Nao. 2003. Gyōmu Kankyō ga Gen'in no Utsubyō ni Rōsai Nintei: Tenkyo Kyohi de Shigoto o Ataerarezu Shikiri de Kakuri (Workers' Compensation Granted for Depression Caused by Work Environment: Refusal of Transfer Led to Deprivation of Job, Secluded by Partition). *Rōdōhōgaku Kenkyū Kaihō (Labor Law Research Report)* 54, no.27: 1–35.

Okada, Yasuo. 1981. *Shisetsu Matsuzawa Byōinshi 1879–1980 (A History of Matsuzawa Hospital 1879–1980)* Tokyo: Iwasaki Gakujutsu Shuppan.

———. 1989. Seishinka Kanja no Jisatsu Jiken: I no Tachiba kara (Suicides Cases of Mentally Ill Patients: From a Medical Point of View). *Jurist Bessatsu: Iryō Kago Hanrei 100 Sen (Jurist Supplement: 100 Cases of Medical Malpractice)*: 90–91.

———. 1999. Nihon ni Okeru Seishinigaku no 100 Nen (One Hundred Years of Japanese Psychiatry). *Kokoro no Kagaku (Human Mind)* 86: 87–91.

———. 2002. *Nihon Seishinka Iryōshi (History of Psychiatry in Japan)*. Tokyo: Igaku Shoin.

Okagami, Kazuo, Iwao Ōshima, and Mototsugu Arai. 1988. *Nihon no Seishinshōgaisha (The Mentally Disabled in Japan)*. Kyoto: Mineruva Shuppan.

Okajima, Yoshirō. 2005. Shi o Nozomu Kanja ni Seishinkai wa Naniga Dekiruka? (What Can Psychiatrists Do for Patients Who Want to Die?). *Seishin Shinkeigaku Zasshi (Journal of Psychiatry and Neurology)* 107, No.9: 936–46.

Okamoto, Kidō. 1999. Kage o Fumareta Onna (A Woman Whose Shadow Was Stepped On). In *Okamoto Kidō Denki Shōsetsu Shū Vol. 3 (Collected Works of Okamoto Kidō Vol. 3)*. Tokyo: Hara Shobō.

Okamura, Chikanobu. 2002. *Karōshi Karōjisatsu Kyūsai no Riron to Jitsumu (Theory and Practice of Providing Relief to Overwork Death and Overwork Suicide)*. Tokyo: Junpōsha.

Okazaki, Yūji, Atsushi Nishida and Masayuki Itō. 2006. Utsubyō de Byōkyū/Kyūshokuchū no Utsubyō no Kanja no "Fukushoku Kanō" Shindan o Megutte (On the "Reinstatement" Diagnosis of Patients Who are on Sick Leave from Work for Depression). *Rinshō Seishinigaku (Journal of Clinical Psychiatry)* 35, no.8: 1059–67.

Okonogi, Keigo. 1971. *Gendai Seishin Bunseki I* (*Modern Psychoanalysis I*). Tokyo: Seishin Shobō.

Ōkuma, Kazuo. 1973. *Rupo Seishin Byōtō* (*Reportage on a Psychiatric Ward*). Tokyo: Asahi Shimbunsha.

Ōkuma, Shigenobu. 1906. Seishinbyō ni Taisuru Zakkan (Impressions on Mental Illness). *Shinkeigaku Zasshi* (*Journal of Neurology*) 4, no.12: 614–25.

Omata, Waichiro. 1998. *Seishin Byōin no Kigen* (*Origins of Mental Hospital*). Tokyo: Ōta Shuppan.

———. 2002. *Doitsu Seishin Byōrigaku no Sengoshi* (*The History of the Postwar German Psychopathology*). Tokyo: Gendai Shokan.

Ong, Aihwa. 1987. *Spirits of Resistance and Capitalist Discipline: Factory Women in Malaysia*. Albany: State University of New York Press.

Oppenheim, Janet. 1991. *"Shattered Nerves": Doctors, Patients, and Depression in Victorian England*. New York: Oxford University Press.

Osborne, Thomas. 1998. Medicine and Ideology. *Economy and Society* 27, No.2–3: 259–73.

———. 1994. Power and Persons: on Ethical Stylisation and Person-Centered Medicine. *Sociology of Health & Illness* 16, no.4: 515–35.

Otsubo, Sumiko and James R. Bartholomew. 1998. Eugenics in Japan: Some Ironies of Modernity, 1883–1945. *Science in Context* 11, no.3–4: 134–46.

Ōtsuki, Yasuyoshi. 1998. Hyōi to Seishinka Rinshō: Rekishi to Bunka no Shiten Kara (Spirit Possession and Clinical Psychiatry: Historical and Cultural Perspectives). In *Rinshō Seishinigaku Kōza* (*Encyclopedia of Clinical Psychiatry*): *Vol. 23 Tabunkakan Seishinigaku* (*Transcultural Psychiatry*), 335–56. Tokyo: Nakayama Shoten.

Ozawa, Chikako. 1996. Japanese Indigenous Psychologies: Concepts of Mental Illness in Light of Different Cultural Epistemologies. *British Medical Anthropology Review* 3, no. 2: 11–21.

Ozawa-de Silva, Chikako. 2002. Beyond the Body/Mind?: Japanese Contemporary Thinkers on Alternative Sociologies of the Body. *Body & Society* 8, no.2: 21–38.

———. 2006. *Psychotherapy and Religion in Japan: The Japanese Introspection Practice of Naikan*. London: Routledge.

———. 2008. Too Lonely to Die Alone: Internet Suicide Pacts and Existential Suffering in Japan. *Culture, Medicine and Psychiatry*, 32: 516–55.

Ozawa, Masahiko. 2010. Shokuba Kankyō mo Aratamenaito Saihatsu (Work Environment Needs To Be Improved As Well). *Asahi Shimbun*, July 27.

Petryna, Adriana. 2002. *Life Exposed: Biological Citizens after Chernobyl*. Princeton, NJ: Princeton University Press.

———. 2004. Biological Citizenship: The Science and Politics of Chernobyl-Exposed Populations. *Osiris* 19: 250–65.

Petryna, Adriana, Andrew Lakoff, and Arthur Kleinman. 2006. *Global Pharmaceuticals: Ethics, Markets, Practices*. Durham: Duke University Press.

Pinguet, Maurice. 1993. *Voluntary Death in Japan*. Translated by Rosemary Morris. Cambridge, UK: Polity Press.

Plath, David W. 1980. *Long Engagements: Maturity in Modern Japan*. Stanford: Stanford University Press.

Porter, Roy. 1985. *Patients and Practitioners: Lay Perception of Medicine in Pre-Industrial Society*. Cambridge: Cambridge University Press.

Rabinbach, Anson. 1990. *The Human Motor: Energy, Fatigue, and the Origins of Modernity*. New York: Basic Books, Harper Collins.

Rabinow, Paul. 1996. Artificiality and Enlightenment: From Sociobiology to Biosociality. In *Essays on the Anthropology of Reason*. Princeton, NJ: Princeton University Press.

Radden, Jennifer. 2000. *The Nature of Melancholy: From Aristotle to Kristeva*. New York: Oxford University Press.

Rai, Shizuko. 1931–32. Baishi Nikki (Shizuko's Diary). *Raisanyō Zensho* (*Collected Works of Raisanyō*). Hiroshima: Raisanyō-sensei Iseki Kenshōkai.

Raikhel, Eugene. 2010. "Post-Soviet Placebos: Epistemology and Authority in Russian Treatments for Alcoholism." *Culture, Medicine and Psychiatry* 34, no. 1: 132–68.

Rhodes, Lorna A. 1995. *Emptying Beds: The Work of an Emergency Psychiatric Unit*. Berkeley: University of California Press.

Rieff, Philip. 1966. *The Triumph of the Therapeutic*. Chicago: University of Chicago Press.

Robertson, Jennifer. 1999. Dying to Tell: Sexuality and Suicide in Imperial Japan. *Signs: Journal of Women in Culture and Society* 25, no.1: 1–36.

Rōdō Keizai Hanrei Sokuhō (*Law Reports on Labor and Economy*). 2007. Kiōreki ga aru Masuikai no Utsubyō Jisatsu (Suicide of an Anesthesiologist) no.1981.

Rohlen, Thomas P. 1974a. *For Harmony and Strength: The Japanese White-Collar Organization in Anthropological Perspective*. Berkeley: University of California Press.

———. 1974b. Spiritual Education in a Japanese Bank. In *Japanese Culture and Behavior: Selected Readings*, eds. T. S. Lebra and W. Lebra. Honolulu: University of Hawaii Press.

Rose, Nikolas. 1985. *The Psychological Complex: Psychology, Politics and Society in England 1869–1939*. London: Routledge and Kegan Paul.

———. 1990. *Governing the Soul: The Shaping of the Private Self*. London/New York: Routledge.

———. 1996. *Inventing Our Selves: Psychology, Power, and Personhood*. Cambridge: Cambridge University Press.

———. 2007. *The Politics of Life Itself: Biomedicine, Power, and Subjectivity in the Twenty-First Century*. Princeton, NJ: Princeton University Press.

Rosenberger, Nancy R. 1992. The Process of Discourse: Usages of a Japanese Medical Term. *Social Science and Medicine* 34, no.3: 237–47.

Rosenhan, David L. 1973. On Being Sane in Insane Places. *Science* 179, no.70: 250–58.

Sakai, Shizu. 1982. *Nihon no Iryōshi* (*History of Japanese Medicine*). Tokyo: Tokyo Shoseki.

Sakaki, Yasuzaburō. 1912. *Kawarimono* (*The Abnormal*). Tokyo: Jitsugyōno Nihonsha.

Sakurai, Hirono, Kunihiko Tsutsumi, Yuko Tomita, and Mitsukuni Murasaki. 1998. Sanji Kyūkyū Senta ni Hansō Sareta Seishinka Tsūinchū no Jisatsu Kito Kanja no Haikei (Research Into Suicide Attempters Under Psychiatric Treatment at a Critical and Emergency Center). *Rinshō Seishinigaku* (*Journal of Clinical Psychiatry*) 27, no.11: 1363–70.

Salzberg, Stephan. 1994. In a Dark Corner: Care For the Mentally Ill in Japan. *Social Science Japan* 2: 12–14.

Sampson, Edward E. 1989. The Deconstruction of the Self. In *Texts of Identity*, eds. John Shotter and Kenneth J. Gergen. London: Sage Publications.

Sanyūtei, Enshō. 1980. *Sakazuki no Tonosama* (*The Lord of Sake Cup*). Tokyo: Shūeisha.

Saris, A. Jamie. 1995. Telling Stories: Life Histories, Illness Narratives, and Institutional Landscapes. *Culture, Medicine and Psychiatry* 19, no.1: 39–72.

Satō, Masahiro. 2009. Sengoki Nihon niokeru Gaishōsei Shinkeishō Gainen no Seiritsu to Suitai 1880-1940 (The Social Construction of Traumatic Neurosis in pre-World War II Japan: 1880-1940). *Kagaku, Gijutsu, Shakai (Science, Technology and Society)* 18: 1–43.

Satō, Tatsuya, and Hajime Mizoguchi. 1997. *Tsūshi Nihon no Shinrigaku (History of Japanese Psychology)*. Kyoto: Kitaōji Shobō.

Sartorius, N., World Health Organization, and WHO Collaborative Study on Standardized Assessment of Depressive Disorders. 1983. *Depressive Disorders in Different Cultures: Report on the WHO Collaborative Study on Standardized Assessment of Depressive Disorders*. Geneva: World Health Organization.

Sawicki, Jana. 1991. *Disciplining Foucault: Feminism, Power, and the Body*. New York/London: Routledge.

Scheff, Thomas J. 1966. *Being Mentally Ill: A Sociological Theory*. Hawthorne, NY: Aldine Publishing Co.

Scheper-Hughes, Nancy. 1992. *Death without Weeping: The Violence of Everyday Life in Brazil*. Berkeley: University of California Press.

Scheper-Huges, Nancy and Margaret Lock. 1987. The Mindful Body: A Prolegomenon to Future Work in Medical Anthropology. *Medical Anthropology Quarterly* 1, no.1: 6–41.

Schmiedebach, Heinz-Peter. 1999. Post-traumatic Neurosis in Nineteenth-century Germany: A Disease in Political, Juridical and Professional Context. *History of Psychiatry* X: 27–57.

Scott, James C. 1985. *Weapons of the Weak: Everyday Forms of Peasant Resistance*. New Haven: Yale University Press.

———. 1990. *Domination and the Arts of Resistance: Hidden Scripts*. New Haven/London: Yale University Press.

Segawa, Nobuhisa. 2001. Minji Sekinin (Civil Liability). *Hanrei Times* 1046: 72–79.

Sekiya, Tōru. 1997. Seishinka Kurinikku no Genjo (The Present Condition of Neuro-Psychiatric Clinics). *Rinsho Seishinigaku (Journal of Clinical Psychiatry)* 26, no.8: 939–46.

Shiba, Shintarō. 1999. *Nihonjin to Iu Utsubyō (Depression Called "Japanese")*. Kyoto: Jinbun Shoin.

Shikano, Masano. 2004. Korera, Minshū, Eisei Gyōsei (Cholera, People, and Hygiene Policies). In *Kinsei Kara Kindai 9 Korera Sōdō (From Premodern to Modern 9: Cholera Epidemics)*, ed. Masanao Shikano. Tokyo: Asahi Shimbunsha.

Shimazaki, Toshiki. 1953. Shinkeishōron Haigo no Mondai (What Lies Behind the Theories of Neurosis). *Seishin Shinkeigaku Zasshi (Journal of Psychiatry and Neurology)* 55, no.4: 511–14.

Shimazaki, Toshiki, and Kiyoshi Ishikawa. 1954. Karl Jaspers no Seishinbunseki Hihan o Megutte (On Karl Jaspers' Critique of Psychoanalysis). *Seishin Shinkeigaku Zasshi (Journal of Psychiatry and Neurology)* 55, no.7: 743–48.

Shimoda, Mitsuzō. 1941. Sōutsubyō no Byōzen Seikaku ni Tsuite (On Premorbid Personality of the Manic Depressive). *Seishin Shinkeigaku Zasshi (Journal of Psychiatry and Neurology)* 45: 101.

———. 1942. *Seishin Eisei Kōwa (Lectures on Mental Hygiene)*. Tokyo: Iwanami Shoten.

Shimoda, Mitsuzō. 1950. Sōutsubyō ni Tsuite (On Manic Depression). *Yonago Igaku Zasshi* (*Yonago Medical Journal*) 2, no.1: 3–4.

Shimbun Akahata Kokumin Undōbu (Newspaper Akahata). 2003. *Shigoto ga Owaranai Kokuhatsu Karōshi* (*I Cannot Finish Work: Overwork Death*). Tokyo: Shinnihon Shuppan.

Shinfuku, Naotake. 1969. *Kamen Depuresshion* (*Masked Depression*). Tokyo: Nihon Meruku Banyu.

Shinfuku, Naotake, Akihide Karasawa, Osamu Yamada, Shigeru Iwasaki, Akira Kanai and Kanji Kawashima. 1973. Saikin 22 nenkan no Utsubyō no Rinshō ni okeru Henka (Changes in Clinical Pictures of Depression: Statistical Study in Cases Observed in Jikei University School of Medicine in these 22 Years). *Seishinigaku* (*Clinical Psychiatry*) 15 no.9: 955–65.

Shirasugi, Etsuo. 1997. Kakke to Edojidai no Hitobito no Shintai Keiken (Kakke and the Bodily Experience of the People in Edo Era). In *Rekishi no Naka no Yamai to Igaku* (*Illness and Medicine in History*), eds. Keiji Yamada and Shigehisa Kuriyama. Kyoto: Shibunkaku Shuppan.

Showalter, Elaine. 1985. *The Female Malady: Women, Madness, and English Culture, 1830–1980*. New York: Pantheon Books.

Silberman, Bernard S. and H. D. Harootunian, eds. 1974. *Japan in Crisis: Essays on Taisho Democracy*. Princeton, NJ: Princeton University Press.

Silverman, David. 1987. *Communication and Medical Practice: Social Relations in the Clinic*. London: Sage.

Sontag, Susan. 1978. *Illness As Metaphor*. New York: Farrar, Straus and Giroux.

Still, Arthur and Irving Velody. 1992. *Rewriting the History of Madness: Studies in Foucault's Histoire De La Folie*. London/New York: Routledge.

Strom, Stephanie. 1999. In Japan, Mired in Recession, Suicides Soar. *New York Times*, July 15.

Suzuki, Akihito. 2003a. A Brain Hospital in Tokyo and Its Private and Public Patients, 1926–1945. *History of Psychiatry*, 14: 337–60.

———. 2003b. Family, the State and the Insane in Japan 1900–1945. In *Psychiatric Confinement in International Perspective*, eds. Roy Porter and David Wright. Cambridge: Cambridge University Press.

———. 2005. Were Asylums Men's Place?: Male Excess in Asylum Population in Japan in the Early Twentieth Century. In *Culture of Psychiatry*, eds. Marijke Gijswijt-Hofstra et al. Amsterdam: University of Amsterdam Press.

Suzuki, Hiroko. 2000. Daigaku Byōin Seishinka no Jikangai Shinryō ni Okeru Jisatsukitosha no Jittai (The Realities of Attempted Suicides in a University Hospital's Emergency Unit). *Igaku no Ayumi* (*Journal of Clinical and Experimental Medicine*) 194, no. 6: 541–44.

Suzuki, Ryū. 1997. Utsubyō no Hikaku Bunkaron (Cultural Comparisons of Depression). In *Kanjō Shōgai: Kiso to Rinshō* (*Affective Disorders: Foundations and Clinical Practice*), eds. Yomishi Kasahara, Masaaki Matsushita, and Hideki Kishimoto. Tokyo: Asakura Shoten.

Szasz, Thomas. 1974. The *Myth of Mental Illness*. New York: Harper & Row.

Tachibana, Nankei. 1927. Hokusō Sadan (Stories from the North Window) Vol. 2. In *Tōzai Yūki* (*Travels in Easten and Western Provinces*). Tokyo: Yūhōdō Shoten.

Tajima, Osamu. 2001. Mental Health Care in Japan: Recognition and Treatment of

Depression and Anxiety Disorders. *Journal of Clinical Psychiatry* 62, Suppl. 13: 39–44.

Takahashi, Mutsuko. 1997. *The Emergence of Welfare Society in Japan*. Aldershot/Brookfield: Avebury.

Takahashi, Ryo. 1974. Treatment for Depression in Japan. In *Depression in Everyday Practice*, ed. P. Kielholz. Bern: Huber.

Takahashi, Satoru. 1998. Senzen ni Okeru Seishin Hakujaku Shinrigaku no Keisei (The Formation of the Prewar Psychology of Retardation). In *Nihon Shinrigakushi no Kenkyū (Studies of the History of Japanese Psychology)*, eds. Shinrigaku Kenkyūkai Rekishi Kenkyūbukai. Kyoto: Hōsei Shuppan.

Takahashi, Takao. 2003. Anrakushi ni Tsuite: Nihonteki Seishikan Kara Toinaosu (On Euthanesia: Reexamining It in Light of Japanese Views on Death and Life). In *Yoki Shi no Sahō (Manners of Good Death)*, eds. Takao Takahashi and Hiroaki Taguchi. Fukuoka: Kyūshū Daigaku Shuppan.

Takahashi, Tōru. 1998. Shinkeishō Gainen no Hensen ni Tsuite (On the Changing Concept of Neurosis). *Seishin Shinkeigaku Zasshi (Journal of Psychiatry and Neurology)* 100, no. 3: 144–46.

Takahashi, Yoshitomo. 1994. Jisatsu Keikō (Suicidal Tendencies). *Rinshō Seishinigaku (Journal of Clinical Psychiatry)* 23, no.1: 55–63.

Takaoka, Takeshi. 2003. *Atarashii Utsubyōron (New Theory of Depression)*. Tokyo: Unbo Shobō.

Takemura, Kenji and Hiroshi Shimura. 1977. Kaihō Ryōhō no Jissen no Moto De Okita Jisatsu no Keiken (Experience of Suicide Cases That Occurred Under the Open-Ward Therapy). In *Seishin Byōin ni Okeru Jisatsu (Suicides in Mental Hospitals)*, ed. Seishin Byōin Kyōkai (Association of Mental Hospitals). Tokyo: Makino Shuppan.

Takemura, Kenji and Hiroshi Shimura. 1987. *Jisatsu no Sain (Signs of Suicide)*. Osaka: Shinryō Shinsha.

Tamura, Kazaburō. 1906. Shinkei no Eisei 1 (Hygiene of Nerves I). *Yomiuri Shimbun*, June 9.

Tanaka, Satoshi. 1992. Dokomade Arukeba Byōki no Nai Kuni: Eisei Tenrankai no Jikūkan (How Far Do We Need to Walk to a Country With No Illness: Space and Time in Hygiene Exhibitions). *Gendai Shisō* 20, no.6: 126–42.

Tashiro, Sanki. 1979. *Tashiro Sanki*. eds. Keisetsu Ōtsuka and Dōmei Yakazu. Tokyo: Meicho Shuppan.

Tatsumi, Nobuo. 1975. Utsubyō no Byōtai Seiri (Pathophysiology of Depression). *Yakkyoku (Pharmacy)* 26, no.9.

Taussig, Michael. 1980. Reification and the Consciousness of the Patient. *Social Science and Medicine* 14B: 3–13.

Tellenbach, Hubertus. 1980 [1961]. *Melancholy: History of the Problem, Endogeneity, Typology, Pathogenesis, Clinical Considerations*. Pittsburgh/Atlantic Highlands, NJ: Duquesne University Press; distributed by Humanities Press.

Terashima, Shōgo. 1969. The Structure of Rejecting Attitudes toward the Mentally Ill in Japan. In *Mental Health Research in Asia and the Pacific*, eds. William Caudill and Tsung-Yi Lin. Honolulu: East-West Center Press.

Todeschini, Maya. 1999a. Illegitimate Sufferers: A-bomb Victims, Medical Science, and the Government. *Daedlus* 128, no.2: 67–100.

Todeschini, Maya. 1999b. Bittersweet Crossroads: Women of Hiroshima and Nagasaki. Ph.D. Dissertation, Harvard University.

Tokyo High Court. 1997. Songai Baishō Seikyū Kōso Jiken (Appeal For Compensation For Damage). 1647/4089.

Tolle, Rainer. 1991. *Seishinigaku (Psychiatry)*. Niigata: Nishimura Shoten.

Tomita, Mikio. 1992. *Seishin Byōin no Teiryū (Undercurrents of Mental Hospitals)*. Tokyo: Seikyūsha.

———. 2000. *Tōdai Byōin Seishinka no 30 Nen (The 30 Years of the Department of Psychiatry at Tokyo University Hospital)* Tokyo: Seikyūsha.

Tsing, Anna Lowenhaupt. 1993. *In the Realm of the Diamond Queen*. Princeton, NJ: Princeton University Press.

Tsubouchi, Shōyō (Yūzō). 1903. Jisatsu Zehi (Pros and Cons of Suicide). *Taiyō* 9, no.9: 56–71.

Tsuchida, Ken. 1979. Tenkankyō Keikenhen (Treatises on Insanity). In *Kure Shūzō*. Tokyo: Seishinigaku Shinkeigaku Koten Kankōkai.

Tsurumi, Wataru. 1993. *Kanzen Jisatsu Manyuaru [The Complete Manual of Suicide]*. Yokohama: Yurindō Publishing.

Turkle, Sherry. 1992. *Psychoanalytic Politics: Jacques Lacan and Freud's French Revolution*. London/New York: Free Association Books; Guilford Press.

Turner, Bryan S. 1996. *The Body & Society* (second ed.). London: Sage Publications.

Turner, Victor W. 1967. *The Forest of Symbols; Aspects of Ndembu Ritual*. Ithaca, NY: Cornell University Press.

Uchimura, Yūshi. 1943. Zappō: Seishin Kōseikai Hakkaishiki Kōen (News: Lecture at the Inauguration of the Mental Welfare Association). *Seishin Shinkeigaku Zasshi (Journal of Psychiatry and Neurology)* 47, no.11: 527.

———. 1954. Nihon Seishinigaku no Kako to Shōrai (Past and Future of Japanese Psychiatry). *Seishin Shinkeigaku Zasshi (Journal of Psychiatry and Neurology)* 55, no.7: 705–16.

Uchimura, Yūshi, Akira Kasamatsu, and Toshiki Shimazaki, eds. 1957. *Seishinigaku Saikin no Shinpo (Recent Developments in Psychiatry)*. Tokyo: Ishiyaku Shuppan.

Udagawa, Genzui. 1995. Oranda Honyaku Naika Senyō (Text on Internal Medicine Translated From Dutch). In *Udagawa Genzui Shū I*, ed. Tsutomu Sugimoto. Tokyo: Waseda Daigaku Shuppankai.

Uematsu, Shichikurō. 1929. Toshi Seikatsu to Shinkeisuijaku (Urban Life and Neurasthenia). In *Sankōkanhō Seishin Eisei Tenrankai Gō (News on Mental Hygiene Exhibition)*, ed. Nihon Sekijūji Sha (Japan Red Cross). Tokyo: Nihon Sekijūji Sha.

———. 1948. *Seishinigaku (Psychiatry)*. Tokyo: Bunkōdō.

Ukai, Hiroshi. 1991. Kindai Nihon ni Okeru Shakai Darwinism no Jūyo to Tenkai (Adoption and Development of Social Darwininsm in Modern Japan). In *Kōza Shinka 2: Shinka Shisō to Shakai (Lectures on Evolution 2: Thoughts on Evolution and Society)*, eds. Atsuhiro Shibatani, Kei Nagano, and Takeshi Yōrō. Tokyo: Tokyo University Press.

Ukigaya, Sachiyo. 2009. Kea to Kyōdosei no Jinruigaku: Hokkaidō Urakawa Sekijūji Byōin Seishinka kara Chiiki e (The Anthropology of Care and Communality: From the Psychiatric Department of Urakawa Red Cross Hospital, Hokkaidō to Community). Tokyo: Seikatsu Shoin.

Usa, Genyū. 1925. Moritashi Shinkeishitsu Ryōhō ni Yoru Chiyu Seiseki (Recovery

Through Morita's Shinkeishitsu Therapy). *Shinkeigaku Zasshi (Journal of Neurology)* 26, no.1: 595–603.

Watanabe, Kinuko. 2002. Karō Jisatsu no Gyōmu Kiinsei (Work As the Cause For Overwork Suicide). *Jurist* 1223: 102–5.

Watanabe, Toshio. 1999. *Shinkeishō no Jidai: Waga Uchi Naru Morita Masatake (Neurosis Era: Morita Masatake in My Interiority).* Tokyo: Gakuyō Bunko.

Watarai, Yoshiichi. 2003. *Meiji no Seishin Isetsu: Shinkeibyō, Shinkeisuijaku, Kamigakari (Heresays on Nerve in Meiji: Nerve Diseases, Neurasthenia, and Spirit Possession).* Tokyo: Iwanami Shoten.

White, Geoffrey M. 1982. The Role of Cultural Explanations in 'Somatization' and 'Psychologization.' *Social Science and Medicine* 16: 1519–30.

White, James W. 1995. *Ikki: Social Coflict and Political Protest in Early Modern Japan.* Ithaca/London: Cornell University Press.

Whyte, Susan Reynolds. 1997. *Questioning Misfortune: the Pragmatics of Uncertainty in Eastern Uganda.* New York: Cambridge University Press.

XYZ. 1902. Shinkeisuijakushō: Sōjūshi, Bunshi, Kanri, Gakusei Shokun no Ichidoku o Yōsu (Neurasthenia: Operators, Writers, Government Officials, and Students, Read This). *Taiyō* 8, no.7.: 134–39.

Yamada, Tomiaki. 2000. Fieldwork no Politics (The Politics of Fieldwork). In *Fieldwork no Keiken (Experiences of Fieldwork),* eds. Hiroaki Yoshii and Atsushi Sakurai. Tokyo: Serika Shobō.

Yamaguchi, Masao. 1990. *Yamai no Uchūshi (Cosmos of Illness).* Tokyo: Ningen to Rekishisha.

Yamazaki, Mitsuo. 2001. Utsubyō wa "Kokoro no Kaze" de Aru (Depression Is a Soul Catching a Cold). *Bungeishunjū* (April).

Yanagita, Kunio. 1967. *Meiji Taishōshi Sesōhen (The History of Meiji & Taishō).* Tokyo: Heibonsha.

Yazaki, Taeko. 1968. Kaifukuki no Utsubyōsha no Seishin Ryōhō (Psychotherapy for the Depressed in the Recovery Phase). *Seishinigaku (Clinical Psychiatry)* 10: 277–84.

Yokoyama, Tomoyuki and Shin Iida. 1998. Utsubyō no Seishin Ryōhō (Psychotherapy for Depression). *Seishinka Chiryōgaku (Journal of Psychiatric Treatment)* 13, suppl.: 87–92.

Yomiuri Shimbun. 1878. Rien De Fusagu Hime ni Tsuketa Kisaku na Onnna, Hime no Kimono Mo Kigaru ni Nusumu (A Friendly Woman Steals the Kimonos of a Lady Depressed Over Divorce). March 23.

———. 1879. Utsubyō no Musume ga Shinbashigawa De Tōshin Jisatsu (A Depressed Girl Throws Herself in Shinbashi River). July 25.

———. 1886. Yamai no Genin Shinkō no Enoki ga Bassai Sare Musume ga Utsubyō ni (The Cause of the Illness: a Girl Develops Depression After a Sacred Enoki Tree Is Cut Down). September 16.

———. 1917. Gakusei no Shinkeisuijaku (Neurasthenia of Students). July 8.

———. 2010. "Utsu Hyakumannin" Kage ni Shinyaku? Hanbaidaka to Kanjasū Hirei (New Medication Behind "One Million People in Depression"? Ratio of Sales to Number of Patients). January 6.

Yoshimatsu, Kazuya. 1987. *Isha to Kanja (Doctors and Patients).* Tokyo: Iwanami Shoten.

Yoshimi, Shunya. 1994. Undōkai no Shisō: Meiji Nihon to Shukusai Bunka (The Atheletics Meet: The Festival Culture of Meiji Japan). *Shisō (Thought)* 845: 137–62.

Young, Allan. 1976. Internalizing and Externalizing Medical Belief Systems: an Ethiopian Example. *Social Science and Medicine* 10: 147–56.

———. 1980. The Discourse on Stress and the Reproduction of Conventional Knowledge. *Social Science and Medicine* 14B: 133–46.

———. 1982a. The Anthropologies of Illness and Sickness. *Annual Review of Anthropology* 11: 257–85.

———. 1982b. Rational Men and the Explanatory Model Approach. *Culture, Medicine and Psychiatry.* 6: 21–34.

———. 1983. Rethinking Ideology. *International Journal of Health Sciences.* 13: 203–19.

———. 1995. *The Harmony of Illusions: Inventing Post-Traumatic Stress Disorder.* Princeton, NJ: Princeton University Press.

Zimmermann, Bénédicte. 2008. Histoire Croisée and the Making of Global History. Based on a paper presented at Global History, Globally. Harvard University, February 8–9, 2008.http://www.iue.it/HEC/ResearchTeaching/20082009-Autumn/SS-reading-Zimmermann.pdf. February 3, 2009.

Zola, Irving K. 1972. Medicine As an Institution of Social Control. *Sociological Review* 20, no.4: 487–504.

Index

abnormality, 5, 21, 37, 45, 53, 86, 172–73
acedia, 28–29n2
acupuncture, 27
adaptation, 71
aesthetics, 4, 14, 15, 24, 108, 128, 170
agency, 186, 199; and biology, 85, 86; lack of, 13; and psychiatry, 7; and suicide, 111, 114, 117–18, 120, 121, 127; and Tellenbach, 73; and Typus Melancholicus, 76. *See also* autonomy; free will; intentionality
alienation, 4; and body, 13, 86, 98, 127, 133, 196; cultural, 103; holistic approach to, 92; and modernity, 79; and overwork and depression narratives, 133; and social change, 179; and social situations, 74, 78; and society, 7; of women, 129n2; and workers, 196, 197
alternative healing, 7. *See also* traditional medicine
Althusser, Louis, 8
antidepressants: advent of new, 4; and biology, 98, 179; brain alteration by, 184; dangers of, 175, 183, 184; discovery of, 71–72; and everyday distress, 178; and fatigue, 198; and hospitalization, 97; inappropriate prescription of, 183–85; as ineffective, 182, 183; introduction of, 6, 16n9; marketing of, 2; and medicalization, 67; and new idioms, 78; overuse and abuse of, 106; as primary treatment, 92, 182; promotion of, 52–53; and psychological cure, 91; public debates about, 153; as quieting dissent, 178; and recession of 2000s, 182; and social pathologies, 175; and suicide, 170; therapeutic failures with, 73; and United States, 198. *See also* pharmaceuticals
antipsychiatry movement: and biological model, 120; and clinical psychology, 52n21; and community health, 8; and failures to cure, 40; and heredity, 48; influence of, 156; and labeling, 78; and Marxism, 7; and medicalization, 77, 78; and neurobiological psychiatry, 104; and psychiatric critiques, 14; and psychiatrists, 181; rise of, 51; and social management, 2; and social problems, 74; and Sōma case, 43
antisocial personality, 46
Applbaum, Kalman, 4, 178
aristocracy, 30
Aristotle, 15
Arnold, David, 41
art therapy, 99
Asia, 197
Association for Hygiene of Greater Japan, 42
autonomic nervous system disorder (jiritsu shinkei shicchōshō), 38, 141, 141n6, 143, 146
autonomy, 4, 121, 190. *See also* agency

Bakhtin, Mikhail M., 12
Barrett, Robert, 12, 35, 36, 94, 127
Basic Law on Suicide Countermeasures (2006), 108, 155, 169
Beard, George, 55, 60, 61
Behague, Dominique Pareja, 198–99
behavioral models, 49n16
Binswanger, Ludwig, 120
biological citizenship, 153
biological determinism, 11, 70, 73, 76, 107
biological management, 6
biological reductionism, 4, 11, 67, 69, 70n4, 124, 177, 178, 182. *See also* reductionism
biological surveillance, 4
biologism, 182
biology, 8, 49, 67–69; and agency, 85, 86; and American psychiatry, 198; and antipsychiatry movement, 120; and case conferences, 101; and depression, 68, 92; and diagnostic interview, 94–97; and economy, 177, 178; and essential difference, 194; and gender, 142; and genetic determinism, 194; individual, 4, 7, 9, 74, 86, 171; and insanity, 29n3; interplay with personality and environment, 99; and JP Medical School, 91; and language, 9–11, 69, 96, 104; and mental illness, 40; and mimic depression, 147; and North American psychiatry, 67; patients' questioning of language of, 13; persuasion about, 86;

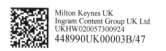